LINACRE STUDIES

Essays on the Life and Work of Thomas Linacre
c. 1460-1524

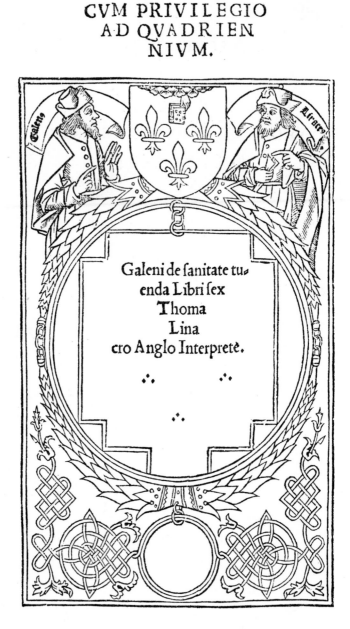

Galeni de sanitate tu-
enda Libri sex
Thoma
Lina
cro Anglo Interprete.

Habetur venale sub pellicano in vico Iacobeo.

Title-page of Linacre's translation of Galen, *De sanitate tuenda*, Paris, 1517
(See pp. xvii, 296–7, 364, & 374 (*Catalogue no. 19*))

LINACRE STUDIES

❋

Essays on the Life and Work of Thomas Linacre
c. 1460-1524

EDITED BY
FRANCIS MADDISON
MARGARET PELLING AND
CHARLES WEBSTER

OXFORD
AT THE CLARENDON PRESS
1977

Oxford University Press, Walton Street, Oxford OX2 6DP

OXFORD LONDON GLASGOW NEW YORK
TORONTO MELBOURNE WELLINGTON CAPE TOWN
IBADAN NAIROBI DAR ES SALAAM LUSAKA ADDIS ABABA
KUALA LUMPUR SINGAPORE JAKARTA HONG KONG TOKYO
DELHI BOMBAY CALCUTTA MADRAS KARACHI

ISBN 0 19 858150 5

Linacre Studies are sponsored by Linacre College, Oxford

*Printed in Great Britain
at the University Press, Oxford
by Vivian Ridler
Printer to the University*

Preface

THE PRESENT VOLUME IS THE RESULT OF A WISH ON
the part of Linacre College to commemorate the distinguished
humanist and physician whose name it bears; it was decided that
the most fitting form of commemoration would be the sponsoring
of publications concerned with Linacre's life, work, and times. This
is the first such publication.

The College is grateful to all the contributors to this volume, and
especially to Dr. Charles Webster, who joined the editorial board
after the project was under way and greatly contributed to its success. Publication was made possible by generous grants from the
Wellcome Foundation and the E. P. A. Cephalosporin Fund, for
which the College records its grateful thanks.

J. B. BAMBOROUGH
Principal

Linacre College
Oxford

Contents

List of Illustrations

The signatures reproduced as figures 3 and 4 are also tooled on the binding of this book

of the Royal College of Physicians in Pall Mall, London; cut down to head and shoulders in 1965, and now at Peckham. *Photograph by John Simons, by courtesy of Mr. and Mrs. A. T. Linacre*

XVIII. *a.* Painting, oils on panel; artist unknown; a fake, or deceptive copy, probably of nineteenth-century origin; the figure is copied from the painting shown on Plate VII, the background from that shown on Plate XVIII.*b.* Wellcome Institute of the History of Medicine, London. *By courtesy of the Director, Wellcome Institute of the History of Medicine*

b. Portrait of George Gisze, 1532, by Hans Holbein, Staatliche Museen Preussicher Kulturbesitz, Gemäldegalerie Berlin (West). *By Courtesy of the Director, Staatliche Museen Preussicher Kulturbesitz*

XIX. *a.* Painting, oils on panel; artist unknown; a fake or deceptive copy, probably of nineteenth-century origin, copied from the painting shown on Plate XIX.*b.* Wellcome Institute of the History of Medicine, London. *By courtesy of the Director, Wellcome Institute of the History of Medicine*

b. Portrait of Dirk Tybis, 1535, by Hans Holbein. Kunsthistorisches Museum, Vienna. *By courtesy of the Director, Kunsthistorisches Museum, Vienna*

XX. *a.* Stained glass panel in oriel window in the Hall, Christ Church, Oxford. *Photograph by John Simons, by courtesy of the Governing Body of Christ Church, Oxford*

b. Woodcut, from the third of the three sets of portrait engravings prefixed to the three parts of Adolphus Clarmundus (= J. C. Ruediger), *Vitae clarissimorum in re literaria virorum*, Wittenberg, 1704.

c. Part of a fresco by Giacomo dal Forno, 1942. Sala dei Quaranta, Università di Padova. *By courtesy of the Rector, Università di Padova*

Editors' Introduction

> . . . I have not met with so much kindness, and so much learning, not hacknied and trivial, but deep, accurate, ancient, Latin and Greek, that but for the curiosity of seeing it, I do not now so much care for Italy. When I hear my Colet, I seem to be listening to Plato himself. In Grocin who does not marvel at such a perfect round of learning? What can be more acute, profound, and delicate than the judgment of Linacre? What has Nature ever created more gentle, more sweet, more happy than the genius of Thomas More? I need not go through the list . . .
>
> Erasmus, from London, to Robert Fisher, 5 December [1499][1]

> . .. tant vous estes saige, prudent, entendu et curieux de vostre santé, et tant bien estez servy de vostre docte médicin, Thomas Linacer.
>
> Rabelais, *Le Quart Livre des faicts et dicts héroïques du bon Pantagruel*, Paris, 1552[2]

ERASMUS PRAISING LINACRE AS AN EXPONENT OF humanist culture in England, Rabelais using Linacre's name for the royal physician in an anachronistic reworking of an old anecdote; these prefigure the later reputation of Thomas Linacre. For his fame is both traditional and eponymous. It is traditional because no considerable reassessment of his life and work, based on an investigation of the scanty biographical material, or on a study of the rich sources for his place in the intellectual history of his time, has been attempted for nearly seventy years; we still rely on Johnson's *Life*, posthumously published in 1835, Osler's Linacre lecture of 1908, or Payne's article in the *Dictionary of National Biography* in 1909.[3] It is eponymous because Linacre's name remains attached to, or has been appropriated by, lectureships and institutions concerned with medicine and humane learning.

In this volume, which is designed to fulfil the need for a modern study of Linacre, we have tried to avoid the hagiographical approach. The contributions have been confined to critical studies of dominant themes related to Linacre's place in humanist studies and Renaissance medicine, and to his historical influence. Consequently, the essays are concerned with many important problems of Renaissance society. We consider that we have been fortunate in our contributors, and thank them for the time and labour they have expended in order to make this volume worth while. Although the contributions are scholarly articles on specialized subjects, these are related, and there is inevitably some overlap of content. Each author has reached his (or her) own conclusions, and the editors have rarely attempted to reconcile any differences, conceiving their function in this respect to be that of removing inconsistencies of detail. We may here mention that, in this volume, the College of Physicians of London is so termed until the year 1682, after which time it may legitimately be called the Royal College of Physicians.[4]

As editors, we are aware that there still remain aspects of Linacre's life which we should have liked to see discussed in this volume. Nothing appears here on the subject of Linacre's medical practice, because nothing is known about it which would distinguish it from that of his contemporaries.[5] It has not been necessary to consider Linacre's religious position in regard to the Reformation, in view of the recent excellent general study by Professor J. M. McConica,[6] but the details of the ecclesiastical preferments received by Linacre, and his assumption of holy orders, would merit further investigation. At least the dates of Linacre's ordination, as subdeacon and as deacon, by the Bishop of London, Richard Fitzjames (d. 1522), are now known.[7] We have inserted such information on these topics as it was possible to discover in printed sources, in the brief Chronology which follows this Introduction.

In the absence of a biographical essay, the Chronology will serve, we hope, as an *aide-mémoire* to those unfamiliar with the details of Linacre's life. Apart from the publication dates of his printed works,[8] and the various property transactions in which he was concerned,[9] the certain facts are few enough.[10] Because we are dealing with a period before the introduction of parish registers, and other potentially relevant records, which might otherwise have been systematically searched, only very good fortune is likely to contribute to the discovery of new information.

★ ★ ★

Regarding Linacre's life, no new material has been found to remove discredit from statements linking him with Derby and the Linacre family of Linacre Hall, Derbyshire.[11] Rather, we are disposed to accept John Caius's description of Linacre as *Cantuariensis*, i.e. of Canterbury,[12] for although Caius was only fourteen years old when Linacre died in 1524, there is good reason to suppose that he would later have been well informed about the facts of Linacre's life.[13] The generally accepted date for Linacre's birth, 1460, has been doubted[14] because of a phrase used by the antiquary John Leland (?1506–52) to describe Linacre, in a statement about William Sellyng's mission to Rome in 1487, on behalf of Henry VII: 'Quo tempore Thomam Linacrum, optimae spei adolescentulum, tanquam ministrum, una secum deduxit . . .' ('At that time, he [sc. Sellyng] took with him as an assistant Thomas Linacre, a young man of the greatest promise').[15] If born in 1460, Linacre would then have been twenty-seven years old and, it is objected, would not have been described as *adolescentulus*. However, confronted with that Ciceronian sentence, we might recall that Cicero described himself as *adolescentulus* in his twenty-seventh year.[16] No doubt Leland knew that usage, but it would be too speculative to argue further that he wished thereby to indicate that Linacre was aged twenty-six or twenty-seven.

There are a number of other miscellaneous facts concerning the life of Linacre, or statements about him, mostly not discussed in the essays in this volume, which will be mentioned here because they have a certain interest, and in order to establish the relevant bibliography in the footnotes.[17] We may begin with the only account to give any details of Linacre's medical practice, though what it tells us is little enough. In a letter written from Basle on 14 March 1525 to Willibrand Pirckheimer (1470–1530), a rich councillor of Nuremberg, Erasmus described how, many years previously, he had been treated for the stone by Linacre:

You shall not know the remedy before I name the author. He was Thomas Linacre, the distinguished physician to the King of England, a man so completely learned in all manner of disciplines, as to be in nothing, I may say, other than over scrupulously attentive.

But more about the author presently; now hear about the remedy. A calculus, arising from drinking beer, was stuck for six weeks in some hollow [of my body]; for the time being, indeed, I was not oppressed by the pain, but my very constitution, agitated and

depressed, warned me that I was in great danger. For I myself wondered what was the matter. I am certainly loth to call for assistance
on my own behalf; and this Linacre was of such a disposition as not
to direct his attention to anything unless pressed. A certain friend
reminded me to arouse the man by some persuasive words. I did so.
There could be nothing more attentive then he. A pharmacist was
summoned. A prescription haveing been prepared in my bedroom, it
was applied by that physician himself. It was applied a second time, and
soon afterwards I awoke to bring forth a calculus like the kernel of a
small almond. In place of this remedy, the Germans use baths.
Nevertheless, this, since it produces the same result, is much more
convenient. Camomile and parsley are wrapped in a linen cloth, and
boiled in a clean, closed vessel, containing pure water, until the
liquid be reduced by half. The hot cloth is taken out of the pot, and
as much moisture as possible is quickly squeezed out; then it is
applied to one's side. If the heat be intolerable, the small bag, in
which are the herbs, is wrapped in a dry linen cloth, so that it can be
held at either end as by handles. And if at first, the side of the body
cannot bear it, because of the heat, I hold it above the place, so that
the warmth benefits the body, until the heat begins to be tolerable.
Soon I make myself ready for sleep; after which, if the pain recurs, I
apply the linen cloth, having boiled it again. I have never done it
twice without the calculus descending to a place near the bladder, in
which the pain is less. However, that protection failed me at first in
the next attack.[18]

In 1514, Linacre, already one of the King's physicians, was attached
to the service of the Princess Mary (1496–1533), as physician, and
allocated two servants; he travelled to Paris in September of that
year, in her entourage.[19] Linacre with two servants perhaps may be
compared, as some indication of his status, to others among Mary's
attendants: Mr. Chamberlain was allocated three servants, Mr.
Treasurer two, and Mr. Hone, schoolmaster, one. Linacre's wages
for four months, paid in September 1514, amounted to £16. 11s. 8d.
In these, and subsequent entries in the published calendar,[20] the
bald facts of Linacre's employment in the Royal household during
the reign of Henry VIII, in attendance upon the Princess, and as
Royal physician, may be traced.

It is to this period of his life that the only surviving personal
description of Linacre refers. In a work published in 1548, George
Lily wrote thus of Linacre at court:

For some time he was placed as tutor to Prince Arthur, son of

Henry the Seventh; however, he devoted all his studies to knowledge of medicine, hitherto scarcely successfully attempted by anyone born in Britain. In this, he so exclusively applied himself that, the care of the King's health having been entrusted to him, he might be seen striding among the nobles of the royal court, wearing a crimson gown reaching to his ankles, and a full cloak of black velvet thrown across his shoulders.[21]

Our visual impression of Linacre must, it seems, rest on that, for no authentic portrait of him exists or is known to have existed.[22] One cannot even argue that the figure entitled 'Linacr*us*', facing 'Galen*us*' in the woodcut title-page of Linacre's translation from Galen, *De sanitate tuenda*, printed at Paris in August 1517 by Guillaume Le Rouge (Rubeus),[23] should be broadly consistent with Linacre's personal appearance (e.g. in having a beard). Although this book was seen through the press by Linacre's friend, Thomas Lupset (1495–1530), aided by Guillaume Budé, whom Linacre had met in Paris in 1514,[24] the similarity of the two figures in the woodcut suggests that portraiture was not attempted.

'To this Dr. Linacer', wrote the Shakespearean scholar, George Steevens (1736–1800), 'we owe the growth of that Prince of Flowers the Damask Rose in England, who brought the plants thereof with him at his return from Italy; and so effectually planted and dispersed them that they are the chief ornament of our Gardens to this Day. See Lord Bacon's *Sylva* from Hackluyt &c.'[25] Bacon's *Sylva* includes no mention of Linacre, but does state that damask roses had not been known in England for more than a hundred years,[26] a remark not incompatible with Hakluyt's statement in 1582: 'And in time of memory things have been brought in that were not here before, as the Damaske rose by Doctour *Linaker* king *Henry* the seuenth and King *Henrie* the eights Physician . . .'[27] The Spanish physician Nicolás Monardes (1493–1578) published in 1551 a Latin treatise on Persian or Alexandrian roses. He there said that among the Italians, French, Germans, and other peoples, frequent use was made of roses, called Damascene because they were believed to have come from Damascus, and that indeed it was almost thirty years since knowledge of them first reached the Spaniards.[28] Again, we encounter a statement that a damask rose or, rather, a *rosa damascena*, was first known in parts of extreme western Europe in the early part of the sixteenth century.

Hakluyt's note is not the first English published reference to the damask rose, but the earlier English references to it do not mention Linacre. The well-known physician William Turner (d. 1568), in the second part (1562) of his important herbal, says that since the time of Mesue (i.e. Mesué *iunior*, a supposed Māsawayh al-Mardīnī (d. 1015)) '. . . there are found diuers other kindes as Damaske rosens/incarnation roses/muske roses/with certayn other kindes whereof is no mention in any olde writer'.[29] The herbal of Henry Lyte (1529?–1607), published in 1578, gives the names of the various types of rose which he distinguishes, in several languages. *Rosa damascena* is not equated with the damask rose: 'The first kinde of garden Roses is called in Italy, *Rosa Damascena*, in this Countrie, *Rosa alba*. . . in English, White Roses . . .', and 'the thirde kinde is called in French, *Rosee de Prouinces* . . . we cal them in English, Roses of Province, and Damaske Roses.'[30]

The parentage of roses now called 'damask' has been clarified by the genetical researches of C. C. Hurst.[31] He distinguishes two 'natural and distinct groups': X *Rosa damascena* (*rubra x phoenicia*)—the *summer* damask rose, corresponding to *Rosa damascena* Blackw. 1757; and X *Rosa bifera* (*rubra x moschata*)—the *autumn* damask rose (X *Rosa bifera* [Poiret]). However, the identification of a damask rose mentioned by a sixteenth-century writer is not only a matter of genetics, but of a confusing and, possibly, confused terminology. We have seen that Lyte said that roses of Provins, the French town 'peopled with apothecaries' profiting by the retention of the scent by the petals of these roses, even when dried, to make various confections, were called damask roses in England. Indeed, the Apothecary's Rose of Provins (*Rosa gallica officinalis* Thory) has been known in England as the Red Damask Rose for more than three centuries, though it is not, botanically, a damask rose.[32] Monardes's Spanish damask rose has been shown to be our Autumn Damask Rose,[33] but although this may be a sixteenth-century introduction into Spain, we cannot be certain that it is the rose referred to by Hakluyt. When we consider that Hakluyt's contemporary, Lyte, takes us into yet another species with his identification of the Italian damask rose (possibly the same as Monardes's) with what we assume is *Rosa alba* L.,[34] we have to recognize that it is quite possible that some variety of damask rose was indeed introduced into England, or made popular, by Linacre, but that we can have little hope of identifying it in modern botanical terms.[35]

But it was not for the practice of botany, nor even of medicine, that Linacre was so esteemed by his contemporaries; it was as a classical scholar and as a grammarian: he 'was (like *William Lilie*) for none of his workes so famous, as for his rudiments or instructions, to the better understanding of the Latine tongue', wrote Thomas Weever, setting the *Rudimenta* above the translations from Galen.[36] And rather more anecdotes and miscellaneous items of information have gathered around Linacre's name in this respect, than concerning his other activities.[37] In 1557, Paolo Giovio published a tale, involving a simple pun, concerning the origin of Linacre's friendship with the humanist Ermolao Barbaro (1453–93):

From there [sc. Florence], having acquired the benefits of many distinctions of varied instruction, because he [sc. Linacre] considered that he should also get to know better the intellects of Rome, and examine the richer libraries there, he hastened to the city. By accident, he formed at the outset a friendship with Hermolaus Barbarus. While he was in the Vatican Library, turning over the pages of Greek codices, Hermolaus came unexpectedly upon the scene, and courteously approaching the bookcase, said, 'Truly, studious guest, you cannot be as much a barbarian (*barbarus*) as I am, since you read so assiduously that most choice book of Plato' (it was the *Phaedrus*). Smiling, Linacre replied, 'You, my consecrated hero, can be none other than the well-known most Latin Patriarch of the Italians'.[38] From that friendship (so accidently begun, so fruitfully developed), he finally returned to Britain, enriched by distinguished volumes . . .[39]

While still in Italy, Linacre's reputation as a Greek and Latin scholar was firmly established. By November 1498, he was a member of the Aldine Νεακαδημία,[40] but already in February of the previous year Aldus Manutius had singled him out for praise in the prefatory letter to the second volume of the *editio princeps* of Aristotle. Describing the trouble taken to establish a correct text, Aldus says that he has important witnesses to this throughout Italy, 'and especially in Venice, Thomas the Englishman, a man most skilled in both Greek and Latin and distinguished in the disciplines of all branches of learning'.[41] More than twenty years later, in 1520, these words were echoed by Antonio Francino, with whom Linacre seems to have become acquainted while in Florence. At the request of Giampiero Machiavelli, a friend of both Francino and Linacre, Francino dedicated to Linacre Julius Pollux's Ονομαστικον, which he had had printed, 'on account of your skill in both languages and in useful learning, and we urge you, if you should ever have the leisure, to translate, with your usual ability, Pollux into Latin'.[42]

A persistent story, which may be traced back to George Lily's 'life' of William Grocyn, 1548, refers to Linacre's involvement in a project to translate Aristotle: 'In fact, sharing the work with Linacre and Latimer, he [sc. Grocyn] undertook the task of translating Aristotle, which, however, soon afterwards, having been presented to a living and having changed his mind, he abandoned.' John Bale (1495–1563), too, mentions that after his return to England, Linacre began to collaborate in a translation of Aristotle:

> And in our time, from Italy to Britain, Thomas Linacre, of Galen a most brilliant translator, who was tutor to Prince Arthur, brought Greek letters, as did his contemporaries, the two Williams, Latimer and Grocyn, who, with a noble but fruitless desire, undertook with Linacre the business of translating Aristotle.[43]

According to William Latimer, Linacre, a man with a sharp mind, had spent even longer in the study of Greek than William Grocyn, who had spent two years without interruption and that under the best masters, Demetrius Chalcondylas and Angelo Poliziano, who were also Linacre's teachers.[44] Erasmus relates that Thomas More, when a young man, learned Greek under the ablest teachers,[45] especially Linacre and Grocyn, and we have More's own testimony that he studied Aristotle in Greek under Linacre's tuition; it is More, too, who confirms that Linacre had completed the translation of two books of the *Meteorologica*.[46]

John Caius placed Linacre among More, Lupset, and Erasmus as authorities in his book on the pronunciation of Greek:

> . . . Indeed, they who lack them (teachers) and are constrained to learn Greek by their own exertions, let them pronounce the Greek letters in the manner of the Latin letters corresponding to the Greek in this table. This system of pronunciation is certainly old and of received use. In teaching the young (as I know myself), these new teachers of the past also shared this view. Truly they knew not how to stand still, but wished to progress by leaps and bounds. Of this opinion were Thomas More, Linacre, Lupset, and Erasmus, who in the proverb, 'Stultior Morycho' [= more foolish than Morychus], pronounced μορύξαι [*sic*] Moryxae, not Moruxai, although he disputed many matters of pronunciaion, which he himself had written rather for the sake of fame, than of usefulness, as careful observation may enable one to know from these and other places . . .'[47]

Whether or not one should infer from this passage that Linacre had adopted the Erasmian pronunciation of Greek is uncertain, for here his name is linked to that of Erasmus in concurring, albeit in a particular circumstance (the teaching of the young) and a specific instance, with a pronunciation not in accordance with Erasmus's opinion concerning the pronunciation of ancient Greek. Most English and continental scholars who had acquired a mastery of Greek pronunciation, pronounced it rather like modern Greek, because the Greek teachers involved in the revival of Greek in Western Europe pronounced it that way. Erasmus, however, sought to determine and to revive the pronunciation of ancient Greek. An attempt to introduce the Erasmian pronunciation at the University of Cambridge led to a serious controversy, and to an exchange of letters in which an anecdote concerning Linacre was related, without much relevance to the argument, though hardly on a flippant occasion. About 1534 or 1535, Sir John Cheke (1514–57) and Sir Thomas Smith (1513–77) began, with great success, to use the Erasmian pronunciation in teaching Greek at Cambridge. In 1540, Cheke was appointed the first Regius professor of Greek at Cambridge, but he was unable to overcome conservative hostility to the new pronunciation, and on 1 June 1542, the Chancellor of the University, Stephen Gardiner, Bishop of Winchester, banned its use. Correspondence between Gardiner on the one hand, and Cheke and Smith on the other, was eventually published, that with Cheke at Basle in 1555.[48] It is Gardiner who first mentions Linacre: 'After Erasmus, there is no point in attacking the Ciceronians. Certainly, Linacer, a most learned man of our age, and of uncommon good judgement in literary matters, could never approve of the Ciceronian style, nor hear it without disgust . . .'[49] To which Cheke retorts:

And here you put before me Linacre, for me to approve of a deed of his, rather than of his other virtues, as if I were to imitate the stamping of the foot, or a gesture of some good orator, and pay no attention to his merits. For whatever moderation he might have had, Linacre, because he applied his mind to Galen, and followed the calm style of speech of Celsus,[50] and the peaceful style of Columella,[51] as is appropriate to that subject, not only could not praise other styles, but could not even hear them without insult to his ears. He ought similarly to please me because when quite beset by advancing and declining years, a man enfeebled by study and by illness, near to death,

he then, though he was a priest, took in his hands for the first time
the New Testament, and read through in it some chapters of Matthew.
When he had gone through the fifth, sixth, and seventh chapters, he
threw away the book with all his might, and swore that either this
were not the Gospel or we were not Christians. However uncommon
a literary judgement might be this deed of his, so much more that of
an Italian rather than of an English priest,[52] if I were to wish to imitate
it and throughout my life pay no attention to Cicero in the way he
kept away from the New Testament, I should lack merit in judgement
and in erudition. No other Latinist of his day did as much in medicine
and, while he confines himself to medicine, then extraordinary praise
is his. But if he creeps out and slanders orators, let him see that he
stick to the last of medicine. For whereas the praise due to him for
translating Galen is almost without parallel, however, if acuteness
of understanding and quickness of mind are discussed, or the serious
and clear treatment of general matters, then, if he were still alive,
although he be most learned and out of the ordinary in his literary
judgement, he would in that yield praise to you, and would himself
take praise for medicine. However, why he was so disgusted on
hearing Cicero, I do not know. We see that examples from Cicero
abound in all those books on the writing of Latin which he himself
compiled. Perhaps, indeed, he did not despise Cicero as much as a
kind of mental peevishness made him wish to be seen to do.[53]

Our anecdotal survey of the life of Linacre should conclude with
a curious episode in his return journey from Italy to England,
recorded in a Latin poem by Janus Vitale, appended to Giovio's
own 'life' of Linacre:

> When Linacre approached the Morini,[54] and his ancestral Britons,
>   Made rich by excellent skills from Italy,
>   A great heap of stones on the lofty crags
>   He piled up at your mouth, lofty Gebenna,[55]
> Then while he was crowning it with flowers and with green
>   branches,
> And while the sacred flame was feeding on the Assyrian wealth[56]
> He said this to you, Italy: 'O holy mother of my studies,
>   Linacre dedicates this temple,
> You, for whom Athens, with learned Pallas, stands up [to honour],
>   Receive from me this reward of constancy'.[57]

To most, this will seem an uncharacteristic action, because we have
become accustomed to think of Linacre as a somewhat formidable
person, unlikely to indulge in a romantic pagan exercise of this

nature. Yet we know as little of his character as of the details of his life. Like so many of his contemporaries, but not all, Linacre appears to us like the silhouette in a shadow-play—the important actions are positive, the outline of the figure subsists, but the details are lacking, of studies, of friendships, of intellectual development, which 'seem to be irretrievably lost to us'.[58] 'Linacre was not given to grandiose statements of principle or belief', writes one of our contributors, who therefore can detect little positive evidence to show that Linacre was a humanist, on at least one definition of a humanist.[59]

Iudicium, judgement, is a word we have met frequently in our survey of some of the biographical references to Linacre; judgement, acute, profound, and delicate, according to Erasmus; his uncommon literary judgement stressed by Cheke, though potentially a hostile witness; and this is in accord with the excessive *severitas* and *gravitas* for which he is blamed by the botanist, Leonhardt Fuchs (1501–66) (who was echoed by the naturalist, Conrad von Gesner (1516–65)) despite the former's preference for Linacre above other translators.[60] And they have more right than we to comment thus on a man formed in a society in which formal rituals and manners were a bastion against recent 'barbarism'.

Those rituals help to conceal from us motive, in correspondence as in dedications. Sincerity is, however, surely patent when Linacre speaks in the preface to the *De sanitate tuenda*, 1517, of an *arcanum naturae* which Galen has brought forth from darkness to light, or praises Fuchs for his translation of Hippocrates, otherwise lost, to the detriment of mankind.[61] And it was sincerity of purpose which lay behind the 'creative genius, which enabled him to convince contemporaries that a learned and well-regulated medical profession would be a more effective agency for the welfare of the commonwealth'.[62] We detect there, too, the perception of fundamental needs, which, in translating Galen, led him to concentrate on practical texts.[63] Possibly less flexible of mind than Erasmus, he was perhaps more prescient and constant of purpose, able to sustain a policy and to carry out plans based on the needs which he saw.

Some have detected in Linacre a 'certain want of imagination',[64] and it was Melanchthon, considering Linacre's grammars, 'who regretted, as a practical teacher, the excessive zeal for completeness which put them out of the reach of most boys' minds',[65] severe criticism in an age which treated children as inefficient adults. Despite George Buchanan's praise of 'meticulous treatment' and 'a certain freshness of approach', in the introduction to his Latin translation of the *Rudimenta*, the original edition of that book contains many careless errors;[66] but, perhaps, these are not attributable to the author.

But there is no doubt that Linacre was a considerable and meticulous scholar. No criticism of him in that respect has come down to us. We may be certain that all those of his contemporaries capable of making the judgement would have shared Erasmus's view, while awaiting the publication of the *De sanitate tuenda*, that he expected nothing from Linacre but what was perfect in all respects.[67] Praise of his scholarship occurs in many of the texts we have had occasion to quote. This very perfectionism, however, was to Erasmus not entirely praiseworthy for it delayed publication of Linacre's work: Linacre suffered from the same fault as Paulus Aemilus (*c.* 1460–1529), author of a much delayed history of France, in finding it difficult to be content with his work, of wishing to retouch and perfect it too often.[68] In 1521, Erasmus wrote to Linacre urging him not to torture the public slowly by depriving them for so long of the opportunity of reading his works, lest it appear that this be cruelty rather than the precaution of modesty. Erasmus wondered if Linacre was frightened of Erasmus's own fault of diversifying his studies too much.[69]

It is Erasmus who gives us a sight of Linacre not allowing friendship to dilute his strict standards of behaviour:

> Our friend Linacre has already thought me wanting in delicacy; for knowing as he did that I left London with hardly six angels in my pocket, and being well aware of my state of health, with the winter coming on, he is still constantly advising me to spare the Archbishop,[70] to spare Mountjoy,[71] and rather to narrow my expenses, and accustom myself to bear poverty with fortitude. A friendly counsel indeed![72]

Later, Erasmus seems to have doubted Linacre's friendship; in 1516 and again in 1517, it appears that More is trying to reassure him, on one occasion commenting on the extraordinary pleasure Linacre had shown on hearing that Erasmus had mentioned his books in a letter to More.[73] Not long before, Erasmus had been exhorting Richard Pace, the Dean of St. Paul's, to retain the friendship of Linacre and of Grocyn, while darkly hinting that each had been guilty of disloyalty; remarks which may reveal more of Erasmus than of Linacre and Grocyn.[74]

The insecure and somewhat erratic Erasmus perhaps contrasts with the more stolid Linacre, whose death on 20 October 1524 evokes simplicity and friendship. His Will of 19 June 1524 deals only with domestic affairs, the simple bequests to two sisters, a brother and two nieces, a 'cousin', a friend, John Plumtre, and his servants. 'I woll that my funeralls and burying shalbe doon in moderat maner . . .'; but the directions for the location of his grave in St. Paul's are specific: '. . . and my body to be buried within the cathedrall churche of Saint Poule of London before the rode of north dore there bitwene the longe forme and the wall directly over agaynst the said rode'.[75] 'Linacre has forsaken the living, to the great sorrow of all teachers', wrote Juan Luis Vives. 'He sincerely wished well to, and helped everyone, and indeed for him the repute of ability and learning was worth more than the suspicion of jealousy . . .'[76] The memory of friendship persisted: the (undated) Will of the aged Cuthbert Tunstall (1474–1559), who strove to implement Linacre's wishes concerning the medical lectureships, requests that he be buried, should he die in London, 'next to the grave of my old friend, Thomas Linacre, the physician'.[77]

There remain his published works, and his foundations, and we may infer that a man who gained the respect and friendship of Aldus Manutius, William Grocyn, Thomas More, Guillaume Budé, and Erasmus undoubtedly merited the epitaph which, more than twenty years after Linacre's death, John Caius had engraved on a brass plate and fixed to the wall near the great north door of old St. Paul's:

Thomas Lynacre, physician to King Henry VIII, and by far the most learned man, in both Greek and Latin, and also in medical matters. He restored to a full life many who, in his time, were weak from illness and who already despaired of recovery. He translated into Latin, with a wonderful and unique eloquence, many of the works of Galen. Shortly before his death, he published, at the request of friends, an excellent work on correct Latin usage. He established in perpetuity two public lectures for the students of medicine at Oxford, and one for those at Cambridge. In this city [sc. London] he strove to establish the College of Physicians, of which he was then elected President. He hated deceit and fraud, was faithful to his friends, and equally beloved by all. Some years before he died, he was ordained priest. An old man, he departed this life, and was greatly missed, on the 20th of October in the year of Our Lord 1524.

Virtue survives the tomb
To Thomas Lynacre, distinguished physician,
John Caius placed [this memorial] in this year 1557[78]

Indeed, his virtues survived, and 'acquired mythological stature'.[79] From Wyer's implied recommendation in the sixteenth-century *Macers Herbal practysyd by Doctor Lynacro*,[80] to the founders of the twentieth-century Linacre House (now College), in this University, who certainly thought that it was established in accordance with Linacre's ideals, the myth has been remarkably durable. Our visual image of Linacre parallels the myth, and those who require icons are as well served by the remains of the nineteenth-century statue which adorned the façade of the Royal College of Physicians, as by any of the traditional portraits.[81] The exploration of the origins and development of Linacre's reputation is the purpose of this book.

★   ★   ★

Since the first discussions in the Governing Body of Linacre College and, later, in an *ad hoc* committee, the form of this collection of essays has changed considerably. At the outset, much help was received from Mr. J. McE. Potter, Wadham College, Oxford, and from the late Charles D. O'Malley, of the University of California at Los Angeles, who gave both advice and biographical material. The Editors have had occasion to seek much assistance at various stages of their work, and they wish to thank particularly for help in the preparation of this volume: Miss Diana Allen, Museum of the History of Science, Oxford University; Mrs. Irene Ashton, Sheffield; Dr. M. Barratt, the Bodleian Library, Oxford; Mr. D. J. Bryden, Whipple Science Museum, Cambridge; Mr. J. N. Bryson, Balliol College, Oxford; Dr. H. K. Cameron, President, Monumental Brass Society; Mr. Bernard Dod, the Clarendon Press, Oxford; Mrs. Mirjam Foot, the British Library, London; Miss Phyllis M. Giles, Fitzwilliam Museum, Cambridge; Miss P. A. Harding, late of Balliol College, Oxford; Lady Ursula Hicks, Linacre College, Oxford; Professor G. L. Huxley, the Queen's University, Belfast; Dr. C. H. Josten, Neuss am Rhein; Mr. Peter Leslie, London; Dr. G. L. Lewis, St. Antony's College, Oxford; Mrs. Constance Linacre, London; Mr. and Mrs. A. T. Linacre, London; Dr. P. A. Lineham, St. John's College, Cambridge; Dr.

Carlo Maccagni, Domus Galileana, Pisa; Mr. R. E. Maddison, Heston; Mrs. Frances O'Malley, University of California at Los Angeles; Dr. Carlo Masera, Rome; Mr. Paul Morgan, the Bodleian Library, Oxford; Miss Anne-Marie Mulligan, Hastings, New Zealand; Dr. P. F. J. Obbema, Bibliotheek der Rijksuniversiteit, Leyden; Mr. L. M. Payne, The Royal College of Physicians, London; Dr. David Phillips, London; Dr. D. McG. Rogers, the Bodleian Library, Oxford; Professor Lucia Rossetti, Università di Padova; Dr. A. B. Scott, the Queen's University, Belfast; Mr. J. S. G. Simmons, All Souls College, Oxford; Mr. John Simons, Museum of the History of Science, Oxford; Dr. Graham Speake, the Clarendon Press, Oxford; Mr. Paul Turner, Linacre College, Oxford; Dott. Vittorio Valli, Università di Padova; Mrs. Rosemary Verey, Cirencester.

FRANCIS MADDISON
Linacre College
Curator, Museum of the History
of Science, Oxford University

MARGARET PELLING
Linacre College
Research Assistant, Wellcome Unit
for the History of Medicine,
Oxford University

CHARLES WEBSTER
Corpus Christi College
Reader in the History of Medicine,
and Director, Wellcome Unit for
the History of Medicine,
Oxford University

Oxford, August 1974

Postscriptum, November 1975

Most of the papers published in this volume were written and submitted to the Editors in 1972 and 1973. Although a few bibliographical additions and corrections have been made during 1975, it has not been possible to bring the bibliographical references thoroughly up to date.

Notes to Editors' Introduction

1. The translation is that of Francis Morgan Nichols, *The Epistles of Erasmus from his Earliest Letters to his Fifty-first Year arranged in Order of Time . . .*, [i], London, 1901, p. 226. The original Latin text is as follows: '. . . tantum autem humanitatis atque eruditionis, non illius protritae ac triuialis, sed reconditae, exactae, antiquae, Latinae Graecaeque, vt iam Italiam nisi visendi gratia haud multum desyderem. Coletum meum cum audio, Platonem ipsum mihi videor audire. In Grocino quis illum absolutum disciplinarum orbem non miretur? Linacri iudicio quid acutius, quid altius, quid emunctius? Thomae Mori ingenio quid vnquam finxit natura vel mollius, vel dulcius, vel felicius? Iam quid ego reliquum catalogum recenseam? . . .'; P. S. Allen *et al.* (eds.), *Opus epistolarum Des. Erasmi Roterodami*, 12 vols., Oxford, 1906–58, i. 273. Robert Fisher was 'the kyng's solicitor at Rome' (see Allen, op. cit. i. 188). In this Introduction, translations from the Latin, not otherwise acknowledged, will be by the Editors.

2. François Rabelais, *Œuvres complètes*, Paris, Éd. du Seuil, 1973, p. 764. This passage occurs in chapter 67 (of the *Quart Livre*), first published in 1552; see Rabelais, op cit., pp. 29–30 and 560. The words are supposed to be those of François Villon (1431–*c.* 1465), in exile in England, addressed to Edward V (1470–83)! As a doctor himself, Rabelais presumably knew Linacre's translations of Galen.

3. John Noble Johnson, *The Life of Thomas Linacre*, ed. by Robert Graves, London, 1835. Johnson (1787–1823), M.A., Magdalen Hall, Oxford, 1810, M.D., 1814, was physician to Westminster Hospital, 1818–22. His editor, Robert James Graves (1796–1853) was also a physician, President of the Irish College of Physicians, 1843–4, F.R.S., 1849. There are biographies of both men in *D.N.B.* Though verbose and often speculative, Johnson's *Life* remains the most useful guide, and a basic source of facts. On publication, it seems to have excited little interest; the copy in the Bodleian Library bears the following note, by the publisher, Ed. Lumley of Chancery Lane: 'As this book did not sell I destroyed all but a few for presents only.' William Osler, *Thomas Linacre* (Linacre Lecture, 1908), Cambridge, 1908. J. F. Payne, 'Linacre, Thomas', *D.N.B.*, 1909. Joseph Frank Payne (1840–1910), Magdalen College, Oxford, a prominent physician and Fellow of the Royal College of Physicians, had contributed a longer biographical introduction to an early photographically produced facsimile edition of one of Linacre's translations:

Galeni Pergamensis de Temperamentis, et de Inaequali Intemperie libri tres Thoma Linacro Anglo interprete . . . Reproduced in exact Facsimile, with an Introduction by Joseph Frank Payne . . . Cambridge, 1881, pp. 5–48. There is a biography of Payne in *D.N.B.* (Supplement 1901–30). An early workmanlike biography of Linacre appears in *Biographia Britannica or, The Lives of the Most Eminent Persons who have flourished in Great Britain and Ireland,* v, London, 1790, pp. 2970–4. The only recent medical historian to devote serious general studies to Linacre was the late Charles D. O'Malley: see in particular his *English Medical Humanists. Thomas Linacre and John Caius* (Logan Clendening Lectures on the History and Philosophy of Medicine, 12th ser.), Lawrence, Ka., 1965, and 'Thomas Linacre', *Dictionary of Scientific Biography,* ed. by C. C. Gillispie, viii, New York, 1973, pp. 360–1. For several studies of Linacre as a humanist, and other brief modern papers, see Margaret Pelling, 'Published References to Thomas Linacre', below, pp. 337–53, esp. 347 ff. See also, generally, George B. Parks, *The English Traveler in Italy,* i, *The Middle Ages (to 1525),* Rome, 1954, pp. 456–62 and *passim*; A. B. Emden, *A Biographical Register of the University of Oxford to A.D. 1500,* ii, Oxford, 1958, 1147–9, who lists twenty-five different spellings of Linacre's surname and the appellation 'Thomas Anglicus' (see above, p. xix, and below, p. xl n. 41); Sir George Clark, *A History of the Royal College of Physicians of London,* 2 vols., Oxford, 1964, esp. i, ch. III, 'Thomas Linacre'; and [D. M. Rogers], *Erasmus and his English Friend'. Catalogue of an Exhibition held at the Bodleian Library, to Commemorate the Fifth Centenary of the Birth of Erasmus, May 1969,* Oxford, forthcoming.

4. Clark, op. cit. i. 337.

5. Apart from Henry VIII and, presumably, other members of the royal family, Linacre's patients included Erasmus, Wolsey, William Warham, and Richard Foxe (Johnson, op. cit., *passim*). How long Linacre continued the active practice of medicine is not known, but Payne, Introduction to *Galen* (cited above, p. xxviii n. 3), p. 25, drew attention to a passage, in Linacre's dedication of his translation of *De naturalibus facultatibus,* London, 1523, sig. [A1ᵛ], to the Archbishop of Canterbury, Warham, which might be relevant. The passage refers to the leisure which a living (owed to Warham) had brought him: 'pro ocio in quod me (honorifico collato sacerdotio) ex negocio primus uindicasti'. On Linacre's ordination, see p. xiv, and p. xxxi n. 7.

We have but a few glimpses of Linacre's medical practice; the only account of a medical treatment by Linacre is quoted on pp. xv–xvi and n. 18. On 5 June [1516], Erasmus, having put off a sea voyage on account of a slight fever, wrote to Linacre, from St. Omer, asking for details of the medicine which he took by Linacre's prescription when last in London, his boy having left the prescription at the apothecary's: '. . . Febricula subito oborta fuit in causa quo minus me nauigationi commiserim, praesertim dissuadente medico Ghisberto [= the town physician of St. Omer]. Maiorem in modum te rogo vt pharmacum quod, cum proxime essem Londini sumpsi te autore, denuo descriptum mihi transmittas; nam puer schedulam apud pharmaco-polam reliquit. Erit id mihi longe gratissimum' (Allen, op. cit. ii. 247; translation in Nichols, op. cit. ii, London, 1904, p. 274). Erasmus was suffer-ing from the stone, the same condition from which, according to Erasmus,

Linacre died (see Erasmus's letter, written at Basle, to Juan Luis Vives, 27 December 1524, in which he says he would feel more bitterly about the death of Linacre, did he not consider from what torments he was withdrawn: 'Linacri mortem acerbius ferrem, ni reputarem quantis cruciatibus subductus sit' (Allen, op. cit. v. 612)). A letter from Erasmus, 27 August 1526, also written from Basle, to the physician and astronomer Guillaume Cop (d. 1532), in which he describes his own illness in detail, and equates it with that from which Linacre died: '. . . Apparet tamen exhulcerationem aut scabiem esse organorum vrinalium. Aiunt Thomam Linacrum hoc malo mortuum esse' (Allen, op. cit. vi. 380), is followed by an even longer letter (?October 1526) seeking medical advice, written to John Francis, one of the founders of the College of Physicians, again saying that Linacre perished of this disease: 'Sic habet morbus, quorsum euasurus nouit Dominus. Vereor ne, si accedat agitatio aut aliud simile, vertatur in excoriationem vesicae; quo malo nihil esse potest cruciabilius. Hoc cruciatu perisse narrant Thomam Linacrum' (Allen, op. cit. vi. 424). Erasmus's diagnosis of Linacre's terminal condition is not supported by George Lily (d. 1559), who says that Linacre died of a ruptured hernia: 'ad extremum disruptae herniae confectus'; George Lily, 'Virorum aliquot in Britannia, qui nostro seculo eruditione, & doctrina clari, memorabilesq*ue* fuerunt, Elogia', in Paolo Giovio, *Descriptio Britanniae, Scotiae, Hyberniae, et Orchadum* [Venice, 1548], f. 49ᵛ. (Cf. below, p. xxxii n. 14; Johnson, op. cit., p. 297 n., 'nephritic paroxysm', and Osler, op. cit., p. 34, 'stone of the bladder'.)

Linacre appears to have set some store by cramp-rings, which were blessed at a special ceremony by the kings and queens of England, 'for the cure of epilepsy and other spasmodic disorders'; convulsions, epilepsy, cramp, and rheumatism being considered broadly related. The royal blessing ceremony appears to be peculiarly English, deriving from a ring which was one of the sacred relics in the shrine of Edward the Confessor in Westminster Abbey; Raymond Crawfurd, 'The Blessing of Cramp-Rings. A Chapter in the History of the Treatment of Epilepsy' in *Studies in the History and Method of Science*, ed. Charles Singer, [i], Oxford, 1917, pp. 165–87, esp. 165, 173, 174, 180, 183. On 10 June [1518], Linacre wrote to Guillaume Budé in Paris, thanking him for help with a book (see below, p. xxxvi n. 24), and telling him that he had sent him some rings, consecrated by the King, as a charm against spasms: ἔπεμψα δέ σοι δακτυλίους τινάς, οὓς ἤδη σοι δοθέντας πείθομαι. ἀτελὲς πάνυ, εἰ πρὸς τὴν τιμὴν αὐτῶν ἀποβλέπεις, δῶρον, εἰ δὲ πρὸς τὴν δύναμιν, οὐκ ἀνεπιτήδειον ἴσως τῆς ἡμῶν φιλίας ἐνέχυρον. δακτύλιος γὰρ καὶ γαμούντων καὶ διδασκάλων καὶ εὐωχησομένων βεβαιοῖ πίστιν. οὗτοι δὲ καὶ παρὰ τοῦ βασιλέως ἡμῶν ἀφιερωθέντες, ἀλεξιτήριον σπασμῶν ἁπάντων εἶναι νομίζονται. ὥσθ' ἱερούς ὄντας, ἱεροῦ χρήματος, οὐκ ἀλλότριον ἤτοι δεσμόν, εἶναι ἢ μνημόσυνον· σύ δ' οὖν αὐτούς, ὅπως ἂν ἔχωσιν, μετ' εὐνοίας πεμφθέντας, εὐνοϊκῶς ἀποδέξῃ. ἔρρωσο Κελτῶν λογιώτατε; Guillaume Budé, *Epistolae*, Basle, 1521, p. 26 (slightly corrected) and Johnson, op. cit., pp. 254 and 310 (who gives a faulty Greek text). Budé's reply, on 8 July following, hints perhaps at scepticism for he says that he has distributed several of the eighteen rings of silver and one of gold to the wives of his friends and relatives, delivering them with an air of ostentation and swearing that they were appeasers of evil, calumny and slander! Budé, op. cit., p. 24, and Johnson, op. cit., p. 250. In this context, Johnson, op. cit., pp. 254–5, appears to have misdated, and therefore misunderstood, Budé's letter to Linacre of 9 September, which we would date to the year 1517, not 1518. The phrase 'Magnas habeo tibi gratias ob munus tuum iucundum...' must refer to an earlier gift; Budé, op. cit., p. 27, and see below, p. xxxvi n. 24. Linacre also sent cramp-rings to Christophorus Longolius (*c.* 1498–1522; 'une sorte de Pic de la Mirandole français' (see Allen, op. cit. iii. 427–3)). On 7 May 1521 Longolius wrote to Linacre from Padua, thanking him for the present brought to him by Reginald Pole, but saying he would rather have had a letter than gold rings or bracelets: 'Pergratum mihi fuit munusculum tuum, quod quasi quoddam coniunctionis atque amicitiae nostrae monumentum Reginaldus Polus hodie mihi reddidit . . . Quod si tuae erga me uoluntatis pignus aliquod apud me esse uolebas, qui tam multa in ipsa Britannia anno superiore dedisses, misisses potius literarum aliquid, quae nobis cum omnibus uiriolis & annulis iucundiores certe fuissent, tum uero certius de tuo in me animo uberiusque testimonium attulissent. Nunc aurum misisti, αἰθόμενον quidem illud πῦρ ἄτε, sed quo neque tu homo philosophus planè abundas, neque magnopere capior: literas non misisti, quas & tibi conscribere fuit facilimum & mihi legere longe iucundissimum. Atque ut intelligas ea me sentire quae scribam, ego uero contra ad te mitto pro annulo epistolam, simul & defensionum nostrarum libellum nunc primum ex sententia nostra editum . . .'; Christophorus Longolius, *Orationes*, Florence, 1524, fols. 108ᵛ–109ʳ.

6. James Kelsey McConica, *English Humanists and Reformation Politics under Henry VIII and Edward VI*, Oxford, 1965. Because he appears untainted by the Reformation, Roman Catholic physicians have sometimes seen in Linacre the archetype of their profession; hence, for example, the journal title, *The Linacre Quarterly*; see Pelling, op. cit., *passim*.

7. Linacre was ordained subdeacon on 22 December 1515 and deacon on 7 April 1520; Register of Fitzjames, London, fols. 170ᵛ and 180–1, recorded in an interleaved copy of Emden, op. cit., with additions by the author, Bodleian Library, Oxford. Linacre's preferments are recorded by Johnson, op. cit., pp. 191–4; see also Thomas Tanner, *Bibliotheca Britannico-Hibernica*, London, 1748, p. 482; *Letters and Papers, Foreign and Domestic, of the Reign of Henry VIII*, ii, ed. J. S. Brewer, London, 1864, pp. 1147, 1240; *Historical Manuscripts Commission, Calendar of the Manuscripts of the Dean and Chapter of Wells*, ii, London, 1914, p. 219; John Le Neve, *Fasti Ecclesiae Anglicanae 1300–1541*, iv, 'Northern Province', comp. by B. Jones, London, 1963, pp. 12, 72, and viii, 'Bath and Wells', comp. by B. Jones London, 1964, p. 47; and Hants Record Office, B/1/A1. 2. fol. 5ᵛ (Visitation Book), cited in interleaved copy of Emden, mentioned above. Tanner, loc. cit., does appear to be referring to ordination and not to collation to a benefice (cf. Payne, Introduction to *Galen*, cited above, (p. xxix n. 3), p. 21, and Johnson, op. cit., p. 193), where he gives 22 December 1520, but has seemingly conflated the dates given above. It may here be recalled that when Andrea Ammonio wrote from London to Erasmus on 19 May [1511]: 'D. Linacer sacerdotio auctus est, pro quo omnes Musas fortunae gratias egisse arbitror' (Allen, op. cit. i. 458), Fortune, whom

Ammonio deemed all the Muses should thank, had provided Linacre with livings, but he was not yet ordained, despite the use of the word *sacerdotio*. Linacre's ordination so late in life occasioned John Weever's pithy description of him as 'this old Physitian, and young Priest'; John Weever, *Ancient Funerall Monuments . . .*, London, 1631, p. 370 (for Linacre's memorial, which records his late ordination, see pp. xxv–xxvi and p. xlviii n. 78).

8. See Giles Barber, 'Thomas Linacre: A Bibliographical Survey of his Works', below, pp. 290–336.

9. See John M. Fletcher, 'Linacre's Lands and Lectureships', pp. 107–97.

10. Most of these facts are found in the early references to Linacre, cited in this Introduction, wherein we have tried to avoid captious criticism of worthy and sincere writers who had no cause to lie, though they may have been mistaken, and we have treated as plausible a number of controversial statements. The earliest 'life' of Linacre is either that by Lily, op. cit. (1548), fol. 49[r–v], or that in John Bale, *Illustrium maioris Britanniae scriptorum, hoc est, Angliae Cambriae, ac Scotiae summarium*, Ipswich, 1548, fols. 216[v]–217[r]; Payne, op. cit., p. 47.

An early commemorative lecture, written for an unexplained 'officij ratio', is that given in the summer of 1560 at the University of Leipzig by Michael Barth, and published the following November: *Oratio de Thoma Linacro Britanno conscripta et habita in Academia Lipsica a Michaele Barth Annaebergensi. Lipsiae Idib. November. Anno M.D.LX.*

11. Raphael Holinshed, *Chronicles*, London, 1587, iii. fols. 977, says Linacre was 'borne in Darbie', and this is repeated by Weever, loc. cit., and Thomas Fuller, *The History of the Worthies of England*, London, 1662, p. 235 [*sic, recte* 231]. See Josephine W. Bennett, 'John Morer's Will: Thomas Linacre and Prior Sellyng's Greek Teaching', *Studies in the Renaissance*, xv (1968), 70–91, at 72–3, n. 9.

12. Or the neighbourhood of Canterbury, or possibly of the diocese of Canterbury. See John Caius, *Historiae Cantabrigiensis Academiae ab vrbe conditae, Liber primus . . .*, London, 1574 ('Liber secundus' starts on p. 115 without a separate title-page, p. 126 (this work is the second part of *De Antiquitate Cantabrigiensis Academiae Libri duo . . .* London, 1574, of which there was an earlier edition in 1568 without the *Historia*)). The passage referring to Linacre reads: 'Ac medicinae stipendium magni illius viri, & literis clarissimi medici Thomae Linacri Cantuariensis, & hic et Oxoniae institutum fuit.'

13. See the discussion in Bennett, op. cit., p. 72.

14. e.g. by Bennett, op. cit., pp. 71–2. The date, 1460, is poorly documented. Johnson, op. cit., p. 1, refers to John Freind, *The History of Physick; from the Time of Galen to the Beginning of the Sixteenth Century. Chiefly with regard to Practice*, 2 vols., London, 1725–6, ii, app. 8. Freind's account of Linacre, ii. 400–15, is partly based on this appendix (pp. 33–44 of a separate pagination) which is a reprint of a Latin letter, dated 19 October (XIV Cal. Nov.) 1725, to Freind from the learned French bibliographer, Michel Maittaire (1668–1747),

long resident in England as a result of the revocation of the Edict of Nantes. The letter is entirely devoted to information about Linacre's life and work, and the date of Linacre's birth, given at the beginning of the letter, is solely derived from the date of death and Linacre's age when he died, given on p. 40: 'Constat Linacrum obiisse anno salutis Christianae 1524, aetatis suae 64, in D. Pauli Aede apud Londinenses sepultum'; a footnote gives the source as '*Baile*. Diction.' The first edition (1697) of Pierre Bayle's *Dictionaire historique et critique* has no article on Linacre, but subsequent editions do, and Maittaire could have used either the second edition, Rotterdam, 1702 (ii. 1825), or the third, Rotterdam, 1720 (ii. 1718–19). Bayle, who calls Linacre '. . . l'un des plus savans personnages du XVI siecle . . .', says that he died in 1524 at the age of sixty-four, citing Lily, Blount, and Moréri. Lily (op. cit. on p. xxx n. 5 above, i.e. in a work published in Paolo Giovio's *Descriptio*, 1548) does not mention Linacre's age at death, nor the date of his birth. Thomas Pope Blount, *Censura celebriorum authorum*, London, 1690, p. 376, indeed notes that Linacre died at the age of sixty-four; he gives no source but, presumably, like Louis Moréri, *Le Grand Dictionaire historique*, Lyons, 1674, p. 1289; 2nd edn., Lyons, 1681, ii. 422, and other editions up to the 9th, Amsterdam, 1702, iii. 350, Blount derives his information from another work by Paolo Giovio, *Elogia doctorum virorum ab avorum memoria publicatis ingenii monumentis illustrium*, Antwerp, 1557, ch. LIII, 135: 'Sexagesimo autem, & quarto aetatis anno, ex dolore disruptae herniae vita excedens, honestam domum Londini Medicorum Collegio dedicauit'; this passage is also found in Petrus Castellanus, *Vitae illustrium medicorum*, Antwerp, 1617, pp. 177–8 (Castellanus (Duchatel) (1585–1682), a Flemish physician and antiquary, reprints the whole of the 'life' of Linacre by Giovio). Moréri also cites Pitseus, Erasmus, Budé, and Van der Linden as sources for his biographical account of Linacre. The first of these, John Pits, *Relationum historicarum de rebus Anglicis*, Paris, 1619, i. 698–700, does not inform us about the date of Linacre's birth, nor has any such information been traced in the writings of the other three authors mentioned.

So far as we have been able to discover, Giovio remains the sole ultimate authority for the statement that Linacre died at the age of sixty-four, and hence was born in 1460. Moreover, Giovio added this statement to his *Elogia* of 1557, because, as we have seen, Lily, a contributor to Giovio's *Descriptio* of 1548, makes no such remark. Cf. Bennett, loc. cit., for references to Edward Hasted, *The History and Topographical Survey of the County of Kent*, Canterbury, 1779–99, concerning Linacre's date of birth and origins. A clue to the date of Linacre's birth is given in a letter from Erasmus to Ambrosius Leo (Ambrogio Leone of Nola), physician to Aldus Manutius's household in Venice. In a letter to him (quoted below, pp. xl and xli n. 43), Erasmus refers to Linacre as being 'of your profession and, if I am not wrong, the same age': '. . . tuae professionis ac, ni fallor, aetatis'. Leo was born in 1459 and died in 1525 (see Charles B. Schmitt, 'Thomas Linacre and Italy', below, pp. 36–75, at p. 73).

15. John Leland, *Commentarii de scriptoribus Britannicis*, ed. by Anthony Hall, Oxford, 1709, p. 483. This is the first publication of this work of Leland.

Bennett, loc. cit., considers the authority of Leland's statement to be under-mined by the fact that it goes on to mention Sellyng's friend, Poliziano, wrongly, as being at Bologna.

16. Cicero, *Orator ad Brutum*, xxx; Cicero, b. 106 B.C., is here referring to his speech, *Pro Roscio Amerino*, delivered in 80 B.C. Sallust, *Catilina*, xlix, so described Caesar when the latter was thirty-three or thirty-five.

17. Some items of biographical information need not long detain us: Weever, loc. cit. on p. xxxii n. 7 above, has a marginal note, '*Tho. Linaker* phisition, and his wife'; clearly an error; Weever mentions no wife in the accompanying text. A letter written from Padua by William Latimer to Aldus Manutius, 4 November [?1498], asks Aldus to assist in the return of a borrowed bed to one Thomas, presumably Linacre; see P. S. Allen, 'Linacre and Latimer in Italy', *English Historical Review*, xviii (1903), 513–17, at 517. A letter from William Grocyn in London to Aldus, 27 August 1499, printed by Aldus in *Astronomici veteres*, Venice, October 1499 (which contains Linacre's Proclus; see below, Barber, op. cit., pp. 291–2), makes it clear that Linacre was back in London by that date; Allen, *E.H.R.*, p. 517.

On 28 November 1503, Linacre was a witness to the Will of Sir Reginald Bray (d. 1503), stepfather of Henry VII, statesman, and architect (he prob-ably designed Henry VII's chapel, Westminster); Geo. F. Tudor Sherwood, 'Early Berkshire Wills, from the P.C.C., on to 1558', *Berks, Bucks, & Oxon. Archaeological Society Journal*, i, no. 1 (1895), 89–92, at 90. B.J., 'A Letter and Linacre', *The Cantuarian*, xxvi, no. 5 (April 1956), 410 (and facing plate, but the document there reproduced, presumably in error, is not the document discussed), gives a transcript of an undated fragment of a letter (in the Chapter Archives in the Cathedral Library, Canterbury; apparently from the binding of a sixteenth-century ecclesiastical court register), written to the Prior of Canterbury Cathedral, possibly by the Vicar of Mersham, Kent (of which parish Linacre was Rector in 1509). The writer asks the Prior to pay £6 to 'M. Lynacr' on the writer's behalf and promises to reimburse the Prior 'at a reasonabull day'. The author of the article thinks that the £6 was for books, but we do not think the transcribed text makes this clear.

In 1520, Linacre was executor of the Will of his friend, William Grocyn. See Montagu Burrows, 'Linacre's Catalogue of Books belonging to William Grocyn', part V of *Collectanea. Second Series*, ed. Montagu Burrows, Oxford Historical Society, xvi, 1890, 319–80.

18. 'Remedium non prius scies quam indicem autorem. Is erat Thomas Linacrus, Regis Anglorum medicus primarius, vir vt in omni genere disci-plinarum exacte doctus, ita nusquam non superstitiosae, pene dixerim, diligentiae.

Sed de autore mox plura; nunc accipe remedium. Calculus e potu ceruisiae conceptus haeserat in sinu quopiam sex hebdomadas; interim non vrgebat quidem dolor, sed ipsa natura solicita ac deiecta monebat subesse magnum periculum. Nam ipse dubitabam quid esset mali. Equidem pro meo genio sum frigidus postulator officii; et Linacrus hoc erat ingenio vt nisi extimula-tus non admodum aduerteret animum. Submonuit amicus quidam vt in-

cantamentis aliquot verborum expergefacerem hominem. Feci. Nihil eo dili-
gentius. Accersitus pharmocopola. Decoctum in cubiculo meo pharmacum,
admotum ipso praesente medico. Bis admotum fuerat, et mox a somno
sum enixus calculum parem nucleo amygdalino. Huius remedii vice Germani
vtuntur balneis. Verum hoc quum idem efficiat, multo parabilius est. Cama-
millas ac petroselinum inuoluo linteo, decoquo in vase puro, aqua munda
ferme vsque ad dimidium. Linteum, vt est feruens, eximo ex olla, et humore
celeriter quantum potest expresso, admoueo lateri. Si feruor est intolerabilis,
sacculum in quo sunt herbae, obuoluo linteo sicco, sic vt velut ansis hinc
atque hinc teneri possit. Et si initio latus non fert contactum ob feuorem,
suspendo supra locum, vt vapor afficiat corpus donec feruor coeperit esse
tolerabilis. Mox compono me ad somnum; post quem si recrudescat dolor,
referuefactum linteum admoueo. Id a me nunquam bis factum est quin calculus descenderit ad loca vicina vesicae, in quibus dolor est mitior. Id tamen
praesidium fefellit me primum in proximo nixu' (Allen, op. cit. vi. 46–7).

A medical consultation with Linacre is referred to by George Lily, describing the death of his father, William Lily, High-Master of St Paul's School,
London: 'With the plague raging in London, his wife with whom he had
always most conscientiously lived in loving harmony killed by it, and at the
same time and from the same cause almost completely deprived of numerous
offspring, even to his fifteenth descendant, he was in the end to perish of a
small "wart" (*verrucula*). A wart, which a long time before had developed on
his hip, was accidentally scratched. Afterwards it had opened up painfully,
involving veins and arteries in a monstrous tumour, and had grown malig-
nantly. Much troubled, some physicians promising him for the condition an
easy cure by surgery, and many wholly dissuading him from it, Linacre
especially declaring the most certain danger to his life, he decided to be
operated upon. A week later he died, a quinquagenarian, to the great grief
of his fellow citizens among whom during his lifetime he was very popular';
'Ad postremum, desaeuiente Londini peste, coniuge, qua cum amabili semper
concordia sanctissime uixerat, absumpta, & numerosa simul sobole, quam ex
eadem ad decimam quintam usque prolem susceperat, penè orbatus, ex
uerrucula, quae diu antea coxae adnata, temerè scalpendo, recrudescentibus
postea doloribus, ad ingentem strumam uenas, arteriasque implicantem,
malignè concreuerat, multum uexatus, ex chirurgia medicis aliquot facilem
eius morbi curationem sibi promittentibus, licet plerisque id omnino dissua-
dentibus, & Linacro inprimis certissimum uitae periculum ei praedicente,
secari uoluit, unde, & septimo post die quinquagenarius interiit, cum magno
ciuium suorum desiderio, quibus dum uixit gratissimus extitit'; Lily, op. cit.,
fols. 47ᵛ–48ʳ.

19. Royal physician since the King's accession in 1509; see Bennett, op. cit.,
p. 72. According to George Lily, loc. cit. on p. xxx n. 5 above, Linacre had
been physician to Henry VII. Mary had been betrothed since 1508 to the
Prince of Castile (the future Emperor Charles V), but was in fact married in
1514 at Abbeville to Louis XII of France.

20. *Letters and Papers, Foreign and Domestic, of the reign of Henry VIII*, i, ed.
J. S. Brewer, 2nd ed. rev. by R. H. Brodie, London, 1920, pp. 1159–62, item

2656, and *passim*; ii, ed. J. S. Brewer, London, 1864, pt. 2 'King's Book of Payments', 1465, and *passim*.

21. Lily, op. cit., fol. 49ʳ: 'Arthuro Principi, Henrici Septimi regis filio aliquandiu preceptor datus, praecipuè autem ad medicinae scientia*m* uix ulli adhuc in Britannia nato foeliciter tentatam, studium omne conuertit: In hac demum ita se exercuit, ut commendata sibi Henrici regis sanitatis tutela, & talari toga purpurea amictus, uillosi serici nigri stola lata in humeros proiecta, inter aulae regiae proceres co*n*spicuus incederet.' George Lily (d. 1559) was the son of William Lily (1468?–1522), High Master of St. Paul's School, London, so his statements about Linacre may be the result of personal observation or, at least, first-hand information.

22. See Maureen Hill, 'The Iconography of Thomas Linacre', below, pp. 354–74.

23. See Frontispiece, Barber, op. cit., below, pp. 296–7, and Hill, op. cit., p. 364.

24. Thomas More wrote to Erasmus on 15 December [1516]: 'As soon as Christmas is over, Linacre is going to send what he is translating from Galen to Paris, to be printed there. Lupset will go with it, and stay to correct the Press'; Nichols, op. cit. ii. 447. The Latin text is as follows: 'Linacer protinus a Natali quae vertit e Galeno mittet Luteciam excudenda, comite Lupseto qui calcographis castigator aderit'; Allen, op. cit. ii. 420. On 9 September [1517], Budé wrote to Linacre saying that he had read in Linacre's Galen, which he praised, what Lupset had asked him to read: 'Legi in tuo Galeno (diui boni quàm splendido futuro mox opere) ea quae me legere Lupsetus uester uoluit . . .'; Budé, op. cit., p. 27 (as stated on p. xxxi n. 5 above, we consider, on internal evidence, that this letter should be dated to 1517; in fact, of the other two letters between Budé and Linacre there printed, the earlier letter is obviously placed second, so the three letters are printed in an order which is the reverse of the date sequence). On 15 September of that year, Lupset himself wrote from Paris to Erasmus, saying that he had completed Linacre's work, *De sanitate tuenda*: 'Absoluimus his diebus opus Linacri de sanitate tuenda' (Allen, iii. 90). Linacre wrote to Budé on 10 June [1518] (letter quoted above, p. xxx n. 5; Budé, op. cit., pp. 25–6), thanking him for assistance with a book, and sending him a gift of cramp-rings. In a very long reply dated 8 July [1518] (also noted above, p. xxx n. 5), Budé says that he cannot regret the labour or time spent on this book: 'At enim librum de sanitate tuenda à te uersum ut legerem, & tibi quoquo modo obsequerer, nec laboris nec temporis rationem habui: quasi uero in hoc tibi operam potius q*uam* mihi ac literis dederim, aut id tibi tempus gratuitum donarim, in quo quantum ipse proficerim, me nunq*uam* poenitebit'; Budé, op. cit. 23.

25. In a holograph note in the margin of the first page of the biography of Linacre in Steevens's own copy of Fuller, op. cit. (Bodleian Library, Oxford, shelf-mark: Malone 3), p. 235 [*sic, recte* 231]. On Linacre and the damask rose, cf. also Hasted, op. cit. iv. 743, n. w, which as far as it refers to Linacre is derived from Hakluyt (see below, p. xxxvii n. 27).

26. Francis Bacon, Lord Verulam, *Sylva sylvarum: or A Naturall Historie . . . Published after the Authors death. By William Rawley . . .*, London, t.p.: 1626;

engraved title: 1627, cent. VII, 165: 'The *Comming* of *Trees* and *Plants* in certaine *Regions*, and not in others, is sometimes Casuall: For many haue beene translated, and haue prospered well; As *Damaske-Roses*, that haue not been knowne in England aboue a hundred yeares, and now are so common.' Steevens seems to have thought that Bacon derived his information from Hakluyt. A copy of a later edition of Bacon's *Sylva*, London, t.p.: 1635; engraved title: 1631 (Bodleian Library, Oxford, shelf-mark: T. 11. 20. Th.) contains manuscript notes by Christopher Wren (1591–1658), Dean of Windsor. A note by the Dean on the sentence beginning, 'As *Damaske-Roses . . .*', remarks, 'yet now, they, & many other sorts of Roses are infinitely encreased'; lists the following types of rose: damask, red, white, York and Lancaster, cinnamon, musk, yellow, Flanders; and concludes, 'The Cause is yᵉ infinite multiplication of Gardens, since 1552, wᵗ time Cardan beeing in England complaines of the Negligence in Planting Gardens throwout yᵉ kingdom:'

27. Richard Hakluyt, *The Principal Nauigations, Voiages, Traffiques and Discoueries of the English Nation . . .*, 3 vols., London, 1598–1600, ii. pt. 1, 165. The statement occurs in the context of an interesting and apparently well-informed passage which is worth quoting here. This passage comes under the heading, 'Other some things to be remembered', in 'Remembrances for master S. to giue him the better occasion to informe himselfe of some things in *England*, and after of some other things in Turkie, to the great profite of the Common weale of this Countrey. Written by the foresayd master *Richard Hakluyt*, for a principall English Factor at *Constantinople* 1582': '. . . If the like loue [referring to the bringing out at great risk of saffron by a pilgrim] in this our age were in our people that now become great trauellers, many knowledges, and many trades, and many herbes and plants might be brought into this realme that might doe the realme good. And the Romans hauing that care, brought from all coasts of the world into *Italie* all arts and sciences, and all kinds of beasts and fowles, and all herbs, trees, busks and plants that might yeeld profit or pleasure to their countrey of *Italie*. And if this care had not bene heretofore in our ancesters, then had our life bene sauage now. . . . And in time of memory things haue bene brought in that were not here before, as the Damaske rose by Doctour *Linaker* king *Henry* the seuenth and king *Henrie* the eights Physician, the Turky cocks and hennes about fifty yeres past, the Artichowe in time of king *Henry* the eight, and of later time was procured out of *Italy* the Muske rose plant, the plum called the *Perdigwena*, and two kinds more by the Lord *Cromwell* after his trauell, and the Abricot by a French Priest one *Wolfe* Gardiner to king *Henry* the eight: and now within these foure yeeres there haue bene brought into *England* from *Vienna* in *Austria* diuers kinds of flowers called *Tulipas*, and those and other procured thither a little before from *Constantinople* by an excellent man called M. *Carolus Clusius . . .*'

28. 'Harum rosarum apud Italos, Gallos, Germanos, diuersasque gentes, nunc est frequens vsus, quas Damascenas vocant, quoniam ex Damasco nobilissima Syriae vrbe credunt deuenisse. Apud nos vero, triginta ferè sunt anni, de qua notitiam attingimus'; Nicolás Monardes, *De secanda vena in pleuriti inter Graecos & Arabes concordia. Item . . . De rosa et partibus eius, De succi rosarum*

temperatura, nec non de rosis Persicis, quas Alexandrinas vocant, Antwerp, 1551, sig. hvi^r–v. There can be little doubt that the phrase, 'Apud nos . . ', refers to Monardes's fellow countrymen, for Monardes, who was born in Seville, returned there, after studying medicine at Alcalá de Henares, and spent the remainder of his life in that city; see Felipe Picatoste y Rodríguez, *Apuntes para una biblioteca científica española del siglo XVI,* Madrid, 1891, pp. 199–201.

29. *The seconde parte of Uuilliam Turners herball* . . ., Cologne, 1562, fol. 116^v. The first part of Turner's herbal was published under the title, *A new Herball* . . ., London, 1551, and this has led to one of several confusions in the *O.E.D.*'s article on the damask rose.

30. Henry Lyte, *A Nieuue Herball, or Historie of Plantes:* . . . *First set foorth in the Doutche or Almaigne tongue, by that learned D. Rembert Dodoens* . . . *And nowe first translated out of French into English* . . ., London, 1578, p. 655.

31. See C. C. Hurst, 'Notes on the Origin and Evolution of our Garden Roses', in Graham Stuart Thomas, *The Old Shrub Roses,* London, 4th edn., repr. 1971, pp. 59 ff., especially 61–9.

32. Ibid., pp. 61–2. It was so named because it was thought to have been introduced from Damascus by a Crusader, Thibault Le Chansonnier (b. 1201).

33. Ibid., p. 68. This is the rose long favoured for the production of rose water, and attar of roses.

34. Cf. ibid., pp. 69–70.

35. If Dean Wren's terminology and classification (p. xxxvii n. 26, above) be valid for the previous century, then we should conclude, by a process of elimination, that Hakluyt was referring either to the Apothecary's Rose of Provins, or to the Autumn Damask Rose.

36. Weaver, loc. cit. It has frequently been suggested (e.g. in the often interesting, but sometimes inaccurate, biographical study of Linacre in John Aikin, *Biographical Memoirs of Medicine in Great Britain from the Revival of Literature to the Time of Harvey,* London, 1780, pp. 28–47, at 41–3, doubtless the source for J. F. C. Hecker, *The Epidemics of the Middle Ages,* transl. by B. G. Babington (Sydenham Society publ.), London, 1844, p. 186 n.a.; Payne, Introduction to *Galen,* cited above (p. xxviii n. 3), p. 17; Payne, Letter to the Editor, *British Medical Journal,* 1909, ii. 1010; Osler, op. cit., pp. 33–4) that Erasmus's satire on grammarians in the *Praise of Folly* includes a description of Linacre. The passage begins: 'I know one "jack-of-all-trades", scholar of Greek and Latin, mathematician, philosopher, doctor, "all in princely style", a man already in his sixties, who has thrown up everything else and spent twenty years vexing and tormenting himself over grammar. He supposes he'd be perfectly happy if he were allowed to live long enough to define precisely how the eight sections of a speech should be distinguished, something in which no one writing in Greek or Latin has ever managed to be entirely successful. And if anyone treats a conjunction as a word with the force of an adverb, it's a thing to go to war about . . .'; Erasmus, *Praise of*

Folly and Letter to Martin Dorp 1515, translated by Betty Radice, with introduction and notes by A. H. T. Levi, Harmondsworth, 1971, p. 146. The Latin text is as follows: 'Noui quendam πολυτεχνότατον, Graecum, Latinum, Mathematicum, philosophum, medicum, καὶ ταῦτα βασιλικὸν, iam sexagenarium, qui caeteris rebus omissis, annis plus uiginti, se torquet ac discruciat in grammatica, prorsus felicem se fore ratus, si tamdiu liceat uiuere, donec certo statuat, quomodo distinguendae sint octo partes orationis, quod hactenus nemo Graecorum aut Latinorum ad plenum praestare valuit. Perinde quasi res sit bello quoque uindicanda, si quis coniunctionem faciat dictionem ad aduerbiorum ius pertinentem'; Erasmus, . . . *Moriae encomium, pro castigatissimo castigatius, unà cum Listrij commentarijs, & alijs complusculis libellis, non minus eruditis quam festiuis*, Basle, Froben, 1519, p. 166. The passage continues in a very unflattering vein (*pace* Payne, Introduction to *Galen*, p. 17), and is not, moreover, in any way an accurate description of Linacre. We have not been able to consult many of the editions of the *Moriae encomium*, but can state that this passage does not occur in the earliest editions we have seen (e.g. Strasbourg, 1511, and the Basle (Froben) edition of 1515, which was the first to contain the commentary by Gerard Lijster). Osler suggested that Linacre might be 'the scholar who gave [Robert] Browning the idea of [the poem,] the "Grammarian's Funeral"' (Osler, op. cit., p. 34; Munro Smith, note quoted editorially in the *British Medical Journal* (1909), ii. 710; Payne, loc. cit.; A. Malloch, 'Browning's Copy of Linacre's Latin Grammar', *Proceedings of the Charaka Club* (New York), viii, 1935, 171–6), but Browning might have been inspired by the passage in Erasmus, see William Clyde DeVane, *A Browning Handbook*, 2nd edn., New York, 1955, pp. 269–72. Cf. also below, Barber, op. cit., p. 306.

37. Edward Surtz and J. H. Hexter (eds.), *The Complete Works of St. Thomas More*, iv, New Haven, Conn., and London, 1965, p. 467, appear to have misunderstood Johnson, op. cit., n. on 27–34, and say that Johnson 'credits Linacre with introducing or reviving the theory of the kinship of Welsh with Greek'. Neither in Johnson, nor elsewhere, have we encountered any evidence that Linacre's classical interests extended to this topic.

38. This refers to the appointment, by Innocent VIII, of Ermolao Barbaro as Patriarch of Aquileia; see Antoine de Varillas, *Anecdotes de Florence ou l'histoire secrète de la Maison de Medicis*, The Hague, 1685, pp. 189–91.

39. Giovio, *Elogia*, 135–6 (also Castellanus, op. cit., pp. 177–8): 'Inde verò multis variae doctrinae ornamentis adauctus, quum Romana quoque ingenia certius agnoscenda, ac opulentiores bibliothecas inspiciendas existimaret, ad vrbem contendit. In primo autem appulsu forte accidit, vt Hermolao Barbaro amicitia iungeretur. Nam ingresso Vaticanam bibliothecam, & Graecos codices euoluenti, superuenit Hermolaus, ad pluteumque humaniter accedens, Non tu herclè, inquit, studiose hospes, vti ego planè sum, Barbarus esse potes, quod lectissimum Platonis librum (is erat Phaedrus) diligenter euoluas. Ad id Linacrus laeto ore respondit, Nec tu sacrate heros, alius esse iam potes, quàm ille fama notus Patriarcha Italorum Latinissimus. Ab hac amicitia (vti casu euenit, feliciter conflata) egregijs demum voluminibus ditatus in

Britanniam redijt . . .' Johnson, op. cit., p. 127, is, not unreasonably, inclined
to believe that this story was invented (or, at least, considerably elaborated)
by Giovio, who 'has added one more to the number of writers in the sixteenth
century, who were unable to resist the opportunity of playing upon a word,
which abstractedly, implied very different qualities from those by which its
possessor was distinguished'!

40. See Schmitt, op. cit., below, pp. 68–70; also Carlos Castellani, *La Stampa
in Venezia dalla sua origine alla morte di Aldo Manuzio seniore*, repr. of edn. of
1889, with introduction by Giorgio E. Ferrari, Trieste, 1973, pp. 42 n. 2; 51
n. 1; 52 n. 2; and 53, which includes a list of members of the Νεακαδημία.

41. Aristoteles, [Opera graeca una cum scriptis Theophrasti, et Philonis
Libro de mundo atque Historia philosophica Galeno adscripta], 5 vols.,
Venice, 1495–8, ii (February 1497), sig. ★ IIʳ: 'Aristótelis uero & quae nunc
legenda damus, & quae mox deo fauente daturi sumus, multum certe elabo-
raui, ut, tum querendis optimis & antiquis libris atque eadem in re multi-
plicibus tum conferendis castigandísque exemplaribus quae dilaceranda
impressoribus traderentur, periréntique ut pariens uipera, in manus hominum
uenirent emendatissima. Id ita sit nec ne sunt mihi grauissimi testes in tota
ferè Italia, et praecipue Venetiis Thomas Anglicus, homo & graece & latine
peritissimus, praecellénsque in doctrinarum omnium disciplinis.' Payne, Introduction to *Galen*, pp. 10–11, mentions that a copy of this edition of Aristotle,
printed on vellum, now in the library of New College, Oxford (shelf-mark:
Ω 7. 1–6), once belonged to Linacre and bears his signature. For a list of books
known to have belonged to Linacre, see Emden, op. cit. ii. 1148, and Barber,
op. cit., below, pp. 331–6.

42. Julius Pollux, Ονομαστικον/*Vocabularium*, Florence, 1520, [2]; cf. Johnson,
op. cit., pp. 241–5, Schmitt, op. cit., pp. 71–2, and Barber, op. cit., pp. 330–1.

43. Lily, op. cit., on Grocyn, fol. 48ᵛ: 'Aristotelis uerò, unà cum Linacro,
& Latemerio communicato labore interpretandi prouinciam est aggressus,
quam tamen paulò post, oblato sibi sacerdotii honore, mutato consilio
deseruit.' The 'living' might refer to Grocyn's appointment in 1506 as
Master of All Hallows, Maidstone, Kent. John Bale, *Scriptorium illustrium
maioris Brytanniae, quam nunc Angliam & Scotiam uocant: Catalogus*, Basle, [1557
9] (this is the 2nd edition of Bale, op. cit. in n. 10 above), pt. ii, 18: 'Attulere
& in Brytanniam ab Italia literas Graecas aetate nostra, Thomas Linacrus,
Galeni nitidissimus interpres: qui Arthuri principis praeceptor fuit. Aequales-
que eius duo Guilhelmi, Latomerus [*sic*] atque Grocyn, qui nobili, sed irrito
uoto, uertendi Aristoteles negocium cum Linacro susceperunt.' In so far as
this enterprise was ever seriously embarked upon, it appears that one of
Linacre's tasks was to translate the *Meteorologica*. A letter from Erasmus, at
Louvain, 15 October [1518], to Ambrosius Leo (see p. xxxiii n. 14), says
that there is in England a most learned man, Thomas Linacre, of whom Leo
may formerly have heard through the praises of Aldus, a doctor like Leo and,
if he is not wrong, of the same age; Linacre's published works are mentioned
and Erasmus goes on, 'we expect shortly Aristotle's meteorological books,

first corrected with a labour that cannot be estimated, and then translated with the utmost success'; he concludes with lavish praise of Linacre: 'Est apud Britannos vir vndiquaque doctissimus Thomas Linacrus, tibi iam olim ex Aldi nostraque praedicatione cognitus, tuae professionis ac, ni fallor, aetatis. Is idem agit quod tu, multis annis eliminatas lucubrationes suas vicissim aedit in lumen. Prodiit Galenus περὶ τῶν ὑγιεινῶν tanta fide, tanta luce, tanto Romani sermonis nitore redditus, vt nihil vsquam desyderet lector Latinus; imo nihil non melius reperiat quam apud Graecos habeatur. Successerunt libri Therapeutices, quos scis quales antehac habuerimus. Expectamus proxima foetura libros Aristotelis Meteorologicos, non aestimandis sudoribus primum emendatos, deinde felicissime versos. Sunt illi permulta in scriniis magno vsui futura studiosis. His monumentis vir ille consulit immortalitati sui nominis, his ornat suam Angliam, his aulam regiam illustrat, atque ipsum in primis Principem, cui medicus est primarius' (Allen, op. cit. iii. 403–4); cf. the quotation from More, given in n. 46 below.

44. Latimer, writing from Oxford, 30 January [1517, not 1518 as in Nichols, op. cit. iii (London, 1918), 240–1]: 'Nam et Grocinum memini, virum (vt scis) multifaria doctrina, magno quoque et exercitato ingenio, his ipsis literis duos continuos annos, etiam post prima illa rudimenta, solidam operam dedisse; idque sub summis doctoribus, Demetrio Chalcondilo et Angelo Politiano. Linacrum item, acri ingenio virum, totidem aut etiam plureis annos sub iisdem praeceptoribus impendisse' (Allen, op. cit. ii. 441–2).

45. Erasmus at Antwerp, 25 June 1520, to Germanus Brixius (Brice) (d. 1538): 'A puero feliciter imbibit Latinas literas, Graecas iuuenis; idque sub doctissimis praeceptoribus, cum aliis, tum praecipue Thoma Linacro et Gulielmo Grocino' (Allen, op. cit. iv. 294).

46. Thomas More, . . . *Lucubrationes* . . ., Basle, 1563, pp. 365–428, '. . . Thomas Morus Martino Dorpio S.D. Apologia pro Moria Erasmi, qua etiam docetur quàm necessaria sit linguae Graecae cognito', at 416–17: 'Sed hoc opus [sc. the *Meteorologica,* of which More has discussed the value] tamen spero propediem fore, ut à Thoma Linacro nostrate, illustrissimi Regis nostri medico, Latinis donetur auribus, utpote cuius iam nu*n*c duos libros absoluit: perfecissetq́ue nimirum opus, atqu*e* ediddisset uniuersum, nisi Galenus eum exorasset, ut quu*m* dux atqu*e* imperator Medicae rei sit, uel seposito interim Aristotele, Latinus eius opera prior ipse redderetur. Prodibit ergo Aristoteles aliquanto serius, sed prodibit tamen nihilo incultior; praeterea nec incomitatus. nam Alexa*n*dri Aphrodisaei commentarios, in idem opus unà uertit, initurus apud Latinos om*n*es immortalem gratia*m*: in quoru*m* non uulgarem utilitate*m*, Philosophi praestantissimi operi ta*m* egregio praesta*n*tissimu*m* interpretem sic adiunxerit, ut eius labore demum ab Latinis possit intelligi: quod hactenus à nemine (ut ego certè suspicor) qui Graecè nescierit intellectum est. Nam quum ipse iam olim ide*m* Aristotelis opus audirem Graecè, eodem mihi perlegente atqu*e* interpretante Linacro, libuit interdu*m* experiendi gratia uulgatam etiam translationem inspicere: è cuius lectione mentem illicò subijt euisdem Philosophi de Physicis suis dictu*m*.' Bale, op. cit., p. 650 (also in edition of 1548) includes 'Aristotelis meteora, Lib. 4.' in his

bibliography of Linacre's works (see p. xlvi n. 58 below). Cf. also Allen, op. cit. iii. 403–4 n.

47. John Caius, *De pronunciatione Graece & Latinae linguae cum scriptione noua libellus*, London, 1574, p. 20: '. . . Qui verò illis (professoribus) destituuntur, & proprio marte linguam Graecam discere coguntur, pronuncient elementa Graeca more Latinorum Graecis in hac tabula respondentium. Quae certè pronunciandi ratio vetus est, & recepta vsu. Huius opinionis quoque olim per iuuentutem (quod ipse noui) erant isti praeceptores noui. Verùm loco stare nesciuerunt, sed gressus glomerare superbos voluerunt. In ea quoque erat et Thomus Morus, Linacrus, Lupsetus, & Erasmus, qui in prouerbio, Stultior Morycho, μορύξαι transfert Moryxae, non moruxai, etsi de pronunciatione multa disputauerat, quae gloria studio potius, quam usus gratia se scripsisse, ex hijs & alijs locis scire licet diligenter obseruandi . . .' A slightly confusing orthography may be clarified by opposing the two pronunciations in a modern broad phonetic transcription: [morixe] not [moryxai]; Caius goes on to give other examples: [gimnasium] not [gymnasium], [sirakuse] not [syrakusai], and so on.

Erasmus had discussed the proverb, *Stultior Morycho*, in the Aldine revised edition of his *Adagia* (*Adagiorum chiliadestres, ac centuriae fere totidem*, Venice, 1508, fol. 177ᵛ, no. DCCCXVIII), and it occurs again in the *Moriae encomium* (see *Praise of Folly*, trans. and ed. by Radice and Levi, p. 83, for an explanation of the proverb).

48. An excellent account of the controversy, as well as a discussion of Cheke's and Smith's views on the reform of English spelling and the evidence for English pronunciation derivable from their works, will be found in E. J. Dobson, *English Pronunciation 1500–1700*, 2nd edn., 2 vols., Oxford, 1968, i. 38–62; see also the articles in *D.N.B.* on Cheke and Smith.

49. John Cheke, *De pronuntiatione Graecae potissimum linguae disputationes cum Stephano Vuintoniensi Episcopo, septem contrarijs epistolis comprehensae, magna quadam & elegantia & eruditione refertae*, Basle, 1555, pp. 176–7: 'Post Erasmum in Ciceronianos, non attinet plura dicere. Certè Linacer homo nostro seculo doctissimus, & iudicio in literis singulari, Ciceronis dictionem numquam probare potuit, nec sine fastidio audire.' The letters do not bear year dates, but this letter is dated 10 July, and the last in the series 2 October. A passage in Erasmus's *Ciceronianus*, wherein Linacre is said to have so disliked Cicero that he would rather have been like Quintilian, to have sought an Attic brevity and elegance, and for didactic purposes to have striven to copy Aristotle and Quintilian, may be considered the source of Gardiner's remarks rather than independent confirmation of them: 'BVL[EPHORVS = Erasmus]. Nunc igitur in Britanniam, quae quum multos habeat Tullianae dictionis candidatos, tantum eos nominabo qui scriptis innotescere uoluerunt. [Mention of Grocyn.] Sed Thomam Linacrum non uerebor proponere? NOS[OPONVS = 'the zealous Ciceronian, who, to preserve a perfect purity of mind, breakfasts off ten currants' (J. Huizinga, *Erasmus of Rotterdam*, trans. by F. Hopman, London, 1952, p. 172)]. Noui uirum undiquaque doctissimum, sed sic affectum erga Ciceronem, ut etiam si potuisset utrumlibet,

prius habuisset esse Quintiliano similis quàm Ciceroni, non ita multo in hunc aequior, quàm est Graecorum uulgus. Vrbanitatem nusquàm affectat, ab affectibus abstinet religiosius q*u*am ullus Atticus, breuiloquentiam et ele-ga*n*tiam amat, ad docendu*m* inte*n*tus, Aristotelem & Quintilianu*m* studuit exprimere. Huic igitur uiro per me quantum uoles laudum tribuas licebit; Tullianus dici non potest, qui studuerit esse dissimilis. BVL. Restat Ricardus Paceus . . .'; Erasmus, *De recta Latini Graecíque sermonis pronuntiatione* . . . *Dialogus*. . . . *Dialogus cui titulus: Ciceronianus, siue, De optimo genere dicendi. Cum alijs nonnullis* . . ., Basle, 1528, pp. 371–2.

50. Aulus Cornelius Celsus, lived under Tiberius (reigned A.D. 14–37), encyclopaedist who wrote on agriculture, medicine, and philosophy. Only eight books of his on medicine survive, and these were published at Florence in 1478, the first classical medical work to be printed.

51. Lucius Junius Moderatus Columella, wrote *c.* A.D. 65 a treatise on agri-culture, *De re rustica*.

52. John Pits, a Catholic, refers to Cheke as hostile to Catholics: 'Ioannes Chekus Catholicas religionis & Catholicorum hominum aduersarius . . .' (Pits, op. cit. on p. xxxiii n. 14 above, i. 699); not perhaps without reason, as Cheke was driven into exile in 1554, following Mary's accession to the throne, was captured in 1556, and brought back to England.

53. Cheke, op. cit., pp. 281–3 (partly reprinted, with minor changes, in Bale, *Catalogus* (cited on p. xl n. 43 above), p. 651): 'Atq*ue* hic mihi Linacrum pro-ponis, cuius factum potius quàm reliquas illius uirtutes si approbarem, uereor ne perinde facerem ut si supplosionem pedis, aut gestu*m* alicuius boni ora-toris imitarer, uirtutes eius relinquerem. nam qu*ae* h*ae*c in Linacio animi modestia esse potuit, quia cogitationes animi in Galenu*m* inte*n*debat, seque-baturq*ue* quietu*m* Celsi, & sedatum Columell*ae* dicendi genus, quod in ea arte ualere debet, idcirco alias res non laudare modò, sed ne ferre quidem sine auriu*m* co*n*uicio posset. In quo mihi perinde placere debet, atque in eo cum prouecta ad modum inclinatáq*ue* aetate esset, homo studijs morbisque fractus, & morti uicinus, cu*m* sacerdos esset, iam tum nouu*m* Testame*n*tum primò in manus cepisse, et ex eo aliquot Matth*ae*i capita perlegisse: & cum quintu*m*, sextum septimumq́ue percucurrisset, abiecto iterum quantu*m* potuit totis uiribus libro, iurasse, aut hoc non fuisse Eua*n*gelium, aut nos non esse Chri-stianos quod eius factum quanquam iudicio in literis singulari esset, quu*m* Italo sacerdote q*u*am Anglo aptius fuerat, si imitari uellem, & si sic omnem uitam uel à Cicerone, quemadmodu*m* ille a nouo Testame*n*to abstinuit, iudicio & eruditione meritò carere*m*. Et fecit in medicina tantum qua*n*tum alius Latinus illius *ae*tatis quisquam: & quandiu in medicina se continet, tandiu laude*m* singularem habet: sin foràs serpat, et oratores carpat, uideat ne ultra medicinae crepidam progrediatur. Nam quanquam in transferendis Galeni libris laus eius est propè singularis: tamen si de acumine & celeritate ingenij disputatur, aut de rebus popularibus grauiter & disertè tractandis, in eo si nunc uiueret, quanqua*m* doctissimus & iudicio in literis singulari esset, tibi laudem co*n*cederet, medicinam ipse assumeret. Et tamen cur tam fastidiosus esset in audiendo Cicerone, nescio: illud uidemus, omnes quos ille

libros de Latini sermonis structura composuit, exemplis Ciceronis abun-
dare: ut non tam fortasse reuera neglexerit, quàm animi quada*m* morositate
uideri uoluit neglexisse.' This seems rather a contrived anecdote to have
invented merely to labour a debating point, or out of dislike of Linacre. If
there be any truth in it, Linacre appears not to have heeded Erasmus's comments on the success of his new edition of the Greek text of the New Testament with a new Latin translation (Basle, 1516), made in the letter to Linacre
of 5 June [1516] (cited above, p. xxix n. 5). Erasmus there remarks that his
New Testament gives such satisfaction to the learned, even among those in
holy orders, that the unlettered are silent for shame: 'Nouum Testamentum
adeo placet ubique doctis, etiam ex ordine theologorum, vt indocti pudore
obticescant.' A copy of Cheke, op. cit., which belonged to the jurist, John
Selden (1584-1654) (Bodleian Library, Oxford, shelf-mark: Seld. 8°C. 12 Art.),
has the name 'Linacre' written in the margin against each of the two passages
quoted here, presumably because Selden was to make use of the anecdote in
his *De synedriis & praefecturis iuridicis veterum ebraeorum libri tres*, London, 1650–
5, p. 480. Selden is there discussing oaths and says that he thinks the reason
why Linacre threw away the New Testament was hardly trivial ('. . . haud
exiguam existimo fuisse causam . . .'), because he had read in chapter V
of St. Matthew's gospel Christ's prohibition of swearing. Since by reading
chapters V, VI, and VII, Linacre would have read the whole of the Sermon
on the Mount, this must be accounted an unduly narrow interpretation
of the story, comparing unfavourably with the obvious one given by Fuller,
op. cit., p. 236 [*sic, recte* 232].

54. A people in Gallia Belgica.

55. Sc. at the mouth of a mountain pass, leading to Geneva (Gebenna), probably the Little St. Bernard (Allen, op. cit., in *E.H.R.* 514).

56. Sc. incense.

57. Giovio, *Elogia*, 137:

> Dum Linacrus adit Morinos, patriosq*ue* Britannos,
>   Artibus egregiis diues ab Italia,
> Ingentem molem saxorum in rupibus altis,
>   Congerit ad fauces alte Gebenna tuas,
> Floribus hinc, viridiq*ue* struem dum fronde coronat,
>   Et sacer Assyrias pascitur ignes opes;
> Hoc tibi, ait, mater studiorum, ô sancta meorum
>   Templum Linacrus dedicat, Italia;
> Tu modo cui docta assurgunt cum Pallade Athenae
>   Hoc de me precium sedulitatis habe.

This poem was reprinted by Ranutius Gherus (J. Gruteus), *Delitiae CC.
italorum huius superiorisque aeui illustrium*, Frankfurt, 1608, ii. 1439. Those with
a taste for this type of verse may care to read a longer Latin poem (of twenty-
five lines), by Jacobus Latomus (Masson), which Giovio also appends (op.
cit., pp. 137–8; also reprinted by Gherus, *Delitiae CC. poetarum belgicorum . . .*,
Frankfurt, 1614, iii). Latomus's poem also refers to Linacre's shrine

constructed on leaving Italy, makes the nymphs of the Arno accuse Linacre
of preferring those of England, and includes the line, apostrophizing Linacre:
'Totus noster homo es: sed Angla mens est.' Giovio's *Elogia* is thus the
original, and only early source, for the anecdote about Linacre meeting Ermolao Barbaro, for Linacre's age at death, and for the story about the shrine.

58. Schmitt, op. cit., below, p. 42. Very little of Linacre's personal correspondence has survived, and what has tells us little about him as a person.
The items of correspondence, as opposed to dedications of published works,
may conveniently be summarized here:

1. Erasmus, Paris, to Linacre, [*c.* 12 June] 1506; Allen, op. cit. i. 426–7.
2. Linacre to John Claymond, President of Magdalen College, Oxford,
   1507 to 1516 (because Claymond was President of Magdalen during
   that period only), Corpus Christi College, Oxford, MS. 318, fol. 135;
   Robert Weiss, 'Notes on Thomas Linacre', *Miscellanea Giovanni Mercati*,
   iv (Studi e testi, 124), Vatican City, 1946, pp. 378–9. See Plate I.
3. Linacre to Giampiero (Johannes Petrus) Machiavelli, Florence, 13
   December 1512 or 1513, British Library, London, MS. Add. 12107
   fol. 10. Refers to manuscripts which Machiavelli was having transcribed in Florence for Linacre, and shows that Linacre was in touch
   with Giovanni Cavalcanti, a Florentine businessman living in London,
   who had dealings with Henry VIII about the supply of saltpetre, and
   who may have helped on the financial side of Linacre's bibliophilic
   activities; Weiss, op. cit., who prints the letter at pp. 379–80. See
   Plate II.
4. Erasmus, St. Omer, to Linacre, 5 June [1516] (see above, p. xxix n. 5
   and p. xliv n. 53).
5. Guillaume Budé, Paris, to Linacre, 9 September [1517] (see above,
   p. xxxi n. 5 and p. xxxvi n. 24).
6. Linacre to Budé, Paris, 10 June [1518] (see above, p. xxx n. 5 and p. xxxvi
   n. 24).
7. Budé, Paris, to Linacre, 8 July [1518] (see above, pp. xxx- xxxi n. 5 and
   p. xxxvi n. 24).
8. Christophorus Longolius, Padua, to Linacre, 7 May 1521 (see above,
   pp. xxxi n. 5).
9. Erasmus, Bruges, to Linacre, 24 August 1521 (see p. xlvii n. 69).
10. Nicolao Leonicus Tomeo, Greek professor, tutor of Reginald Pole
    at Padua, to Linacre, 19 January 1524, Biblioteca Vaticana, Cod.
    Rossianus Lat. 997, fol. 21. Sends Linacre a copy of his edition of
    Aristotle's *Parva naturalia* in order to have his critical and considered
    judgement upon it; wishes to have Linacre's well-known commentaries
    on medical matters; desires to have something of his own on the
    shelves of Linacre's celebrated library; praises Lupset and Pole who
    send greetings. Paraphrased and partly quoted in Cardinal [F.A.]
    Gasquet, *Cardinal Pole and his Early Friends* (London, 1927), pp. 51–2.

Some of the more interesting contemporary, or near-contemporary, references
to Linacre are discussed in this Introduction; many others, in the correspondence and works of Erasmus and elsewhere, are listed in Pelling, op. cit.,

below, pp. 338 ff. See also G. M[arc'Hadour], 'Thomas More and Thomas Linacre', *Moreana*, iv (1967), 63–7. Dedications of Linacre's works are reprinted by Johnson, op. cit., pp. 310–30. Bale, in his 'life' of Linacre, gives a bibliography of Linacre's works which includes the following two tantalizing entries:

> 'Epistolas [*sic*] ad diuersos   Lib. 1. Cum multi tibi quotidie, uir.
> Diversi generis carmina   Lib. 1.'

(quoted from Bale, op. cit. (1557–9), pt. i, p. 650; the first edition (1548, cited on p. xxxii n. 10 above), f. 217^r, omits the word 'uir' in the incipit; no bibliography is found in Bale's note on Linacre in *Index Britanniae Scriptorum . . . John Bale's Index of British and Other Writers*, ed. Reginald Lane Poole and Mary Bateson (Anecdota Oxoniensia . . . Mediaeval and Modern Series, ix), Oxford, 1902, p. 442). Neither of these two items in the bibliography has been identified. Because Bale gives no incipit for the *Diuersi generis carmina*, nor for another item, *Aristotelis meteora*, Lib. 4., he may in these instances be citing works he had heard of, but not seen. (Certainly four books of a translation of Aristotle's *Meterologica* were never published, even if completed; see above, p. xx, pp. xl–xli n. 43, and p. xli n. 46.) The presence of the incipit against the one book of the *Epistolae* (the title of which is reminiscent of the *Epistolae D. Erasmi Roterodami ad diuersos, & aliquot aliorum ad illum*, Basle, 1521) suggests strongly that Bale had indeed seen some such volume, not necessarily printed. It is perhaps significant that although Bale thoroughly revised his 'life' of Linacre for the 1557–9 edition of his work (and corrected therein the date of Linacre's death), he did not see fit to alter this entry in his bibliography and in fact added a missing word to the incipit.

59. Richard J. Durling, 'Linacre and Medical Humanism', below, pp. 76–106 at pp. 76–7.

60. Ibid., p. 105. We have quoted the passage from Erasmus at the beginning of this Introduction; on another occasion, however, Erasmus said of Linacre that he was 'a man of not so much accurate as severe judgement': 'Vir non exacti tantum, sed severi judicii' (quoted from Aikin, op. cit., p. 37, because we have not located its original source); cf. Erasmus [Antwerp, *c.* 19 June 1516], to Budé: 'Atque ipse quoque Linacrus, vir exacti quidem sed seueri iudicii et qui non temere probet quemlibet, Budaeo nihil non tribuit' (Allen, op. cit. ii. 252).

61. Walter Pagel, 'Medical Humanism—A Historical Necessity in the Era of the Renaissance', below, pp. 375–86, at p. 385.

62. Charles Webster, 'Thomas Linacre and the Foundation of the College of Physicians', below, pp. 198–222 at p. 200; cf. R. G. Lewis, 'The Linacre Lectureships subsequent to their Foundation', below, pp. 223–64 at p. 224: 'It was precisely because of the difficulty of establishing regular lectures in medicine at Oxford and Cambridge that Linacre set out to do so.'

63. Webster, op. cit., below, p. 208.

64. D. F. S. Thomson, 'Linacre's Grammars', below, pp. 24–35, at p. 32.

65. Ibid., p. 31.

66. Ibid., pp. 26, 28–9.

67. Erasmus to Budé, 21 February [1516/17]: 'Thomae Linacri lucubrationes ex officina Badiana propediem exituras dici non potest quam gaudeam. Nihil ab eo viro expecto non absolutissimum omnibus numeris' (Allen, op. cit. ii. 479); see Barber, op. cit., below, p. 296, and Durling, op. cit., below, p. 103.

68. Erasmus, *Apophthegmatum, siue dictorum Libri sex, ex optimis quibusque linguae autoribus Plutarcho praesertim excerptorum* . . . , Basle, 1531, p. 653, 'Morosa diligentia': 'Nec multum abfuit ab hoc uitio Thomas Linacrus Anglus, uir undequaque doctissimus.'

69. Erasmus at Bruges, 24 August 1521, to Linacre: 'At tu, si mihi permittis vt libere tecum agam, sine fine premis tuas omnium eruditissimas lucubrationes, vt periculum sit, ne pro cauto modestoque crudelis habearis, qui studia huius seculi tam lenta torqueas expectatione tuorum laborum, ac tam diu fraudes desideratissimo fructu tuorum voluminum. Fortasse terret te nostrum exemplum. Sed etiam atque etiam vide [ne], dum studiosius vitas nostram culpam, in diuersum deflectas' (Allen, op. cit. iv. 570–1). These passages from Erasmus are the foundation in Bayle, op. cit., 3rd edn., Rotterdam, 1720, ii. 1718–19, for a long and interesting excursus on the failure of authors to publish: 'Le défaut dont on blâme le notre Linacer n'est fort commun parmi les Auteurs, & néanmoins on peut dire qu'à certains égards il ne l'est trop; car pour l'ordinaire ce ne sont pas les mauvais Auteurs, ou les Ecrivains médiocres, qui en sont coupables, ce sont les plus excellentes plumes.'

70. William Warham (1450?–1532), Archbishop of Canterbury.

71. William Blount (d. 1534), 4th Baron Mountjoy, who brought Erasmus to England in 1498.

72. Translation from Nichols, op. cit. [i], 36, of a letter written by Erasmus in Cambridge to John Colet, 29 October [1511]: 'Iam etiam Linacro nostro videor parum verecundus, qui cum sciret me Londino discedere vix sex instructum nobilibus, et valetudinem optime norit, ad haec instantem hyemem, tamen sedulo monet vti parcam Archiepiscopo, vti parcam domino Montioio; sed ipse potius me contraham et assuescam fortiter ferre paupertatem. O amicum consilium!' (Allen, op. cit. i. 478–9).

73. Letters from More, in London, to Erasmus [17 February 1516]: 'Linacre thinks and speaks well of Erasmus' (Allen, op. cit. ii. 198); 15 December [1516]: 'Nescis quam sit gauisus ea mentione librorum suorum, quam in epistola tua fecisti quam nuper scripsisti ad me; crede mihi, is toto pectore tuus est' (ibid. ii. 420); 13 January [1517]: 'Non credas quam vehemens amator tui, quam acer propugnator studiorum tuorum sit Linacer' (ibid. ii. 430).

74. Erasmus, at Basle, 4 September [1515], to Pace: '. . . Linacrum fac in amicitia retineas et, si fieri potest, etiam Grocinum. Non haec scribo quod vel metuam aliquid vel quicquam ab illis expectem commodi, sed quod tules

viros perpetuo velim amicos. Non egent illi meis praeconiis, illud tamen ausim dicere, nec inter Anglos esse qui de illis vel senserit magnificentius vel praedicauerit honorificentius quam Erasmus. Et non libet meminisse quid vterque, haud scio quorum instinctu, in nos molitus fuerit; id quod ipsa re comperi, non suspicione conieci, quanquam olim iam idem olfeceram. Sed homines sumus; ego semper ero mei similis, et huic iniuriae tot opponam illorum benefacta. Linacri feci honorificam mentionem in scholiis Hieronymianis. Nil magnum sit, si contemnam contemptus, si oderim odio habitus' (Allen, op. cit. ii. 139).

75. Fletcher, op. cit., below, pp. 164–5; Johnson, op. cit., p. 343.

76. Vives, in London, to Erasmus, 13 November 1524: 'Linacer reliquit homines, magno doctorum omnium moerere. Quibus omnibus bene cupiebat et fauebat ex animo; plusque apud eum valebat opinio ingenii et eruditionis quam suspicio simultatum: συνιεῖς ὀπὶ πάντα' (Allen, op. cit. v. 577).

77. Fletcher, op. cit., below, p. 146 and n. 2.

78. The place and text of the memorial are recorded by Sir William Dugdale, *The History of St. Pauls Cathedral in London*, . . . London, 1658, p. 56; whose transcription of the inscription we copy here:

> Thomas Lynacrus, Regis Henrici viii. medicus; vir & Graecè & Latinè, atque in re medicâ longè eruditissimus: Multos aetate sua languentes, & qui jam animam desponderant, vitae restituit: Multa Galeni opera in Latinam linguam, mirâ & singulari facundiâ vertit: Egregium opus de emendatâ structurâ Latini sermonis, amicorum rogata [*sic, recte* rogatu], paulò ante mortem edidit. Medicinae studiosis Oxoniae Publicas lectiones duas, Cantabrigiæ unam, in perpetuum stabilivit. In hac urbe Collegium Medicorum fieri suâ industriâ curavit, cujus & Praesidens proximus electus est. Fraudes dolosque mirè perosus; fidus amicis; omnibus ordinibus juxta clarus [*sic, recte* charus]: aliquot annos antequam obieret Presbyter factus. Plenus annis ex hac vitâ migravit, multùm desideratus, Anno Domini 1524. die 20, Octobris.
>
> Vivit post Funera virtus
Thomæ Lynacro clarissimo Medico
Johannes Caius posuit, anno 1557.

79. Cf. Lane Poole and Bateson, op. cit., p. 442, for Bale's version obtained from Edward Braynewode, and a note on the corrections we have adopted.

79. Margaret Pelling, 'The Refoundation of the Linacre Lectureships in the Nineteenth Century', below, pp. 265–89, at p. 265.

80. Barber, op. cit., below, p. 330.

81. Hill, op. cit., below, p. 366 and *passim*.

The Life of Thomas Linacre: a Brief Chronology*

?1460	Thomas Linacre born, probably in the diocese of Canterbury	
1481	At Oxford by this date: stays there until his departure for Italy	
1484	Elected Fellow of All Souls College, Oxford	
1487, ? April	Leaves England for Italy, probably in the company of William Sellyng and envoys from Henry VII to Innocent VIII	
1487, early May	Arrival in Italy; perhaps stops at Florence instead of going to Rome	
c. 1488	First becomes acquainted with William Latimer	Two years' study in Florence with Angelo Poliziano and Demetrios Chalcondylas
1489, 16 November	Will of John Morer describes Linacre as *studentus Florence*	
1490, end of summer	Leaves Florence for Rome	
1490, 4 November	Admitted to the English Hospice of St. Thomas of Canterbury at Rome	
1491, 3 May	Named a *custos* of the English Hospice	
c. 1492 or 1493	Leaves Rome for the Venetian Republic, ? for Padua	
1495	On the bursary books of All Souls College	
1496, 30 August	Takes degree *in medicinis* at Padua	
1497	Aldus Manutius praises Linacre in his prefatory letter to the *editio princeps* of Aristotle, 1497	
1498, November	By this date in Venice: member of the Aldine Νεακαδημία	

* This chronology is solely intended to serve as an *aide-mémoire*, and is based, as far as possible, on dates which are accepted by contributors to this volume. The information concerning Linacre's ecclesiastical appointments has been extracted from Johnson's *Life* (see p. xxviii n. 3), occasionally corrected, and supplemented from an interleaved copy of Emden, *Biographical Register of the University of Oxford* (see p. xxix n. 3 and p. xxxi n.7). A few non-controversial dates have been obtained from other sources. Only the dates of first publication of Linacre's works are noted.

1499, 27 August	Letter from William Grocyn in London, to Aldus, refers to Linacre's recent return to that city
1499, 15 October	Publication of Linacre's translation of pseudo-Proclus, *De sphaera*; Linacre charged with the education of Prince Arthur (1486–1502)
1499, 5 November	By this time acquainted with Erasmus, then in England
c. 1500	Thomas More studies Greek in London, with Linacre
1503	Linacre is a witness to the Will of Sir Reginald Bray, Lord High Treasurer
1509	Appointed a physician to King Henry VIII
1509, October	Collated by the primate, William Warham, to the rectory of Mersham, Kent, from which he can have received no emolument as he resigned in little more than a month from his collation
1509, 14 December	Admitted a canon, and installed by proxy in the prebend of Easton in Gordano in the cathedral of Wells, Somerset
c. 1510	Linacre delivers a 'shagglyng' lecture in the University of Oxford
1511	Admitted to the church of Hawkhurst, Kent, on presentation of the Abbot and convent of Battle, Sussex, a rectory retained until his death
ante 1511, 13 September	Linacre offers a Latin grammar, prepared by him, for use at St. Paul's School, London; the grammar rejected by John Colet
1514	Linacre attached to the service of Princess Mary (1496–1533: i.e. Mary of France) as physician, is allocated two servants, and in September travels in her entourage to Paris, where he becomes acquainted with Guillaume Budé
c. 1515	First publication of Linacre's *Progymnasmata grammatices vulgaria*
1515	Linacre's translation from the Greek of *De sanitate tuenda* prepared by this date
1515, 14 January	Linacre transfers to Thomas More and others lands in Kent for reasons which are not clear
1515, 22 December	Linacre ordained subdeacon
1517, 24 August	Nominated to a canonry and prebend in the collegiate church of St. Stephen, Westminster, in succession to the Italian humanist, Andrea Ammonio of Lucca; publication of *De sanitate tuenda*, dedi-

	cated to Henry VIII in a letter dated 16 June 1517
1518	Appointed canon and prebendary of South Newbald in York cathedral
1518, 6 March	Presented to the rectory of Holsworthy, Devon
1518, 23 September	Foundation of College of Physicians, by royal Letters Patent incorporating The President and College of Physicians of London, on the petition of three Royal physicians, including Linacre, three other physicians, and one layman (Wolsey)
1519, 9 April	Linacre admitted Precentor of York cathedral
1519, 23 April	No longer prebendary of South Newbald in York cathedral
1519, June	Publication in Paris of Linacre's translation, *Methodus medendi*
1519, 1 September	Linacre enters into an obligation concerning the manor of Traces, Kent, his first and most substantial acquisition of lands towards the endowment of the lectureships
1519, November	Resigns as Precentor of York
1520	Becomes Rector of Wigan, Lancashire; executor of the Will of William Grocyn and prepares a catalogue of Grocyn's books
1520, 7 April	Linacre ordained deacon
1520, 8 November	Linacre party to an indenture relating to lands at Traces
1521, 24 August	Erasmus refers to Linacre's declining health
post 1521, September	Publication at Cambridge of Linacre's translations, *De temperamentis* and *De inaequali intemperie*
1521, towards end	Letter, from Oxford University to Linacre, refers to Linacre as *novum Latinae linguae parentem*, and refers to Thomas Lupset's lectures on Linacre's Proclus
? 1522 or 1524	Publication of Linacre's translation, *De pulsuum usu*
1522	Linacre's preface to Galen, *De motu musculorum*, translated by Leoniceno, which was published in London; relinquishes rectorship of Freshwater, I. of W., held for a brief period
1522, March–November	Recorded on 8 March that Linacre is to have canonry in St. Stephen's, Westminster (*vice* T. Warren; *cf. sub* 1517, 24 August, above), but resigns prebend by 29 November (see *Calendar of State Papers (Domestic)*)

1522, 30 September ⎤ 1523, 8 January ⎦ –	Purchase, etc., of house in Knight Rider Street, London	
? 1523	First publication of Linacre's *Rudimenta grammatices*	
1523	Charter of College of Physicians ratified by Act of Parliament; College given authority to govern medical practice throughout England; Oxford University writes to Linacre urging him to implement his plans for setting up lectureships	
post 1523, 25 May	Publication of Linacre's translation, *De naturalibus facultatibus*; in dedication (dated 25 May), Linacre refers to his ill-health	–Linacre first President of the College of Physicians, the corporate meetings of which were later held in his house in Knight Rider Street
ante 1523, October	Appointed tutor to future Queen Mary I (then aged 7)	
1524, 14 June	Agreement between Linacre and the Master and Fellows of St. John's College, Cambridge, concerning a free lecture on physic	
1524, 19 June	Date of Linacre's Will making personal bequests only	
1524, 19 August	Agreement between Linacre and others, and the Master of St. John's College, Cambridge, concerning the lecture on physic	—Period of acquisition of lands by Linacre, transactions involving Thomas More, Cuthbert Tunstal, and others influential in Court and humanistic circles; also some sales of property owned by Linacre. (Not all transactions are noted here)
1524, 12 October	Royal consent obtained by the Mercers' Company for Linacre's estates to pass into mortmain (the licence referred to the proposed lectureship at Cambridge, as well as the two at Oxford)	
1524, 18 October	Date of further Will of Linacre, dealing with disposition of estates and the form of lectureships he sought to establish thereby	
1524, 20 October	Death of Linacre; two sisters, Joan and Alice still living, also a brother, Thomas, two nieces, Agnes and Margaret, and a 'cousin', Robert Wright of Chester; shortly before his death had exchanged rectorship of Holsworthy for annual pension of £28	
1524	Publication posthumously of Linacre's translations, *De symptomatum differentiis* and *De symptomatum causis*	
1524, December	First and last publication in England of Linacre's *De emendata structura Latini sermonis*	
1526	Publication of Linacre's translation of Paulus Aegineta, *De victus ratione quolibet anni tempore utili*	

ante 1528, 2 July	Appointment, as Linacre lecturer at Cambridge, of Christopher Jackson, who was elected a Fellow of St. John's College, Cambridge, in April 1525 and who died before 2 July 1528
1528, December	Publication of Linacre's translation of Paulus Aegineta, *De diebus criticis*
1533	Publication in Paris of George Buchanan's Latin translation of Linacre's *Rudimenta*
1540, 6 May	Indenture concluded between Cuthbert Tunstal and the Principal of Brasenose College, Oxford, and the Warden of All Souls College, Oxford, to set up the lectureships. (These arrangements were not implemented)
1542, 25 September	Mercers' Company hears a request from Tunstal for the chest of Linacre's papers, and agrees to the request, thereby marking the end of the Company's association with the Linacre endowment
1549, 1 December	Tunstal formally donates Linacre's lands to Merton College, Oxford
1549, 5 December	Merton College names its representative to receive the property
1549, 10 December	Indenture made between Tunstal and the Warden and Fellows of Merton College concerning the regulation of the Linacre lectureships
1550, 25 July	Issue of Letters Patent by the Warden and Fellows of Merton College recognizing their obligations
1559, 24 November	George James admitted as first Linacre lecturer (junior), at Oxford

Thomas Linacre, Cornelio Vitelli, and Humanistic Studies at Oxford

CECIL H. CLOUGH[*]

THOMAS LINACRE HAS A NOTABLE PLACE AMONG those English humanists who in the last quarter of the fifteenth century resided for some years in Italy. In his case documentary evidence is sufficient to provide the bare bones of his sojourn there from 1487 until some ten years later. Little is known, though, of his earlier life, the concern of this study: contemporary evidence, as one would expect, is both scanty and enigmatic. It is certain that Linacre was at Oxford by 1481, and he remained there apparently until he went to Italy, but since a vital register is lost, the nature of humanistic studies at Oxford in this period remains a subject for speculation.[1] My object is to consider such evidence as exists, and, if I may anticipate my conclusion, I suggest anew a connection at Oxford between Linacre and the Italian humanist Cornelio Vitelli of Cortona.

Linacre's studies during his first years in Italy provide a starting-point for a consideration of his Oxford days, as they suggest how advanced his humanistic studies there had been, and above all throw

---

[*] School of History, University of Liverpool.

[1] For Linacre in England probably in 1497–8, see George N. Clark, *A History of the Royal College of Physicians of London*, 2 vols., Oxford, 1964, i. 42 n. 3; A. B. Emden, *A Biographical Register of the University of Oxford to A.D. 1500*, 3 vols., Oxford, 1957–9, ii. 1148, indicates Linacre was in London by 1499. The University Register [of Congregation], 1464–1504, is missing; see the Editor's Preface, *The Register of the University of Oxford, 1449–1463, 1505–1571*, ed. C. W. Boase, Oxford Historical Society, i, 1885, pp. v–vii, and the introduction to *The Register of Congregation, 1448–1463*, ed. W. A. Pantin and W. T. Mitchell, ibid., N.S. xxii, Oxford, 1972, pp. xvii–xix; for the nature of this latter Register see ibid., pp. xiv–xvii.

some light on the Greek he had learnt in England. William Latimer, who became Linacre's friend, and was first acquainted with him about 1498 in Padua, stated in a letter to Erasmus, written in January 1517 while Linacre was still alive, that Linacre had studied some two years in Florence under Angelo Poliziano and Demetrius Chalcondylas.[1] This letter was printed first in Froben's collection (Basle, 1519), and may have been the source for George Lyly's statement to the same effect, though more probably the authority was George's father, William, who had been with Linacre in Italy.[2] George Lyly certainly was the source for Giovio's information, and for John Bale's.[3] Latimer mentioned no date, but John Leland (*c.* 1503–52) writing some twenty years later said that Linacre left

[1] For the contact between Linacre and Latimer see P. S. Allen, 'Linacre and Latimer in Italy', *English Historical Review*, xviii, 1903, 516–17; D. Erasmus, *Opus epistolarum*, ed. P. S. Allen, 12 vols., Oxford, 1906–58, ii. 441–2, letter 520 dated 30 January [1517]: 'Nam et Grocinum memini, virum (vt scis) multifaria doctrina, magno quoque et exercitato ingenio, his ipsis literis duos continuos annos, etiam post prima illa rudimenta, solidam operam dedisse; idque sub summis doctoribus, Demetrio Chalcondilo et Angelo Politiano. Linacrum item, acri ingenio virum, totidem aut etiam plureis annos sub iisdem praeceptoribus impendisse.'

[2] Allen's note in Allen, ii. 438. For William Lyly see below, p. 3 and p. 6 n. 3.

[3] G. Lyly, 'Ad Paulum Iovium Episcopum Nucer. Virorum aliquot in Britannia, qui nostro seculo eruditione, et doctrina clari, memorabilesque fuerunt, Elogia', in P. Giovio, *Descriptio Britanniae, Scotiae* . . ., Venice, 1548, fol. 49ʳ: '. . . Thomas Linacrus perdiscendi studio ex Britannia in Italiam uenit, Florentiae Demetrio, et Politiano praeceptoribus usus, atque a Laurentio Mediceae familiae principe uiro, preclari ingenii admiratione, familiariter acceptus . . .' The reference to Lorenzo de' Medici may derive from Linacre's dedication of Galen to Giovanni de' Medici, see below, p. 4 n. 6. Even so, George Lyly was the son of William, who was with Linacre in the English Hospice in Rome, see B. Newns in Appendix 26, 'List of *Confratres* admitted to the Hospice', to his paper 'The Hospice of St. Thomas . . .' in 'The English Hospice in Rome', *The Venerabile*, xxi, 1962, 190; William Lyly was Grocyn's godson. P. Giovio, *Elogia virorum literis illustrium*, Basle, 1577, p. 119: 'Thomas Linacrus ex Insula Britannia ad perdiscendas Graecas literas in Italiam profectus, Florentiae Demetrium & Politianum audiuit, eaque enituit morum suauitate, atque modestia, vt a magno Laurentio liberis suis, familiari studiorum consuetudine, quanquam aetate maior, socius adderetur . . .' J. Bale, *Scriptorum illustrium maioris Brytanniae* . . . *Catalogus*, Basle, 1559, p. 560; for Bale see T. D. Kendrick, *British Antiquity*, London, 1950, pp. 69–72, and May McKisack, *Medieval History in the Tudor Age*, Oxford, 1971, pp. 11–25. See also F. O. Mencken, *Historia vitae et in literas meritorum Angeli Politiani*, Leipzig, 1736, pp. 81–2.

England for Italy with William Sellyng, and accordingly he presumably went in the company of English envoys sent by King Henry VII to Pope Innocent VIII, in order to secure a dispensation for the royal marriage to Elizabeth of York; Sellyng was one of these envoys.[1] The company reached Rome on 8 May 1487; Linacre, one supposes, had journeyed with it as far as Florence, and therefore he may have left England in April, and reached Florence probably in early May.[2] Sellyng was Prior of Christ Church, Canterbury, and, as will be considered, apparently he was Linacre's patron, so Leland's information concerning the circumstances of Linacre's departure for Florence is, if not proven, at least substantiated. Leland, it is worth noting, was taught by William Lyly, who, as already mentioned, was personally acquainted with Linacre in Italy, and possibly Leland had details of Linacre from his master, or subsequently from George Lyly, William's son. Sellyng it was who delivered the formal address before Pope Innocent VIII.[3] He was a Benedictine, who in 1464 had been given leave to study abroad, and thereafter studied at the universities of Padua and Bologna; at the latter he took the degree of Doctor of Divinity on 22 March 1466.[4] On Leland's authority, Sellyng had acquired some knowledge of Greek at Bologna, possibly from Andronicus Calliustus, professor of Greek there.[5] Leland also stated that Sellyng 'was familiar in

[1] J. Leland, *Commentarii de scriptoribus Britannicis*, ed. A. Hall, 2 vols., Oxford, 1709, ii. 483: 'Quo tempore, Thomam Linacrum, optimae spei adolescentulum, tanquam ministrum, una secum deduxit; ac Bononiam in itinere forte revisens Politiano, veteri amico suo illum commendatissimum reliquit erudiendum.' Leland's use of 'adolescentulum' for Linacre conveys a misleading impression of Linacre's age at the time he went to Italy, as Bennett (cited on p. 4 n. 3), p. 72, remarked. In 1487 Linacre was about 26 or 27, see p. 8 n. 4 below. Be it noted that the subject of 'deduxit' is Sellyng. For Leland see Kendrick, *British Antiquity*, pp. 45–64, and McKisack, *Medieval History* . . ., pp. 1–11. For the embassy, see next note.

[2] U. Balzani, 'Un'ambasciata inglese a Roma', in *Archivio della R. Società Romana di Storia Patria*, iii, 1880, pp. 182–3, merely gives the date of arrival in Rome on the basis of Burckhard; cf. J. Burckhard, 'Liber Notarum', ed. E. Celani, in L. Muratori, *Rerum Italicarum scriptores*, N.S., XXXII, part i, 1, 1903, pp. 195–6.

[3] For Leland see the sources cited in n. 1 above. For the draft of Sellyng's oration, see p. 9 n. 5.

[4] R. Weiss, *Humanism in England during the Fifteenth Century* (3rd edn.), Oxford, 1967, p. 154.

[5] Leland, *Commentarii de scriptoribus* . . ., ii. 482–3; cf. Weiss, *Humanism in England* . . ., p. 154.

Bonomy [Bologna] with Politiano, and was the Setter forth of Linacre to Politiano'.[1] Poliziano was never at Bologna University, but he was at Padua, and perhaps it was there that Sellyng became acquainted with him.[2] One can accept that Leland was correct concerning Sellyng's contact with Poliziano, and that it was Sellyng who was influential in causing Linacre to study under him; his error was merely in locating in Bologna Sellyng's acquaintance with Poliziano. There is supporting evidence that Sellyng was Linacre's patron in the will of John Morer, rector of Tenterden, Kent, drawn up on Palm Sunday, 1489.[3] In his will Morer left Linacre a bequest of £10, which Prior Sellyng was to see he received within a year.[4] The will also reveals Morer's belief that Linacre was then studying in Florence,[5] and since Morer knew Sellyng it is possible that Sellyng was the source of this information, if not Linacre himself. Linacre's dedication to Giovanni de' Medici (when Pope Leo X) of his Latin version of Galen's *De temperamentis* (Cambridge, 1521) has been the authority for the claim that Linacre and Giovanni had been youthful fellow pupils of Poliziano. The passage, which is both vague and obscure, does not mention Poliziano, or throw any light on Linacre's Greek studies.[6]

---

[1] J. Leland, *The Itinerary*, ed. T. Hearne, 9 vols. (3rd edn.), Oxford, 1769, vi. 7; cf. the *Commentarii*, quoted in p. 3 n. 1 above.

[2] Cf. R. Weiss, 'Un allievo inglese del Poliziano: Thomas Linacre', in *Il Poliziano e il suo tempo: Atti del IV Convegno Internazionale di Studi sul Rinascimento (Firenze, 23–26 settembre, 1954)*, Florence, 1957, p. 323 n. 7.

[3] The Will was given in synopsis by H. R. Plomer, 'Books mentioned in Wills', *Transactions of the Bibliographical Society*, vii, 1904, 108–9, 118. It is printed in full by Josephine W. Bennett, 'John Morer's Will: Thomas Linacre and Prior Sellyng's Greek Teaching', *Studies in the Renaissance*, xv, 1968, 89–91; for its location, see ibid., p. 70 n. 2. W. Osler, *Thomas Linacre*, Cambridge, 1908, p. 5, speculated that Linacre was possibly a relative of Sellyng; J. E. Sandys, *A History of Classical Scholarship*, Cambridge, 3 vols., 1908, ii. 225, stated that Linacre was Sellyng's nephew, but gave no authority.

[4] Bennett, p. 90: 'Item lego domino Thome Lynaker studenti Fflorence X li legalis mo*n*ete tradendas intra med*u*m annu*m* post mortem mea*m* honorabili patri domno priori ecclesie Cant. et per eundem seu assignatos suos eid*em* dno Thome mittend*um*.' Italics indicate the expansion of contractions where contractions are indicated in the text, see ibid., p. 89 n.

[5] Ibid., p. 90.

[6] For this printing see E. P. Goldschmidt, *The First Cambridge Press in its European Setting*, Cambridge, 1955, p. 12; Linacre's presentation copy to King Henry VIII of this edition, printed on vellum, is in the Bodleian Library, Oxford, shelf-number Arch. Ae. 71. The passage of the dedication (fol. 1ᵛ)

Angelo Poliziano gave public lectures in the Studio fiorentino from November 1480 until the summer of 1494; his appointment was for a period of two years, and was renewed biennially. On the occasion of one such renewal it was indicated that his duties were 'leggere nello Studio fiorentino quattro lezioni sia greche sia latine, cioè due la mattina e due nel Pomeriggio, quali egli avvisi essere più utili e fruttuose alla gioventù fiorentina', and subsequently 'leggere nello Studio fiorentino facoltà poetica ed oratoria e interpretare gli autori greci'. By 1489 his stipend was the high one of 300 florins a year.[1] Annually from 1486 to 1490 Poliziano gave a course of lectures on Homer's *Iliad* and *Odyssey*, and one entitled 'historia omnium vatum' of Greek and Latin authors.[2] Seemingly it was in the

reads: '. . . Accedit quod quu*m* recens in me collatae no*n* vulgaris munificentiae tuae, qua me quoqu*e* sicut reliquos quicunqu*e* te olim comitabamur in ludum beare es dignatus, non immemore*m* me aliquo salte*m* officij genere declarare volui: vnu*m* hoc inter facultates meas quo id efficere conarer literarium perspexi genus. quod et mihi cui pene praeter literas nihil est, et tibi qui in literis es emine*n*tissimus maxime visu*m* sit congrue*n*s . . .' (Italics indicate the expansion of contractions where contractions are indicated in the text.) This has been freely translated to mean that Giovanni de' Medici and Linacre were contemporary pupils of Poliziano, see J. F. Payne, Introduction to the facsimile reprint of the 1521 edition, Cambridge, 1881, p. 23; R. Weiss, 'Notes on Thomas Linacre' in *Miscellanea G. Mercati*, 4 vols., Vatican City, 1946, iv. 374 n. 7, and repeated in his 'Un allievo . . .', p. 233; Goldschmidt, p. 12. In fact Giovanni de' Medici was only taught by Poliziano for a few months, c. April–May, 1479, see G. B. Picotti, *La prima educazione e l'indole del futuro Leone X*, Potenza, 1919, pp. 12–13. It may have been this dedication that was the source for Lyly's claim that Linacre had been in the 'familia' of Lorenzo de' Medici, see p. 2 n. 3 above.

My friend Mr. S. F. Ryle has suggested the following translation, which depends on reading as a comma the colon printed after 'volui': '. . . In addition since I wished to make clear, by some form of service at least, that I was not unmindful of the extreme generosity that you have recently shown towards me, and by which you have condescended to favour me as you have the others of us who were once your fellow-students, I realised that literature was the only kind [of service] through which my talents would allow me to attempt to do so: since I have virtually no distinction in anything other than literature . . .' All one can say is that the reference to Linacre's literary skill seems to confirm *in ludum* as being some pursuit of learning. This latter, shared by Linacre and Giovanni de' Medici, may have been Poliziano's public lectures in Florence, or other public lectures.

[1] I. del Lungo, 'Angelo Poliziano: Il "Greco" dello Studio fiorentino', in A. Poliziano, *Le Selve e La Strega*, ed. I. del Lungo, Florence, 1925, pp. 231–2. Cf. Ida Maïer, *Ange Politien: La formation d'un poète humaniste (1469–1480)*, Geneva, 1966, pp. 423–35.   [2] Del Lungo, pp. 236–7; Maïer, pp. 427–30.

academic year 1489–90 that he gave a private course on Pliny, as is indicated by his annotated copy of Pliny's *Naturalis historia* (Rome, C. Sweynheym and A. Pannartz, 1473). The relevant jotting says: 'Anno dein MCCCCLXXXX, pridie Kalendas Maias: Cum tribus vetustissimis codicibus contuleram Idem Politianus: hoc ipsum exemplar . . . Quin hoc ipso anno privatim Britannis quibusdam et Lusitanis qui se Florentiam contulerant literarum studio: cupientibus atque a me petentibus enarraui septimestri spatio θεῷ χάρϊν.'[1] Poliziano did not name the English and Portuguese students who attended these private lessons on Pliny's *Natural History*, but it is likely that among them were Linacre, and William Grocyn, another Oxford graduate, who was in Florence in the period 1488–91.[2] On 4 November 1490 Linacre was staying at the English Hospice in Rome, and for the year from 3 May 1491 was its 'Custos', so probably he had been residing there continuously, and in order to hear the lectures of Pomponio Leto and of Sulpizio Verulano.[3] One can conclude, however, that Linacre was in Florence for three years, and that he could have attended Poliziano's public course of two years'

[1] For the Pliny, shelf-number Auct. Q.1.2, in the Bodleian Library, Oxford, see Ida Maïer, *Les Manuscrits d'Ange Politien*, Geneva, 1965, pp. 351–2. The jotting is found in Pliny on fol. 401ᵛ, and is printed by Maïer, op. cit., p. 352, and cf. also Maïer, *Ange Politien . . .*, p. 388 n. 20. Del Lungo, pp. 233, 238, provides less precise information and a less accurate text.

[2] Weiss, *Humanism in England . . .*, p. 173 n. 10, and cf. S. Jayne, *John Colet and Marsilio Ficino*, Oxford, 1963, p. 6; see also p. 2 n. 1 above, and cf. Weiss, 'Un allievo . . .', pp. 232–3, and G. B. Parks, *The English Traveler to Italy*, Rome, 1954, i. 461–2.

[3] 'Liber' 17, fol. 18ᵛ, in the archives of the English College, Rome, gives the date of admission for both Linacre and Lyly as 4 November 1490; fol. 19ʳ gives the date of Linacre's election as Warden as 3 May 1491, and indicates his term of office was until 3 May 1492; I am indebted to Mr. Paul Chavasse, the archivist of the College, and to Professor A. R. Myers for help with this minute book. V. Flynn, 'Englishmen in Rome during the Renaissance', *Modern Philology*, xxxvi, 1938, 136–7, also gives these dates. Weiss in 'Notes on T. Linacre', p. 374, and 'Un allievo . . .', p. 333, provides the date 4 November 1490; however, Parks, p. 457, gives 1489 as the year, and is followed by Emden, ii. 1148; Newns, 'List of *Confratres . . .*', p. 190, gives the date wrongly as '3. 5. 1490', but the correct date is given by J. Allen, 'Introductory: Continuity 1362–1962', in the same issue of *The Venerabile*, xxi, 1962, 5. Merely the year, 1491, is mentioned by Allen, op. cit., for Linacre's Wardenship, and by A. Kenny in Appendix 28 'The officials of St. Thomas's Hospice' to his paper 'From Hospice to College', likewise in *The Venerabile*, cited above, p. 267. Parks, p. 457, gives the date as May 1491, and says his Wardenship was 'presumably for one year'.

duration during this time, as well as the private one on Pliny. On 12 July 1486 Chalcondylas began a course 'ad legendum in Studio florentino et interpretandum phylosophiam greco sermone', which was continued, or merely repeated, in 1487 and 1488.[1] Chalcondylas, whose stipend was 200 florins annually, was a Platonist, and while the content of his lectures is not known, one can suspect that Plato occupied a prominent place.[2] In the case of the lectures of both Poliziano and Chalcondylas a sound grasp of Greek was necessary.

No near-contemporary of Linacre actually states that Linacre had acquired some Greek before he reached Italy.[3] That he had acquired some knowledge of the language at Oxford need not, however, cause surprise as, on the authority of Erasmus, Grocyn who was at least ten years Linacre's senior had acquired some Greek at Oxford, probably before 1476.[4] Morer's will, mentioned above, may furnish further evidence of Linacre's Greek studies in England, for besides the bequest of £10, Morer left five books to Linacre:[5] 'viz. Senten*ci*arium impress*um*, Thucidem historiarum Peloponenc*ium* impress*um*, Tull*ium* in nova Rethorica in pergamen*to* script*um*. Item eidem duos libros grecos vn*um* impress*um*, alter*um* pergamen*to* script*um*'.

Bishop Peter of Aquila's *In libros sententiarum* was printed in Speier in 1480;[6] Valla's translation of Thucydides was printed in Treviso, probably in 1483;[7] *Tullium in nova Rethorica* was the *Ad Herennium*,[8] which is now not attributed to Cicero. One can expect that the notary who drew up the will was incapable of writing the Greek titles, and presumably Morer had only two works in Greek,

[1] G. Cammelli, *I dotti bizantini e le origini dell'umanesimo*, iii, *D. Calcondila*, Florence, 1954, 64–5.

[2] Ibid., pp. 65–6, for the stipend; p. 61, for his Platonic interests.

[3] Bennett, p. 72, says: 'although Leland says again that he [Linacre] studied Greek before he went to Italy'; but the footnote source given is Leland, as cited in p. 3 n. 1 above, and this does not provide the information, which I have not found elsewhere in Leland, cf. J. Leland, *Antiquarii de rebus Britannicis collectanea*, ed. T. Hearne, 6 vols., Oxford, 1715, v, 'Encomia illustrium virorum', found in Appendix I, pp. 81–184, and see pp. 85, 112, 129, 136 for references to Linacre.

[4] Weiss, *Humanism in England . . .*, p. 174; see also Latimer's letter to Erasmus, quoted in p. 2 n. 1, which implies Grocyn's Greek studies in England were at a sufficiently advanced level to enable him to attend the courses of Poliziano and Chalcondylas.

[5] Bennett, pp. 90–1. For the meaning of the italics see p. 4 n. 4 above.

[6] Bennett, p. 71.

[7] Ibid.; *Short-Title Catalogue of Books printed in Italy . . . now in the British Museum*, London, 1958, p. 672.   [8] Bennett, pp. 71, 82.

one printed, one in manuscript. The first book to be printed entirely in Greek characters was Constantine Lascaris's *Grammar* (1476), but by 1489 others had appeared, and it is impossible to identify the book or the manuscript in Greek bequeathed by Morer.[1] Morer's will contained other bequests of his books, and he appears to have selected the titles to suit the taste of the various beneficiaries: accordingly he chose the books he believed most likely to interest Linacre.[2] Morer may, therefore, have known of Linacre's Greek studies in England from personal contact with him; the other possibility from the evidence of the will is that, since Morer knew in 1489 that Linacre was in Florence, he may have only then become aware of his Greek studies.

The earliest known record of Linacre is his election to a fellowship at All Souls College, Oxford, in 1484.[3] By the terms of election a member had to be of at least three years' standing in the University, so it appears that Linacre came up to Oxford in 1481, or earlier. In 1484 his age was about twenty-four, and as entry to the University was often at sixteen, he may have matriculated into an Oxford college several years before 1481.[4] His place of origin is not given in the record of election in 1484, but members of the All Souls foundation were to be from the diocese of Canterbury.[5] It is possible, therefore, that Linacre's first college at Oxford was Canterbury, where Sellyng himself had commenced as a student by 1454.[6] Accepting that Sellyng was Linacre's patron, one can speculate that the connection originated in the diocese of Canterbury. Sellyng as prior of Christ Church since 1472 was likely to have known the best scholars of the attached grammar school, and hence possibly Linacre attended that school; the school attached to St. Augustine's *extra muros*, Canterbury, however, also under Sellyng's care, is another possibility.[7]

---

[1] Bennet, p. 82. Some of the material from Linacre's library is indicated by Weiss, 'Notes on T. Linacre', p. 377.

[2] Bennett, pp. 87–8, for this conclusion and the supporting evidence.

[3] Ibid., p. 73.

[4] Ibid. When Linacre died on 20 October 1524 he was in his 64th year, and therefore was born in 1460 or 1461, see Clark, i. 37.

[5] Bennett, p. 73; cf. Clark, i. 37.

[6] Weiss, *Humanism in England . . .*, p. 153.

[7] For Sellyng appointed Prior see ibid., pp. 155–6, and for St. Augustine's see Bennett, p. 85. Emden, ii. 1147, says he was 'possibly a scholar of the Almonry School or of the Archbishop's School, Canterbury'.

Morer was some thirty years Linacre's senior, and it is tempting to consider how he came to be so well acquainted with Linacre as to leave him such a generous bequest—indeed no other individual was left anything comparable. Morer had been a Fellow of New College, Oxford, 1446–65; in 1465 he obtained the living of All Hallows the Great, London, but two years later exchanged it for the office of Chancellor to the Bishop of Bath and Wells. His career was tied to the patronage of the Nevilles, and Edward IV's victory in 1471 truncated his advancement. From that date until 4 October 1479, when Morer obtained the living of St. Mildred's, Tenterden, through Sellyng's patronage, his activities are uncertain.[1] He left some books to Eton College, and he may have been a Fellow there 1471–3.[2] Morer also left books to the grammar schools of Christ Church and St. Augustine's, Canterbury, and his interest suggests that he taught at these schools, presumably in the period 1473–9;[3] one can believe, in such a case, that the living of Tenterden was something of a reward for his services in teaching in Canterbury. It follows from this that Linacre, who was likely to have been a student in one of these two schools in the 1470s, may have been taught by Morer.[4] In other words Linacre was probably left the bequest by Morer because he had been his favourite pupil. Given Morer's interest in the humanities, as is testified by the books listed in his will, it is likely that he encouraged Linacre's early humanistic studies. That Morer had any deep knowledge of Greek seems doubtful, and it would be rash to speculate that he taught Linacre even the rudiments of it, though he may have encouraged in his pupil the desire to study Greek when opportunity offered.

What is known of the study of Greek at Oxford in the second half of the fifteenth century? The late Professor Roberto Weiss was aware of the autograph draft of Sellyng's Latin oration delivered in Rome in 1487, which bears a note asserting: 'quandam oracionem quam ego W. Sel. composui Oxonie sub Stephano Surigono'.[5] From

[1] Bennett, pp. 82–5.

[2] Ibid., pp. 83, 84 n. 65, 87.

[3] Ibid., pp. 89–90, cf. p. 85.

[4] Cf. ibid., pp. 85–7, where it is also suggested, rather rashly perhaps, that 'teacher and precocious pupil could have begun the study of Greek together', at Oxford, in the period 1479–82.

[5] MS. Cott. Cleop. E.III, in the British Museum, ink foliation 123–5 and published by Balzani (cited in p. 3 n. 2 above), pp. 198–206; the note is on fol. 125r, for which see Balzani, pp. 197, 202 n. 1; R. Weiss, 'Humanism

this Weiss argued 'one can infer that Stephanus Surigonus was one of his [Sellyng's] teachers at Oxford, and that he was taught by him Latin eloquence'.[1] As mentioned above, Sellyng was at Oxford by 1454, perhaps remaining there until 1464; Surigone, who came from Milan, could have been in Oxford during some of this time, and even later, for he appeared in Cologne only in 1471. Accordingly Weiss speculated: 'It is not likely that Surigone taught Greek in Oxford officially, but he very probably knew that language, and it is quite possible that he taught it informally while there.'[2] The importance of this for Linacre is that if Surigone had left Oxford by 1471 at the latest he could not have been Linacre's teacher there by some years.

Clearly, in comparison with the scholars at whose feet Linacre sat in Italy, his teacher at Oxford was considered of little importance. No source mentions him by name. Linacre's study of Greek was likely to have been undertaken after his first degree, and hence in the years 1484–7. His main courses even in this period, however, would have centred on the authors writing in classical Latin. All one can do to identify the teacher who gave such instruction, given the loss of the vital register, is to hazard a reasoned guess. Following the tradition that originates with Linacre's biographer John Noble Johnson, Cardinal Gasquet had few doubts on the matter, believing that at Oxford Linacre's Greek studies had been fostered 'in the lecture room of Cornelio Vitelli'.[3] It was Professor Weiss who claimed this was impossible, since he believed Vitelli only reached Oxford late in 1489 or early in 1490.[4] In 1488 Vitelli had reached Paris where, at first, he taught privately. His request to give a

in Oxford', a letter to the Editor, published in *The Times Literary Supplement*, no. 1823, vol. xxxvi, 9 January 1937, p. 28, and see also idem, *Humanism in England* . . ., p. 156.

[1] Weiss, 'Humanism in Oxford', p. 28; cf. also idem, *Humanism in England*. . ., p. 153.

[2] Weiss, 'Humanism in Oxford', p. 28.

[3] J. N. Johnson, *The Life of Thomas Linacre*, ed. R. Graves, London, 1835, pp. 13, 151 n. This is a very rare book, a fact explained by the publisher's note on the fly-leaf of the copy in the Bodleian Library, shelf-number 35.570: 'As this book did not sell I destroyed all but a few for presents only. Ed. Lumley'; for the tradition see also p. 17 n. 3 and p. 19 n. 1 below. F. A. Gasquet, *Cardinal Pole and his Early Friends*, London, 1927, pp. 51–2.

[4] R. Weiss, 'Cornelio Vitelli in France and England', *Journal of the Warburg Institute*, ii, 1939, 223; idem, *Humanism in England* . . ., p. 173; idem, 'Il debito degli umanisti inglesi verso l'Italia', *Lettere Italiane*, vii, 1955, 307.

course of lectures on the poets was authorized by the University on 5 September 1489, but his quarrels with rival scholars seemingly precipitated his departure for England. When precisely Vitelli reached England is not known. In the autumn of 1489 Robert Gaguin had written an indiscreet Latin poem which appeared to criticize King Henry VII of England, who had received coolly the French King's embassy to negotiate a peace alliance, that Gaguin himself headed. King Henry's secretary, Pietro Carmeliano of the Fava family of the Valle Sabbia near Brescia, replied with a Latin poem that attacked Gaguin, as did Bernard André and John Skelton, the poet laureate, both likewise of the Court circle. One can suppose these writings were intended as propaganda and to exert a form of diplomatic pressure on the French. Vitelli contributed a biting epigram directed against Gaguin, his former friend in Paris, and possibly it was this that forced him to leave Paris; on the other hand Vitelli may have been safe in England, perhaps at London, when he wrote.[1] Apparently by the autumn term of 1490 a man called 'Cornelius', presumably Cornelio Vitelli, was renting a room in Exeter College, Oxford, and he continued to pay rent until the summer of 1492.[2] The fact that he paid rent indicates that he was a *commensalis*, not a Fellow of the College.[3] On Christmas Day, probably in 1490, 'Cornelius', specified as Italian, was a guest of the Vice-President of Magdalen College at dinner; in the record he is termed

[1] Weiss, 'C. Vitelli . . .', pp. 223–4; p. 223 n. 10 stated: 'A paper on this subject is being prepared by the present writer', but it never appeared in print; a draft of it does not appear to be among the Weiss papers in the Warburg Institute Library, and perhaps the project was abandoned in the light of H. L. R. Edwards, 'Robert Gaguin and the English poets, 1489–90', in *Modern Language Review*, xxxii, 1937, pp. 430–4; cf. also M. Pollet, *John Skelton*, trans., London, 1971, pp. 20, 211, with errors.

[2] MS. rolls of 'Computi', 1490–1500, Exeter College Archives. These consist of sheets of vellum, and the references to Cornelio are found on that headed in pencil '1491–92'. On these sheets items were jotted down at various times, sometimes without a date, and hence precise dating is not always possible, as is the case for Cornelio's rent payment. He paid for his chamber 20*s.*, which covered five terms' rent; it is uncertain, but probable, that these were the three of 1491, one (the first) of 1492, one (the last) of 1490. In the summer of 1492 Cornelio paid a further 4*s.* for his chamber for the previous term. One may suppose he had been given credit in 1491, since he had just arrived. See *Register . . . [of] Exeter College, Oxford*, ed. C. W. Boase, Oxford Historical Society, xxvii, 1894, p. lxxii (Marchant, cited in p. 19 n. 1, errs in giving p. xviii); also Weiss, 'C. Vitelli . . .', p. 225 n. 5.

[3] Weiss, 'C. Vitelli . . .', p. 225.

'orator', which implies he held, or had held, a university post as *lector*.[1]

Professor Weiss's case is weak only in the assumption that Vitelli could not have been in England before 1488. He seems, indeed, in his wanderings, as in his quarrelling, to have been typical of his times.[2] On 1 February 1487 he began a course of lectures at Louvain University, replacing Lodovico Bruno, who had held the chair of poetry. He was still at Louvain on 24 November, and presumably left for Paris in 1488,[3] perhaps dissatisfied with the terms of renewal of his contract at the end of a year's service offered by Louvain.

Vitelli was a native of Cortona, a town that had been subject to Florence since 1414.[4] The genealogy of the Vitelli family of Cortona

---

[1] MS. with the spine title: 'Bursary Book, Magd. Coll. Oxon., 1490–99', in Magdalen College Archives, where the reference to 'Cornelius' is on fol. 17ʳ (pencil foliation). The day of his visit is given 'In die Natali Domini', but without the year, which can only be guessed at. The manuscript consists of paper fascicles, which probably had been loose until they were bound, seemingly in the late eighteenth century. The chronological order of the fascicles appears to have been established for binding on the basis of the evidence of scholars' names, whose dates of residence were known from other records; handwriting and watermark evidence may have given some guidance. All one can say is that the date 1490 for Cornelio's visit is probably correct. *A Register of the Members of St. Mary Magdalen College, Oxford*, ed. W. D. Macray, N.S., 7 vols., 1894–1911, i, London, 1894, pp. 22–3, gives the information under '1490–1', meaning 1490, and Weiss, 'C. Vitelli . . .', p. 225, has mistakenly dated the visit as 1491. A. Wood, *The History and Antiquities of the University of Oxford*, subtitled: *Annals*, ed. J. Gutch, 2 vols., Oxford, 1792–6, i. 646, refers to this visit under 1488, on the evidence of 'the weekly Accounts of the Steward of Magdalen College'. These latter were presumably the fascicles of the Bursary Book above, which were probably unbound when Wood saw them, and the date was his speculation; and, indeed, the fascicle that mentions Cornelio bears on its first folio the date 'circa 1487', which subsequently has been cancelled and '1490' added. Wood was followed by H. Maxwell-Lyte, *A History of the University of Oxford . . .*, London, 1886, pp. 386–7; Emden, iii. 1951, errs in giving the date October 1491, taken from Macray.

[2] Cf. Surigone himself; see Weiss, *Humanism in England . . .*, p. 139.

[3] For Louvain see É. Daxhelet, 'Notes sur l'humaniste italien C. Vitelli', *Bulletin de l'Institut historique belge de Rome*, xv, 1935, 88–9; for Vitelli's arrival in Paris see Weiss, 'C. Vitelli . . .', pp. 220–1.

[4] Vitelli himself said he was of Cortona, see Daxhelet, p. 83 n. 2; cf. P. Vergil's error, mentioned below, p. 20, which probably derived from misreading 'Corythius'. Similar misreadings are indicated by Daxhelet, and by N. Fabbrini, 'Vite d'illustri cortonesi' (written at the end of the nineteenth century), MS. 705, Bibl. Comunale, Cortona, II, fol. 83ᵛ. For Vitelli see the

does not mention any Cornelio, and one possibility is that this was a name he adopted, perhaps after his student days, for its classical echoes: similar changes were effected by at least two of his circle, Boccardo (died 1506) and Calderini (*c.* 1446–78).[1] One can merely guess that Cornelio's birth was in the 1440s or early 1450s; his friends appear to have been of this generation, be it noted. Francesco Patrizi (1413–94) of Siena probably about 1480 wrote an epigram which refers to Vitelli as 'Cornelio da Bologna'; certainly the epigram, which mentions this Cornelio in the same context as it does Niccolò Perotti (*c.* 1430–80), could not relate to anyone other than Cornelio Vitelli.[2] Perhaps the explanation is that Cornelio Vitelli had been a student at Bologna, or taught privately there. Vitelli claimed that Francesco Filelfo, who died in 1481, had been his teacher, and while it is possible that Vitelli had been to Milan, it is most likely that he heard Filelfo in Rome whither the latter was summoned by Pope Sixtus IV in 1474 and where he taught from 12 January until 19 June 1475, and from 4 January until 23 April 1476. In Rome, too, Vitelli probably attended the lectures of Domizio

references provided by G. M. Mazzuchelli, 'Alfabeto di scrittori italiani', 3 vols., ii (L–Z), MS. Vat. lat. 9289, fol. 339ᵛ, and iii, MS. Vat. lat. 9290, fol. 272ᵛ, both in the Vatican Library, and M. E. Cosenza, *Biographical and Bibliographical Dictionary of the Italian Humanists of the World of Classical Scholarship in Italy, 1300–1800*, 6 vols., Boston, Mass., 1962–7, iv, no. 373, v, nos. 1902–3; Emden, iii. 1950–1, with several errors. Paola Supino Martini, 'Un carme di Lorenzo Vitelli sulle origini Troiane di Corneto', *Italia medioevale e umanistica*, xv, 1972, 350.

[1] No details of Cornelio's parentage are found in Fra G. G. Sernini Cacciatti, 'Notizie di uomini illustri cortonesi . . .' (written 1758), MS. 547, Bibl. Comunale, Cortona, pp. 31–2; Fabbrini (cited in p. 12 n. 4), fols. 83ʳ–87ʳ; G. Mancini, *Contributo dei cortonesi alla coltura italiana* (2nd edn.), Florence, 1922, pp. 41–2. G. F. Boccardo took the name Pilade, see G. Tiraboschi, *Storia della letteratura italiana*, 10 vols., Rome, 1782–97, vi. 2, p. 373, and for him see Cosenza, iv, no. 351; Domizio Calderini was baptized Domenico, see G. Mercati, *Per la cronologia della vita e degli scritti de N. Perotti . . .*, Rome, 1925, p. 93 n. 3; for him see J. Dunston, 'Studies on D. Calderini', *Italia medioevale e umanistica*, xi, 1968, 71–150, and C. Dionisotti, 'Calderini, Poliziano e altri', ibid., pp. 151–79.

[2] L. F. Smith, 'A notice of the "Epigrammata" of Francesco Patrizi, Bishop of Gaeta', *Studies in the Renaissance*, xv, 1968, 136, no. 211, for the epigram, and see also pp. 105–8. The late Miss K. T. Butler noted that: 'Cornelio Vitelli came from Bologna to Oxford, where he held the first chair of Greek in that University', but provided no source, see her black file with the spine title: 'Italians and Italian in England', sheet relating to Italians in Oxford no. cxv, which is among the papers of Miss Butler, Girton College Archives, Cambridge.

Calderini on Martial, and perhaps those of his rival Niccolò
Perotti, though there is no certainty that the latter actually did
lecture at this time; probably Perotti's ideas on Martial simply were
made known in consequence of the circulation of his writings.[1]
Vitelli's earliest known work is a Latin epigram, reminiscent of
Ovid and Martial, which he dedicated to Federigo da Montefeltro.[2]
The epigram is undated, but it refers to Federigo as Duke, an
honour he received in 1474, while its transcription in a collection of
similar pieces destined for the ducal library indicates that it existed
by 1475. A possibility is that Vitelli was in Rome in 1474 at the
time Federigo was honoured by the Pope, and that he wrote the
epigram for him in an effort to obtain patronage. If, as seems likely,
he hoped to become tutor to Federigo's infant son Guidobaldo, he
was unsuccessful, for Gianmario Filelfo, Francesco's son, obtained
this post in 1476.[3]

Seemingly on 1 April 1478 Vitelli gave the funeral oration of
Angela *née* Thiene, the wife of Paolo Leoni of Padua. From the

[1] Daxhelet, p. 88 n. 4. Vitelli claimed that Merula's aspersions concerning
Filelfo's scholarship had precipitated Filelfo's death, which took place on
31 July 1481, see C. Rosmini, *Vita di Francesco Filelfo*, 3 vols., Milan, 1808, i.
231–3, 238, 245, 259. The aspersions were published in G. Merula [*Epistola
adversus Franciscum Philelphum*] (no place [Venice, N. Girardengus], no date
[1480?]), of which there is a copy in the British Museum, shelf-number
IA.30054(2), see *Short-Title Catalogue of Books printed in Italy* . . ., p. 435. For
the lectures of Calderini, see Mercati (cited in p. 13 n. 1), p. 87; for the
unlikelihood of Perotti's giving lectures see ibid., pp. 87–9; for Perotti in
general, apart from Mercati, see Sesto Prete, 'Osservazioni e note su N.
Perotti', *Fano, 1969*, Fano [1970], pp. 111–20. Vitelli's possible contact with
Calderini and G. A. Campano may have taken place in Rome at this time; for
Vitelli's defence of Calderini (who had died in 1478, some years before Vitelli
wrote) see below, p. 15; for Campano see Weiss, 'C. Vitelli . . .', p. 219
n. 4. The idea that Vitelli was a member of the Accademia Romana, which
seems to originate with A. Zeno, *Dissertazioni Vossiane*, 2 vols., Venice, 1752, ii.
64, may be a deduction from Vitelli's association with Filelfo and Calderini.

[2] Daxhelet, pp. 84–5, where the claim that the poem was written in con-
solation for the death of Battista Sforza (1472) is corrected; this error appears
to have originated with Mancini, and was perpetuated by Weiss, 'C. Vitelli
. . .', p. 220.

[3] For the dating of this collection of pieces see C. H. Clough, 'Piero della
Francesca . . .', *Apollo*, xci, 1970, 282; for Federigo's honours see idem, 'The
Relations between the English and Urbino Courts, 1474–1508', *Studies in
the Renaissance*, xiv, 1967, 204–5; for G. M. Filelfo see idem, 'Federigo da
Montefeltro's Patronage of the Arts, 1468–1482', *Journal of the Warburg and
Courtauld Institutes*, xxvi, 1973, 133.

preface which is addressed to Pietro, Paolo's son, found in a manuscript of this oration, it is reasonable to assume that Vitelli was Pietro's tutor at this time. By 1481 Vitelli was, it seems, teaching the sons of Venetian patricians in Venice, and his main concern perhaps was the exposition of Martial; it was also at this time that he gave a course of lectures at Padua, possibly privately.[1] He was, furthermore, a close friend of the Brescian, Giovanni Francesco Boccardo, called Pilade, to whom he dedicated his brief *De dierum mensium annorumque observatione*, which contained criticism of the scholarship of Giorgio Merula (1431–94), the professor of eloquence at Venice.[2] The work is undated, but was written about 1481, and printed in Venice by B. de Tortis in the second half of 1481 or early in 1482 together with Vitelli's full-scale attack on Merula: *Cornelii Vitelli Corythii in Defensionem Plinii et D. Calderini contra G. Merula Alexandrium ad Hermolaum Barbarum . . . Epistola.*[3] The *Epistola* refers to Merula as having taught in Venice for six years, which was true in 1481,[4] and was answered by an *apologia* printed in Venice in 1482: *Pro G. Merula Alexandrino adversus quendam Cornflium* [sic] *Vitellium apologia*, the work of Paolo Romuleo, who exposed Vitelli to virulent invective.[5] Another of Vitelli's works likewise appears to have been

---

[1] The oration is item iv in a miscellany, MS. B.P. 515, fols. 1–2ᵛ, Museo Civico, Padua, which is of the late fifteenth century, cf. P. O. Kristeller, *Iter Italicum*, London–Leyden, 1967, ii. 22–3. The evidence concerning 1481 is in Daxhelet, pp. 86–7, 93. Vitelli in his dedication letter to Partenio, which prefaces his *Enarratiuncula*, cited below at p. 16 n. 1, says: '. . . Hac enim proxima aetate, cum libellum illum mihi legendum Venetijs dedisses, negaremque tunc me illum posse evoluere, dixi (vt scis) Laturum mecum Patauium, hac conditione, vt cum primum possem, quid de eo sentirem, ad te scriberem . . .'

[2] Daxhelet, p. 91. The work consists of nine folios; it is found with the *Epistola* in the copies: Ross. 1247, Vatican Library; British Museum, see *Short-Title Catalogue of Books printed in Italy . . .*, p. 734. A manuscript copy by itself is in MS. 1517, Bibl. Angelica, Rome. For Boccardo see R. Weiss, 'Umanisti benacensi del quattrocento', in *Il Lago di Garda: Storia di una comunità lacuale. Atti del Congresso Internazionale promosso dall'Ateneo di Salò*, ed. A. Frugoni and E. Mariano, 2 vols., Salò, 1969, ii. 192 n. 10, 199–200.

[3] Daxhelet, pp. 91–3, for a brief but penetrating examination of the work. For Calderini's attack on Perotti's work on Pliny see Dunston (above, p. 13 n. 1), pp. 119–20.

[4] Daxhelet, p. 86 n. 5, where the evidence is cited.

[5] For a copy in the British Museum, shelf-number IA.25072, see *Short-Title Catalogue of Books printed in Italy . . .*, p. 585; for a manuscript of it see Kristeller, *Iter Italicum*, ii. 63; cf. Weiss, 'C. Vitelli . . .', p. 220. Romuleo appears unknown, cf. Cosenza, iv, no. 1558.

composed in Venice, but this was not published for some forty years. This latter—*Cornelii Vitellii in Eundem Primum [Plinii] enarratiuncula perquam erudita*—shows the author in friendly relations with Antonio Partenio da Lazise (Lazisio) (1456–*c.* 1506), who became professor in Verona in 1485. This work, while it stressed the value of Niccolò Perotti's edition of Pliny, published in 1473, as against that of G. A. Bussi, also brought forward some weaknesses in Perotti's emendations. Vitelli wrote another tract in the form of a letter addressed to Partenio, which considered the corrections further. This piece was judged so useful that from 1490 it was frequently published at the end of Perotti's *Cornucopia*. Apparently it first appeared in print in Venice about 1480 following upon Perotti's exposition of his own case concerning the emendations.[1] The work on Pliny's text was what Patrizi had in mind in his epigram about Cornelio and Perotti. It is perhaps to the period of Vitelli's sojourns in Venice and Padua that one can date his contact both with Girolamo Bologni (1454–1517) of Treviso, who dedicated some verses to him in his 'Promiscuorum libri XXI', and with Raffaello Regio (died 1520).[2] Vitelli's stay in Venice seems very similar to that in

---

[1] The *Enarratiuncula* was first printed in *Marini Becichemi scodrensis elegans ac docta in C. Plinivm praelectio . . .*, Basle, 1519, pp. clxxxiii–cxc; there is a copy in the Vatican Library, shelf-number Barb. K.V.77, see Daxhelet, p. 92 n. 11; C. H. Clough, 'Becichemo', *Dizionario biografico degli italiani*, vii, 1965, 511–15. For the analysis of the work see Daxhelet, pp. 93–4. For the tract in the form of a letter see Weiss, 'C. Vitelli . . .', p. 219 n. 5 (3); a copy in manuscript is indicated by Kristeller, *Iter Italicum*, ii. 53. For the printing *c.* 1480: *Commentariolus in C. Plinii Secundi Prooemium, cum observationibus Cornelii Vitelli in eundem Commentariolum* (no place [Venice?], no date [1480?]), in folio, 10 fols., unnumbered, fol. [8ᵛ]: '[C]Ornelius Vitellius parthenio Benacensi suo salutem'. There is a copy in the Bibl. Nazionale, Naples, shelf-number X.F.21; see D. Reichling, *Appendices ad Hainii–Copingeri Repertorium bibliographicum; additiones et emendationes*, 3 vols., Munich, 1905–11, iii. 140 as H. 12708 (cf. Mercati, cited at p. 13 n. 1, pp. 90–1); cf. Perotti, *Cornucopiae, sive Lingua latinae Commentarij diligentissime recogniti atque ex archetypo emendati . . . Cornelii Vitelij in eum ipsum libellum Sypontini annotationes* [Venetiis, 1513], of which there is a copy in the Vatican Library, shelf-number Racc. gen. Classici II. 305. For Partenio see Cosenza, iv, nos. 1330–1, and Weiss, 'Umanisti benacensi . . .', ii. 197–8, 201–2.

[2] For Patrizi's epigram see above, p. 13. For Bologni see R. Cesarini, 'G. Bologni', *Dizionario biografico degli italiani*, xi, 1969, 327–31, Cosenza, iv, nos. 313–14, and Kristeller, *Iter Italicum*, ii. 18, 285; for Regio see Daxhelet, p. 86, and Cosenza, iv, no. 1519. Kristeller, *Iter Italicum*, ii. 286, indicates two collections of Latin verses which include some addressed to Vitelli, which may not be those of Bologni.

Paris; in both places he became involved in bitter quarrels on matters of current scholarly interest.[1] He left Paris for Oxford; is there any evidence that he had previously left Venice for Oxford?

Leland, who from the 1530s was visiting monastic libraries, wrote that there existed (and the implication may be that he had seen) in the chancery of the bishopric of Bath and Wells the public oration given by Thomas Chaundler in reply to a lecture of Cornelio Vitelli's: 'Extat & ejus Oratio, qua respondet Cornelii Vitollii, praelectoris in Novo collegio Isidis Vadi, orationi primae. In Fontanensi ecclesia Cancellarii officio fungebatur'.[2] Unfortunately both the oration and the lecture are lost, but presumably they had been delivered at Oxford. Leland does not give the date. Professor Weiss believed it to be 1491; his case, which has never been given, appears to rest on the fact that Vitelli was known to be in Oxford in the years 1490–2.[3] Neither does Leland indicate in what capacity Chaundler had replied to Vitelli's lecture; Chaundler had been Chancellor to Thomas Bekynton, Bishop of Bath and Wells from 1452 until 1467, and one can see that one of his orations might have been of

---

[1] The details of the quarrels in Paris are provided by Weiss, 'C. Vitelli . . .', pp. 221–3.

[2] Leland, *Commentarii de scriptoribus Britannicis* (cited in p. 3 n. 1), ii. 457; Weiss, 'C. Vitelli . . .', p. 225 n. 7, errs by giving this reference as p. 547.

[3] For the loss of the oration and lecture cf. Weiss, *Humanism in England . . .*, p. 6. For the date 1491 see idem, 'C. Vitelli . . .', p. 225 n. 7: 'It would be too lengthy to state here the grounds for doubting this date [1475 (for which see p. 19 n. 1), and a visit before 1487]. This point will be fully dealt with in my forthcoming work on English fifteenth-century humanism.' This latter, published as *Humanism in England . . .*, is somewhat ineffectual here, as the text on page 136 has two references both numbered 1, and only a single footnote. The footnote gives first the reference to T. Bekynton, *Official Correspondence*, ed. G. Williams, 2 vols., Rolls series, London, 1872, ii. 315–20, which does not concern Vitelli at all (though it misled Emden, iii. 1951, who cites Vitelli's oration as actually being in Bekynton's correspondence, which it is not). Secondly it refers to Leland, as quoted above, p. 3 n. 1. On p. 173 n. 3 Weiss again merely refers the reader to his 'C. Vitelli . . .' article. The suggestion that Chaundler replied to Vitelli 'in Oxford about 1491' (Weiss, p. 136) errs at least in the year, as Chaundler died in November 1490 (see p. 19 below); cf. Weiss, 'Notes on T. Linacre', p. 374 n. 7. Wood (cited in p. 12 n. 1), i. 645, under 1488 says: 'P. Vergil . . . doth tell us that he [Vitelli] was a lecturer in New College, that is, (I suppose) he read humanity lectures in New College Hall to all that came.' Vergil (see p. 20) does not say this, and Wood possibly had in mind Leland's information; cf. i. 412 where Vergil is quoted correctly.

interest to an associate who remained in the chancery.[1] Chaundler, born about 1417, was Warden of New College from 1454 until 1475, and Chancellor of Oxford University from 1457 until 1461, and again from 1472 until 1479; he had been Vice-Chancellor while serving Bekynton, 1463–7. Chaundler was in friendly correspondence with Sellyng, and for a time rented a room in Canterbury College; in gratitude for his benefactions to this college, moreover, his name was enrolled among its patrons. If Vitelli was a 'praelector' of New College with a free room there, it is hard to see why he paid for a room from Exeter College; again, he is found only once in New College Hall-books, in April 1492 (and this date may not be correct) seemingly when he dined there as a guest.[2] The explanation may be the simple one: he was 'praelector' at New College before his sojourn in Oxford in the years 1490–2. That Vitelli turned against his friend Gaguin for criticizing the English king could have been in consequence of a visit to England, and his desire to ensure that charges of disloyalty could not be levelled against him. Apparently late in March 1490, Sellyng was expected in Paris as an English envoy to negotiate with King Charles VIII in the light of the treaty of Frankfurt. Vitelli might have wanted to catch Sellyng's attention in order that the latter might assist his return to England. Vitelli's writing of the period spent in Venice, 1480–2, gives no hint of his having taught at Oxford, and hence the period 1482–7 seems the more likely for his first visit there. One might have expected Chaundler to have given his oration in his capacity as Warden of New College,

[1] A. Judd, *The Life of T. Bekynton*, Chichester, 1961, p. 112; Bennett, p. 83.
[2] Emden, i. 398–9; Weiss, *Humanism in England* . . ., pp. 134–6, 196; Bennett, p. 78; *Duke Humfrey and English Humanism in the Fifteenth Century: Catalogue of an Exhibition . . . Bodleian Library, Oxford*, Oxford, 1970, pp. 19–21, 58. For Canterbury College see the editor's Preface, *Canterbury College, Oxford*, ed. W. A. Pantin, 3 vols., Oxford Historical Society, N.S. vi–viii, Oxford, 1947–50, i, pp. v–vi. For Vitelli dining in New College in April 1492 see Emden, iii. 1951, who cites 'New College Hall-books, 1491–2'. Neither Dr. Francis Steer, the archivist of New College, nor I have been able to find this reference; Dr. Emden has been unable to throw further light on the problem from his notes. The volume in question is entitled: 'Liber Seneschalla Aulae, 1478–1499', and in New College archives, see F. W. Steer, *The Archives of New College, Oxford*, London, 1974, p. 135 no. 5529; lists for the years 1482–3, 1483–4, 1490–1 are not included. I have not found a 'Cornelius' in the entire volume. I am much indebted to Dr. Steer for all his assistance with this manuscript. The Warden's household accounts for the period 1470–92 do not now exist. For other archival material in New College see p. 19 n. 2.

or as Chancellor of the University, but he terminated these appointments in 1475 and 1479 respectively.[1] From 22 February 1481 until his death on 2 November 1490 he was Dean of Hereford, and so perhaps he was indeed summoned from Hereford to Oxford to deliver his oration to Vitelli—his Latin prose was certainly deemed of outstanding quality.[2]

The most likely period of Linacre's Greek studies at Oxford was 1481 to 1487; with this Vitelli's first years in Oxford would overlap. It may be significant that Vitelli arrived in Louvain in February 1487, and that a few months later Linacre was in Florence—a valid reason in determining Linacre's departure for Italy might have been the loss of his teacher at Oxford, particularly if that teacher were an Italian. Polydore Vergil of Urbino, who arrived in England in 1503,[3] incorporated a passage concerning Cornelio Vitelli into his *Anglica Historia* at some time after the first manuscript draft, which was

[1] For Sellyng's embassy of 1490 see Weiss, *Humanism in England* . . ., p. 156 n. 6. The idea that Vitelli arrived in Oxford in 1475 seems to have originated with M. Burrows, *Collectanea*: ii, Oxford Historical Society, xvi (Oxford, 1890), p. 340, where it is argued that as Chaundler relinquished the Wardenship of New College, Oxford, in 1475, this year must have been the latest date for his speech of welcome to Vitelli as a Praelector of that college; the date is followed by E. C. Marchant, 'C. Vitelli', *The Dictionary of National Biography* xx (1899), 376; W. H. Woodward, *Studies in Education during the Age of the Renaissance*, Cambridge, 1908, p. 107, says 'Vitelli, an Italian scholar, was teaching Greek, as a private tutor, in New College, about 1470–75'.

[2] For him as Dean, cf. A. L. Moir, *Deans of Hereford*, Hereford, 1968, p. 28. The date of his death is indicated on the memorial brass in Hereford Cathedral; see A. J. Winnington-Ingram, *Monumental Brasses in Hereford Cathedral* (3rd edn.), Hereford, 1972, p. 15. The suggestion of a summons from Hereford was advanced in *Medieval England*, ed. A. L. Poole, 2 vols. (2nd edn.), Oxford, 1958, ii. 539. The series of Chapter Act Books for Hereford does not begin until 1512; *Registrum Thome Myllyng, Episcopi Herefordensis (1474–1492)*, ed. A. T. Bannister, Cantilupe Society, Hereford, 1919, printed with the same title and pagination but a different title-page, Canterbury and York Society, xxxvi, London, 1920, refers to Chaundler on pp. 60, 62, 95, 194, 198, but does not establish when Chaundler was absent from the diocese. I am grateful to Miss P. E. Morgan of Hereford Cathedral Library for her help. Shirley Bridges, cited in p. 21 n. 2 below, i. 111, mentions Chaundler at New College on Monday, 7 April and Sunday, 4 May 1483, giving her authority as 'New College Muniments'; material of this date with this information, however, cannot be traced, cf. p. 18 n. 2 above. On 25 March 1486 Chaundler was entertained at Magdalen College, see *A Register* . . ., cited in p. 12 n. 1, N.S. i. 15.

[3] D. Hay, *Polydore Vergil*, Oxford, 1952, p. 2.

begun about 1514, and before the first published version of 1534:
'. . . antea enim Cornelius Vitellius homo Italus Corneti, quod est
maritimum Hetruriae oppidum, natus nobili vir optimus, grati-
osusque omnium primus Oxonii bonas literas docuerat . . .'[1]

The reference to Vitelli's birthplace as Corneto Tarquinia clearly
errs,[2] but the claim that Vitelli was the first who taught 'bonas
literas', meaning Latin and Greek, should not be too lightly dis-
missed. It seems likely that Vitelli left England shortly after 1492
and Vergil appears never to have met him.[3] Vergil, who for a time
was in Wells and could have seen the oration of Chaundler which
Leland saw subsequently, had no reason to exaggerate Vitelli's
importance.[4] In view of the sophistication of humanistic studies in
the first decades of the sixteenth century, he may well have been
providing a just and representative evaluation of Vitelli. Certainly,
despite claims to the contrary, there is no doubt that Vitelli knew
Greek, and had a sound grasp of Greek authors.[5] Sabellico considered him a highly gifted scholar, though intemperate.[6] His stay
in England may have been relatively peaceful, perhaps because there
were no scholars at Oxford of sufficient calibre to be judged by him
as rivals. It is worth remarking, moreover, that Linacre probably
attended Poliziano's courses on Pliny, whose writings were of
special interest to Vitelli. Eventually, if Giovio is to be credited,
Linacre made contact with Ermolao Barbaro, and perhaps Vitelli
paved the way. The anecdote of the first meeting, as told by Giovio,
places the encounter in the Vatican Library in Rome, when Linacre
was reading a text of Plato. At Padua, where he took his degree in
the summer of 1496, Linacre was interested in Aristotle in the
Greek, and this might indicate some influence on the part of Bar-

---

[1] For the date of the first draft see C. H. Clough, 'F. Veterani, P. Vergil's
"Anglica Historia" . . .', *English Historical Review*, lxxxii, 1967, 776–7. The
first edition was printed in Basle, 1534, and the variants between this and
the manuscript first draft are published in P. Vergil, *The 'Anglica Historia'*,
ed. D. Hay, in Camden series, lxxiv, London, 1950, p. 147. For Wood's
misquotation of Vergil see p. 17 n. 3 above.

[2] See p. 22 below.

[3] There is no record of Vitelli at Oxford after 1492, when he ceased to rent
a room from Exeter College.

[4] Vergil was in Wells, acting as proxy for its bishop in 1504; see Hay,
Polydore Vergil, p. 5.

[5] The evidence is provided by Daxhelet, pp. 84, 94; Bennett, p. 74 n. 17,
errs on this point.

[6] Daxhelet, p. 97.

baro.[1] It is worth remembering that in 1481 Vitelli had dedicated his *Epistola* to Barbaro, and a pupil of Vitelli's might have expected some favours from Barbaro in consequence.

It must be said that the circumstances resulting in Vitelli's coming to Oxford about 1482 are not known. Chaundler, though, had been created an apostolic protonotary, giving his oath on 24 April 1480, and clearly had important Italian connections; by 1485 he was termed 'sacre theologie professor', and hence was probably still at Oxford in this capacity.[2] It might be that Chaundler delivered the reply to Vitelli's oration, perhaps about 1483, because he himself had been influential in procuring Vitelli's services at Oxford.

If it is accepted that Vitelli was praelector at New College in the period 1482–7, he certainly did not come to England with that post in 1489–90, and there is no evidence that he subsequently obtained it again. Professor Weiss, indeed, judged that Vitelli arrived in England in 1489–90 in search of royal patronage, and this can be accepted.[3] Henry VII favoured foreigners, and his secretary, Pietro Carmeliano, had rapidly advanced himself from teaching Latin in the Cathedral School of Westminster, a post he had held in 1484.[4] Presumably Vitelli returned to Oxford in 1490 because he was familiar with it, and he rented a room from Exeter College in order to teach privately, as he had done previously in Venice, Padua, and Paris, while waiting for royal patronage, or some University emolument. Neither hope was fulfilled.

[1] Weiss, 'Un allievo . . .', p. 333; for his degree at Padua see Rosemary J. Mitchell, 'Linacre in Italy', *English Historical Review*, l, 1935, 696–8.

[2] Weiss, *Humanism in England . . .*, p. 134; Shirley Bridges (now the Hon. Mrs. Hilary Corke), 'Thomas Chaundler' (unpublished Oxford B.Litt. thesis, 2 vols., 1952, shelf-number d. 8. 19/1, 2, in the Bodleian Library, Oxford), i. 105. Emden, i. 399, gives the date 24 April 1477 for Chaundler becoming an apostolic protonotary. For Chaundler as Professor of Theology, which is not mentioned by Emden, see *The Register of T. Mylling . . .*, p. 95, under 10 January 1485, when Chaundler was summoned to attend convocation at Westminster, and his memorial brass cited p. 19 n. 2. Bridges, 'Thomas Chaundler', i. 109, mentions an inscription written to the same effect, and dated between 1481 and 1485, in New College MS. 242, fol. 1ᵛ. For Chaundler in Oxford see also p. 19 n. 2.

[3] Weiss, 'C. Vitelli . . .', p. 223.

[4] P. Guerrini, 'Pietro Carmeliano da Brescia, Segretario reale d'Inghilterra', *Brixia Sacra*, ix, 1918, offprint pp. 6–7; cf. also R. Weiss, 'Lineamenti di una biografia di Giovanni Gigli . . .', *Rivista di Storia della Chiesa in Italia*, i, 1947 pp. 379–91.

What was the nature of the relationship between Linacre, Vitelli, and William Grocyn, for the latter has been claimed to have taught Linacre Greek?[1] Grocyn was reader in theology from 1483 until 1487, and at Magdalen College;[2] then, with Vitelli's assistance, he could have perfected the Greek he had previously acquired. Probably Grocyn was in Florence attending the same lectures as Linacre in 1488–90.[3] He was back in Oxford by the summer of 1491, and from Hilary Term of that year until Trinity Term, 1493, he rented a room from Exeter College.[4] It can be accepted that he taught privately, with Greek included among the subjects taught.[5] Vitelli, if faced with Grocyn, a former pupil, who was more successful than he in attracting students, may have decided to leave Oxford. A Greek epigram written by Poliziano against a certain 'Cornelius', who had accused him of plagiarism, probably refers to Vitelli; Cornelio's attack had been directed against Poliziano's *Miscellanea* and his translation of Herodotus, and since the latter was printed in Italy in the late summer of 1493, Cornelio's accusations must have been in the last year of Poliziano's life.[6] The implication may be that Vitelli had returned to Italy to teach by then. It is not known when

[1] See p. 23 n. 2 below.

[2] Burrows, *Collectanea*, ii. 344–6; Weiss, *Humanism in England . . .*, p. 173; Emden, ii. 827.

[3] For Grocyn studying in Florence see Latimer's letter to Erasmus quoted in p. 2 n. 1 above; 1488–90 appears to be the only period of two years that Grocyn could have been abroad and studied under Poliziano and Chalcondylas, cf. Weiss, *Humanism in England . . .*, pp. 173–4, n. 10; Parks, *The English Traveler*, pp. 461–2; Emden, ii. 827.

[4] He was back in Oxford by 4 June 1491, see Weiss, *Humanism in England . . .*, pp. 173–4, n. 10; for his renting of the room see Emden, ii. 827, which gives the documentation.

[5] Wood, *The History . . .*, ii. 837: '. . . sure it is, that he [Grocyn], after he had been instructed in Italy by those exquisite Masters Demetrius Chalcondila, and Angelus Politianus, returned into England, and read the Greek tongue several years to the Oxonians; about which time instructing Richard Croke, the Cambridge orator, in the said language . . .', and see his authorities cited. This is presumably the source for Burrows, *Collectanea*, ii. 347, and for Emden, ii. 287, who says Grocyn 'gave first public lectures in Greek in the University', which is rather misleading in its implication that Grocyn held a University post for the express purpose of lecturing in Greek.

[6] Maïer, *Ange Politien . . .*, p. 151 n. 66, where the 'Cornelius' is not identified; for the circulation of Poliziano's *Miscellanea* and the printing of the translation of Herodotus, see ibid., pp. 429, 435; Maïer does not date the Greek epigram. Weiss, 'C. Vitelli . . .', p. 219 n. 4, thought that the 'Cornelius' in question might be Vitelli.

Vitelli died, but he may have been alive *c.* 1500–2, since Bernard André, referring to him then, rather implied he was, and called him 'facundissimus orator Cornelius Vitellius';[1] of course André, writing in England, may have been ill informed of Vitelli's existence.

All in all, while one may be unable to prove that neither Sellyng nor Grocyn gave Linacre any basic instruction in Greek,[2] from strong circumstantial evidence it was Cornelio Vitelli who, as prae-lector at New College, gave him the sound knowledge of that language which he clearly had prior to 1487 and his studies in Florence.

[1] Weiss, 'C. Vitelli . . .', p. 226 nn. 1 and 4.

[2] The evidence concerning Sellyng is marshalled by Bennett (cited in p. 4 n. 3 above), with the conclusion that there is no basis for the tradition that he taught Linacre any Greek; this is to overstate the case. Burrows, *Collectanea*, ii. 345 says: 'That he [Linacre] had already [prior to going to Italy] attended Grocyn at Oxford we may well believe, though actual proof is wanting. The pupil of Selling was of the exact age during his early residence to profit by the Lectures of the Divinity Reader, which one may be sure, were as much in Greek as in Divinity,—perhaps also by those of Vitelli.' It appears as though what Wood says (quoted in p. 17 n. 3) is being applied by Burrows as prior to Grocyn's visit to Italy.

Linacre's Latin Grammars

D. F. S. THOMSON*

THE DIFFUSION OF MANUALS OF INSTRUCTION IN THE universal language of Western scholarship formed no small part of the public responsibility of the earliest printers. It was not then surprising if almost as soon as this task was undertaken and the mysteries of accidence, and of syntax, began in some measure to escape from their lurking-place among the secrets of a craft, the ancient guidance of Donatus or of Priscian—interpreted by versifying grammaticasters of earlier or of later date—was found severely wanting. No doubt intelligent pedagogues had, here or there, modified for the boys' sake the knowledge which they themselves drew from handbooks written for the needs of a much older time; but general discontent with the sources themselves, when they were exposed to view, made it imperative that rules once framed with adult comprehensiveness should be presented afresh, in a manner that suited the childish understanding and did not demand the presence of a tutor.

Yet not all of the new writers were able to divest themselves of the scholar's passion for complete, concise, exact, and verifiable statement. Certain of the grammars that were offered for children's use, though they might employ mnemonic aids, were still excessively verbose, either because they attempted to define a concept or state a rule with unnecessary precision at the moment of its first introduction, or because their apparatus of illustrative examples was so lavish as to overwhelm even the most industrious learner. The fortune of Linacre's best work in this field might have been very different, in his native country at least, had he more firmly repressed

* Department of Classics, University College, University of Toronto.

an inclination—based perhaps on a want of experience in teaching boys—to keep scholarly fullness more steadily in view than the capacity of most pupils for absorbing instruction. This was all the more to be regretted, since Linacre's grammars seem to have been distinctly in advance of those of his contemporaries—at least the great mass of them—in the virtue of correctness (with occasional lapses, as we shall see), while he was highly praised for the purity of his own Latin style, as well as for his apt choice of examples.

Linacre published three grammars; two of them were undated on first publication, and their dates of composition have been disputed. The work I have called his best is certainly his most elaborate: the *De emendata structura Latini sermonis*, published in London in December 1524 by Richard Pynson,[1] and never again printed in England. Two shorter works were composed in English, despite their Latin titles: the *Progymnasmata grammatices vulgaria*, to which widely divergent dates have been assigned,[2] and the *Rudimenta grammatices*, which has been described as an expanded version of the *Progymnasmata*.[3]

[1] London: R. Pynson, 1524. Facsimile in the series English Linguistics 1500–1800, edited by R. C. Alston, No. 83, Scolar Press: Menston, Yorks., 1968. On this edition, see Giles Barber, 'Thomas Linacre: A Bibliographical Survey of his Works', below, pp. 303–4; also W. Osler, *Thomas Linacre*, Linacre Lecture, 1908, Cambridge, 1908, pp. 32 ff. and Plate XI (title-page). Some of the editions are mentioned by Osler, pp. 36, 38. This work was 'reprinted over fifty times in the sixteenth century' (R. C. Alston, Introduction to the facsimile edition: see above). The sixth book (*de figuris*) was recommended for use in Norwich Grammar School in 1566; see T. W. Baldwin, *Shakespere's Small Latine and Lesse Greeke*, Urbana, Ill., 1944, i. 417.

[2] On the apparently unique copy in the British Museum, see Barber, op. cit., pp. 292–5; also Osler, op. cit., pp. 30–1 and Plate IX (introductory verses by Linacre, More, and Lily). On its publication by John Rastell see Barber, op. cit., and A. W. Reed, 'The Regulation of the Book Trade before the Proclamation of 1538', *Transactions of the Bibliographical Society*, xv, 1920, 173–4. Reed suggests a date before Rastell's 1517 voyage; Barber places the date of publication about the year 1515. Reed observes that 'the prefatory verses by Lily point to the existence of another version, vitiated by errors and published anonymously, a pirated or stolen edition, in fact'.

[3] London: R. Pynson, n.d. Facsimile in the series English Linguistics 1500–1800, edited by R. C. Alston, No. 312, Scolar Press: Menston, Yorks., 1971. On the date and other matters, see Barber, op. cit., pp. 300–2; also Osler, op. cit., pp. 31–2 and Plate X (title-page). R. C. Alston, op. cit., Introduction, notes that 'typographical evidence seems to point to a period between Pynson's printing of Horman's *Vulgaria* in 1519 and . . . 1524 the year in which the *De emendata* appeared. Pynson's device on the verso of [M4] is McKerrow No. 53 which is recorded in books issued between 1522 and

Linacre dedicated the *Rudimenta* to his pupil (in 1523) the Princess Mary, and clearly designed or adapted it for her use; various dates have been suggested for its composition and publication, from about 1519 to 1524. George Buchanan, the Scottish humanist, translated the *Rudimenta* into Latin for the use—in Paris—of his pupil Gilbert Kennedy, third Earl of Cassillis; it was published in the following year, 1533, by Robert Estienne, and this issue seems to have attracted notice at once on the Continent, though not in England. Buchanan's prefatory letter to his pupil deserves to be translated and noted as a judicious contemporary estimate of the value of the work:

Last year I went quickly through Linacre's Rudiments, to fix in your memory things you already knew. At that time, I was extraordinarily taken with the author's meticulous treatment (stopping short of mere fuss, however) of the very smallest details, and the clear way in which he arranges his book—so far as the disorderly mass of information pertaining to this subject allows—and also a certain freshness of approach which will (I believe) be welcomed by discerning readers where the theme is so very commonplace.

For these and many other reasons I have decided that it would be worth while to translate the little work into Latin out of the English in which it was first published by its author; either in order to draw attention to Linacre's scholarly competence in this additional branch of learning, or else because boys can profit more by acquiring the rudiments of grammar from the very well-springs of purity, as it were —from Hippocrene itself, indeed—than from the muddied waters of everyday life which are usually thrust under their noses by headmasters in schools; or, lastly, with the intention that young men who enlist in the Muses' service under the best of commanders may thereby listen with greater confidence to advice which (since it rests on the authority of a consummate scholar) they will regard as the oracles of the gods, rather than as mere notions that emanate from human frailty.

Yes, I am fully aware that there will be some who will suppose, even before they have read this work, that it is a pointless addition to the multitude of older authorities; for they are convinced that on this subject nothing can be said at this time that has escaped the

1526.' The full title is *Rudimenta Grammatices Thomae Linacri diligenter castigata denuo* (which of course implies that there had been an earlier version of some kind). For a list of some editions published in France, see G. Neilson (ed.), *George Buchanan, Glasgow Quatercentenary Studies 1906*, Glasgow, 1907, pp. 399 ff.

attention of those old grammarians who have won official approval the schools—or if anything fresh should in fact be added, such as most of what is said in this book on the declension of nouns, or certain tenses and moods of verbs, it is so unimportant that it would be far better if it had been left unwritten.

But this kind of complaint emanates from men of surpassing ignorance; or else from such as are so regrettably under the sway of their personal feelings that when they observe some matters to be stated in a form differing from that in which the same matters were either learnt by them individually or taught to them by those whose words they take for Gospel, they will bring an accusation not merely of irresponsible conduct but almost of blasphemy against those who (as they put it) 'stray from their fathers' footsteps' and have the effrontery to suspend, and even to repeal, rules that were once vouchsafed to mankind with the solemn sanctity of holy law.

Against this kind of arrogant haughtiness on the part of the class I have described, I appeal to all men of learning, and to such as love the humanities. Unless I am mistaken, they will find that their own needs are satisfied by Linacre's longer work [the *De emendata structura Latini sermonis*]. As for the present little book, I should like it to appear under your name, and also, in compliment to yourself, as a gift to be shared with all studious youth. If the young themselves should regard my assistance with favour, I will consider that these labours of mine have brought in a rich and rewarding harvest.

My greetings to you.

George Buchanan's Latin version of the *Rudimenta* has several points of interest:

1. Although he made and published it in Paris, he does not offer, as one of the reasons for translating the work out of the original English, the larger public it may thereby reach on the Continent. Yet in fact, as we know, this is exactly what happened; there were to be many continental editions, whereas the book fell out of use in England.

2. While Buchanan carefully changes the name 'London' to 'Paris' in the illustrative examples, he also carefully substitutes *regnante Jacobo* for *regnante Henrico*—no doubt for the benefit, or to encourage the loyalty, of his Scottish pupil, who in the end turned out less than loyal to the Stewarts, for history tells us that he appears a few years later as Henry's paid agent.

3. The contrast between 'well-springs' and 'muddied waters of everyday life', and the association of the latter with 'headmasters' (*gymnasiarchi*), may perhaps contain a double or triple reference to

William Lily's grammars; for not only was Lily the High Master of St. Paul's School, but he wrote in the vernacular; and not only that, but when he gave a Latin example it was often in the form of a little sentence or phrase of his own concoction rather than a quotation from Cicero such as Linacre was careful to use when he could.

4. In his final paragraph, Buchanan recognizes the existence and character of Linacre's larger work—*opus maius*—the *De emendata structura* (written of course in Latin) as appealing to, and satisfying, the needs of more advanced scholars; this work, also, justified Buchanan's approval by running through many continental editions. In a paraphrase, rather than translation, of the dedicatory letter to the *Rudimenta*, P. Hume Brown has entirely obscured this reference, which had plainly escaped him, for he mistranslates the Latin.[1]

5. For all his praise of Linacre's work, Buchanan again and again quietly corrects mistakes of detail and also principles of procedure which he appears to consider as pedagogically unsound, as we shall observe in a moment. He does so without the slightest evidence of scholarly peevishness, but on the contrary with a kind of magnanimity which I believe to have been characteristic of the man, and rare enough among the humanists of his time.

Although Lily no doubt surpassed Linacre in the arts of promoting his own work and capturing official favour, it is not altogether surprising if (even discounting these activities) history records that Lily's contribution was accepted, and Linacre's rejected, by Colet. Of course the rejection had occurred by 1511, as we know from a letter of Erasmus,[2] and we do not now possess any grammar by Linacre of so early a date; but the *Progymnasmata* (*c.* 1515?) and *Rudimenta* (1523?) probably inherited at least the principles of arrangement, method of illustration, and general approach of Linacre's lost grammar as it was offered to St. Paul's School. If they did, then the following weaknesses of the later grammars at least help to explain the rejection.

1. Linacre seems to have been remarkably careless about the kinds of accuracy which are so important in a grammar written for boys. One can well imagine the Dean's choler rising when he was confronted with *crurium* as the genitive plural of *crus*, or with a debased—apparently misremembered and unchecked—version of a

---

[1] *George Buchanan: Humanist and Reformer*, Edinburgh, 1890, p. 66.

[2] *Opus Epistolarum Des. Erasmi Roterodami*, ed. P. S. Allen, 12 vols., Oxford, 1906–58, i, Ep. 227 (p. 467).

line in Virgil.[1] After all, even clerical philanthropists are human; and a boy who reads at ten years old 'Caesare et Libulo consulibus', even if this should be a mere printer's error, is likely (alas) to remember Libulus, not Bibulus, all his life. These three mistakes, together with those that follow, were (without any fuss) removed from Buchanan's Latin version: *hane* for *have*, *pluia* for *pluvia*, *fos* for *for*, *puella* for *pulla*, *digum* for *dignum*, 'femine' for 'feminine', *amabunut* for *amabunt*, *heu* for *hem*, *veh* for *vah* or *vae*, and so forth. Again, statements such as this: 'the Ablative . . . hath these signs in englysshe, for, fro, with than, and by'; inconsistency in the use of lower-case *v* and *u*; combined with this, punctuation which might well baffle a young pupil, e.g. *cum vellemus, uelletis, lent*; further inconsistency in prefixing *utinam* to the optative subjunctive or omitting it, and similarly in the omission or inclusion of *o* with the vocative case (both of these in the tables of accidence); omission of *finis* from the list of nouns of ambiguous gender; inconsistency in arrangement ('I, me vs and we', where Buchanan has I/me/we/us); headings absorbed into the text in such a way as to make nonsense; misleadingly condensed statements, e.g. *Pridie postridie Calendarum*; lavish use of abbreviations which would puzzle beginners; printers' errors in sentence-division; confusion of categories (of which a mild example is *non facis*, under the Adverb—on all fours with *bene facis* or *male facis*); and much else, including the description of the third conjugation of the verb as the second.

One is accordingly tempted to surmise that on grounds of accuracy alone Colet may have been inclined to regard with disfavour the book that Linacre offered. But there are weaknesses of method as well.

2. Linacre adopts the catechetical method, which Lily abandoned for a more straightforward kind of exposition. To a modern reader, it almost seems as though Linacre supposes the young reader to be perusing, let us say Cicero, and suddenly to encounter an odd phrase which requires to be discussed; for Linacre will give the example first, then the question, and finally the rule or explanation. No doubt this is how the grammarians of the late Roman empire now and then approached their task; nevertheless it was hardly a helpful approach for the young barbarians of northern Europe whom Colet and other Renaissance schoolmasters had to nurture in the elements; and Lily more wisely puts the rule first and then discusses

---

[1] *Aeneid*, ix. 514; Linacre ends the line thus: *casus testudine templi*.

it, at sufficient length to make the point clear, adding one or perhaps two simple examples, usually of his own devising.

3. Linacre has too many illustrations; and because he is careful to use 'real Latin', as a modern teacher might say—taken wherever possible from Cicero or another of the 'best' writers of the classical age—the illustrations themselves sometimes make hard reading for small boys. We have noticed that George Buchanan recommended Linacre as a result of his experience with the *Rudimenta*; but, though Buchanan was an experienced tutor, he makes no mention of this fault. The reason, I think, is simply that Buchanan had much older pupils in mind than Colet, for example; the young Earl of Cassillis was seventeen years old when Buchanan introduced him to the book, eighteen when he dedicated it to him.[1] In the scheme of education devised by Buchanan in later years for the University of St. Andrews, Linacre's *De emendata structura* is prescribed for the use of the third class; at a more elementary level, the grammar recommended by Buchanan is one of Lily's.[2]

4. Linacre abbreviates too much. Here, and in the point which follows, we may justly accuse him of a certain lack either of experience of boys, or of imagination in the matter of entering into their minds, or indeed of both together.

5. He is too terse—considering, again, the needs of mere children —in introducing and discussing new material. By contrast, a writer has spoken correctly enough of the 'diffuse, elementary language' of Lily's *Rudiments*.[3]

To sum up. It has been claimed that Linacre's *Rudimenta* possesses considerable importance inasmuch as it was one of the earliest Latin grammars written in English. The claim might be amply justified if the book had been widely used, or officially adopted, in its country of origin; but we have already seen that this was not so. The merits that this short work owned in the eyes of a contem-

---

[1] Whereas in 'Lily' a phrase meaning 'he is ten years old' is quoted in illustration of a certain point of usage. This may be considered as traditional among grammarians; but it has none the less a certain degree of significance.

[2] See D. A. Millar (ed.), *George Buchanan: A Memorial 1506–1906*, St. Andrews, [1907], p. 414. Buchanan presented a copy of the 1540 edition (heavily annotated; it has been suggested that the annotations may be in his own hand) of his translation into Latin of Linacre's *Rudimenta* to St. Andrews University (ibid., p. 409).

[3] See Vincent J. Flynn, 'The Grammatical Writings of William Lily, ? 1468–? 1523', *Papers of the Bibliographical Society of America*, xxxvii, 1943, 95.

porary are quite clearly set out in the letter by Buchanan which I have earlier translated; those merits were (it might be broadly said) recognized only when Buchanan's own Latin translation appeared in France. Its faults, including faults of omission, are tactfully alluded to by Juan-Luis Vives, the great educational theorist, in his short treatise on the method of teaching Latin grammar, where some attempt is made to supply its deficiencies.[1] As for the six books of the *De emendata structura*, written in Latin, on which Linacre toiled so manfully and so long that he achieved thereby the double immortality of an anonymous—but identifiable—description in Erasmus' *Praise of Folly* and (much later) the protagonist's role in Robert Browning's 'Grammarian's Funeral': their scholarly virtues were such as to arouse the admiration of Melanchthon, who at the same time regretted, as a practical teacher, the excessive zeal for completeness that put them out of the range of most boys' minds. In the long run it was more than anything else the strings of apt illustrations from the classics themselves, coupled with an over-developed taste for brevity in expression, that condemned Linacre's work to be found unacceptable in the junior classroom. His best and most elaborate grammar-book was, one might almost say, composed —though he himself was perhaps hardly conscious of the fact—not so much for the children's sake directly, as *in usum grammaticorum*. Its use in the *Brevissima Institutio*—the latter part of 'Lily's grammar' —which has been amply demonstrated by C. G. Allen,[2] may here be cited. In this scholarly category, its freshness and its relative independence (for all that it still keeps close to Priscian's language and order in many places) broke new ground, and helped to establish a new era. Had it made all the sacrifices that regard for the needs of youth tends to exact from the teacher in the classroom, it could not well have done so.

The *De emendata structura Latini sermonis libri sex* is a 'much more elaborate work', as the editor of the correspondence of Erasmus rightly remarked, than the *Progymnasmata* or *Rudimenta*.[3] The *De emendata structura*, written in Latin, is the work referred to by Erasmus as 'Linacre's Syntax';[4] it is undoubtedly the principal

[1] Letter to Katherine of Aragon, dated 7 October 1523 (prefatory to *De ratione studii puerilis*), in George Buchanan, *Opera omnia*, 2 vols., Edinburgh, 1715, ii, *Rudimenta Grammatices*, etc., p. 28.

[2] 'The Sources of "Lily's Latin Grammar": a Review of the Facts and some Further Suggestions', *The Library*, 5th Series, ix, 1954, 85–100.

[3] Allen, i, Ep. 227, p. 467 n. 6.   [4] Ibid., vii, Ep. 1867, p. 153.

source of Linacre's fame as a grammarian. It belongs to the tradition of Lorenzo Valla's *Elegantiae*: its aim is to purify the student's style by directing him to the practice of the great classical Latin writers, both in prose and in verse. Yet despite Linacre's assertion that he writes for learners, the level of treatment is extremely adult, philosophical, 'scientific' (that is, classificatory), and critical, and quite unsuited to the needs of the youthful adolescent, eager for laws and rules. For example, contradictory opinions are quoted, without being in all cases resolved, from the ancient grammarians—Priscian, Diomedes, Servius—and from modern authorities such as Valla. Linacre indeed assumes that the student for whom he writes is able to consult the works of Festus, Nonius, Donatus, and Servius; for he says that he need not discuss the topic of archaism, since it has been diligently investigated by these grammarians. He also assumes —even outside the section specifically devoted to 'Hellenism'—a degree of familiarity with Greek which was extremely rare in his day, making frequent use of Greek technical terminology and invoking the opinions expressed in Theodore of Gaza's Greek grammar. In other words, the *De emendata structura* reveals, for all its weight of learning, something of the same weakness as the *Rudimenta*: namely a certain want of imagination, at least from the pedagogical point of view. It is further vitiated by carelessness, though not—on the evidence of surviving copies at any rate—as badly as the earlier work; for example, the Virgilian phrase *ibant obscuri* is attributed to the second, instead of the sixth, book of the *Aeneid*. Misprints are fewer than in the *Rudimenta*, but they are not absent; Servius appears as 'Sergius', to take only one example. On the whole, therefore, the doubts of the practical educator Melanchthon[1] (to be echoed later by Milton)[2] about the value of the *De emendata structura* for the instruction of the not wholly mature student appear to be iustified. It may be admitted to be the work of a truly learned man;

---

[1] See the introduction to the 1531 edition of Linacre's *De emendata structura*.

[2] See J. M[ilton], *Accedence commenc't Grammar . . .*, London, 1669, sig. A2ᵛ: 'What will not come under Rule, by reason of too much variety in Declension, Gender, or Construction, is also here omitted, least the course and clearness of method be clog'd with Catalogues instead of Rules, or too much interruption between Rule and Rule: Which *Linaker* setting down the various Idiomes of many verbs, was forc'd to do by Alphabet; and therefore, though very learned, not fit to be read in Schools'. (Facsimile in the series English Linguistics 1500–1800, edited by R. C. Alston, No. 271, Scolar Press, Menston, Yorks, 1971.)

but of one who must be regarded as an antiquarian in the field of language, rather than as a teacher of language. At the same time there is, as Buchanan and others observed, a great quantity of knowledge to be acquired from the study of its six books; even a Latinist of the present day will benefit by browsing through them, especially perhaps the final book. Accordingly a very brief summary of the contents of each book separately may be worth while.

The first book has to do with the traditional 'eight parts' of speech (four of them subject to inflexion, namely nouns—including adjectives—pronouns, verbs, and participles; four of them 'indeclinable', namely prepositions, adverbs, interjections, and conjunctions). In each case a definition is given (with the addition of alternative definitions, where these have been proposed) and the different kinds are named, described, and illustrated by examples. Where there is a debate among grammarians about the appropriate terminology, as for example over *agnomen* and *cognomen*, it is reported in some detail. Of course it is not the author's concern here to inform the student concerning the accidence of nouns, verbs, and so forth: this belongs to the *Rudimenta*.[1]

The second book, on *enallage*, or the substitution of one part of speech for another, is interesting and illuminating, even today. However much one may sometimes be inclined to quarrel with Linacre's basis of classification, his attempt to apply it comprehensively heightens the reader's alertness to the way in which Roman writers exploited and manipulated the resources of their language. The third book begins by saying that it proposes to treat of *emendata structura*, 'which is also called *constructio*', as applied in the relationships among the various parts of speech—a concept to

---

[1] Linacre may have been prompted to undertake a more elaborate, as well as a briefer, work in this field by the example set by Donatus, who 'had composed two short grammatical treatises: the *Ars Minor*, for beginners, and the *Ars Maior*, for students further advanced' (Flynn, op. cit., p. 89). In allusion to the *De emendata structura*, we have already observed that Buchanan, who may perhaps be taken as representing the opinion of his day, used this kind of terminology—*opus maius*. Niccolò Perotti's *Rudimenta Grammatices* had tried to reach both audiences at the same time: 'Is enim libellus huius generis est, ut non modo iis qui circa prima elementa adhuc immorantur, sed ad altiora quoque tendentibus prodesse possit' (Prefatory letter by Calphurnius to the 1488 edition of Perotti; quoted by R. P. Oliver, introduction to *Niccolò Perotti's Version of the Enchiridion of Epictetus* [Urbana, University of Illinois Press, 1954]), p. 11 n. 45.

which the nearest modern equivalent is perhaps one part of the meaning of the German word *Stilistik*. The book thereupon takes for its particular topic the relationship of nouns to pronouns; here the material is grouped under pronouns, which are cited in the margins for easier reference but not arranged overall in alphabetical order.

Book four similarly treats of verbs and participles: for this purpose, verbs are divided into active, passive, and 'neuter', and a list of case-usages is provided. In fact the book goes far beyond the relationship of verb and participle, and is a valuable guide to the usages of particular verbs; much of the material assembled here properly belongs to a stylistic lexicon, rather than to a grammar-book. In the penultimate book the 'indeclinable' parts of speech are considered and illustrated in the same way.

The last book, *de constructionis figuris*, is perhaps the most valuable of them all. It gives an account of the familiar figures and resources of style, backed by quotations from the classics. Not all of Linacre's categories are accepted today; for example, what we now call the *constructio ad sensum* is treated as a variety of *syllepsis*; but the view is always balanced and commonsensical, the number of authorities who are cited is seldom inadequate, and respect grows with the reading. All the same it must be admitted that for all his virtues— memory, judgement, comprehensiveness—Linacre never quite emerges as a professional performer in this field, even if we try to evaluate him by the standards of his own day. For all its lexical bias his book does not give us quite enough information to serve as a dictionary, while it does not prune its matter enough, or eschew controversy with enough firmness, to be a useful guide to the young learner; and lastly it is not organized with the degree of attention to system and planning which, even in that century, tended to mark those books that were designed—in our modern phrase—for 'ready reference'. It must surely be described as a work of love and learning to which the *horae subsecivae* or leisure hours of a medical practitioner were devoted. In its method, so well suited to the classificatory intelligence of its author, it bears something of the stamp of the medical case-book. This kind of mind, and the style of exposition that accords with it, has of course a long and honourable history which may be traced back at least to Aristotle and his pupil Theophrastus. The 'inventory style' (to borrow a phrase from a recent writer)[1] descended to the great naturalists of the nineteenth

---

[1] See *The Times Literary Supplement*, 22 June 1973, p. 710.

century and later; its voice is that of the perennial man of science, albeit the matter in hand may, as here, be of a linguistic and literary kind. It may be claimed, perhaps, that this is what gives Linacre's *opus maius* its unique quality.

Thomas Linacre and Italy

THE PRESENT PAPER BRINGS TOGETHER THE ESSEN-
tial facts concerning Thomas Linacre's connections with Italy. Most
of it will deal with the twelve-year period (1487–99) which he spent
in Florence, Rome, Padua, and Venice. It will be seen that the
amount of information concerning this period is distressingly small,
and his movements on the peninsula cannot be traced in anything
approaching a narrative fashion. The best course is therefore to rely
on well-substantiated information, while eliminating the fanciful
and false reconstructions which have plagued many earlier accounts.[1]
Since the properly documented facts are so few and the gaps in our
knowledge so many, I have taken the occasion from time to time to
supplement the known facts about Linacre with a certain amount
of background material and with various details regarding the men
with whom he came into contact while in Italy. Even though most
of this is well known to specialists in various fields, much of the
information has normally not been specifically connected with
Linacre's name.

It is particularly with regard to Linacre's stay at the University
of Padua that I have attempted to supply a large amount of information which has previously not been easily available. While the
emphasis on the Paduan years is to some extent arbitrary, Linacre's
significance in the later history of medicine in England made it
particularly useful to illuminate his Padua education. Moreover,

---

* Warburg Institute, University of London.
[1] This is not the place to list all the bad literature on Linacre, but it might
be mentioned that one of the most unreliable of all writings on him is one
of the most relied on, viz. the account by J. F. Payne in *Dictionary of National
Biography*, xi. 1145–50. I shall indicate my disagreement with other publica-
ions on Linacre as the occasion arises.

earlier writings on Linacre have been unduly vague on this question. I have not attempted to give a comprehensive account of the University, but some light will be shed on the intellectual atmosphere there at the close of the fifteenth century. To go further at this stage would be somewhat unwise, for the basic materials for a more detailed and more accurate account of that institution are only now being published and within a few years we should be able to understand the situation far better.[1]

I. *Linacre in Florence*

According to a tradition which goes back to at least the sixteenth century, Linacre went to Italy with William Sellyng (*c*. 1448–94), Prior of Christ Church, Canterbury.[2] In the absence of conflicting evidence it seems safest to accept this as the occasion for Linacre's initial visit to Italy. Sellyng arrived in Rome on 8 May 1487 charged with a diplomatic mission to Pope Innocent VIII on behalf of Henry VII.[3] If Linacre travelled with Sellyng, it is difficult to know in what capacity. In any case, Linacre's stay in Rome was relatively short and all trace of it seems to have been lost. According to William Latimer, who should have been in a position to know—though memory is fallible—William Grocyn studied with Demetrios Chalcondylas and Angelo Poliziano for two years and Linacre studied with them 'the same number of years or even longer' (*totidem aut etiam plures annos*).[4] Since we know that Linacre had left Florence for Rome at the end of summer, 1490, and that he was in all probability

[1] See below, p. 43 n. 1.

[2] The first specifically to tie Linacre with Sellyng seems to have been John Leland, *Commentarii de scriptoribus Britannicis*, ed. A. Hall, Oxford, 1709, p. 483. This connection has been repeated by most later writers on Linacre. See especially A. B. Emden, *Bibliographical Register of the University of Oxford to A.D. 1500*, Oxford, 1957–9, iii. 1666–7. Leland's work dates from about 1540.

[3] On this see U. Balzani, 'Un'ambasciata inglese a Roma', *Archivio della Società Romana di Storia Patria*, iii, 1880, 175–211; W. F. Schirmer, *Der englische Frühhumanismus*, Leipzig, 1931; reprinted Tübingen, 1963, pp. 154–62; R. Weiss, *Humanism in England during the Fifteenth Century* (3rd edn.), Oxford, 1967, pp. 153–9. Thus the date of Sellyng's arrival seems to be firmly established as 1487, though much literature on Linacre and Sellyng (e.g. P. S. Allen, 'Linacre and Latimer in Italy', *English Historical Review*, xviii, 1903, 514) gives the date as 1485 or 1486.

[4] *Opus Epistolarum Des. Erasmi Roterodami*, ed. P. S. Allen, 12 vols., Oxford, 1906–58, ii. 441–2. The letter written to Erasmus is from Oxford and is dated 30 January 1517.

present at Poliziano's lessons on Pliny earlier that year, it would seem reasonable to believe that he had arrived in Florence in 1487 or 1488 at the latest.[1] It is perhaps possible that he merely travelled in Sellyng's company to pursue advanced studies, especially in Greek, at Florence and had no direct connection with the diplomatic mission.

Poliziano taught Greek and Latin eloquence at the Studio Fiorentino for the fourteen-year period between his return to the Medici capital in 1480 and his death. While we do not have much detailed information on his teaching activity during these years, his lecture topics are known.[2] After his early vernacular lyric poetry, Poliziano turned increasingly to more scholarly pursuits. His first teaching (1480–5) focused primarily upon works of rhetoric and Latin poetry. He then spent a number of years expounding Homer (1485–90), before turning to the more philosophical interests which marked the closing years of his life. Linacre, along with Grocyn, who was studying with Poliziano during the years 1487–91,[3] was in all probability present at some of the lectures on the *Iliad* and *Odyssey*, as well as at the lectures on the *Historia naturalis* of Pliny given in 1490.[4] Poliziano himself, while not mentioning Grocyn and Linacre by name, referred to the fact that he taught Pliny to several British students present for seven months during 1490.[5] During the initial years of

[1] Linacre's presence in Florence as a student in 1489 is clearly attested to by the will of John Morer, dated 16 November 1489, which reads in part: 'Item lego domino Thome Lynaker studenti Fflorence . . .' This is quoted in J. W. Bennett, 'John Morer's Will: Thomas Linacre and Prior Sellyng's Greek Teaching', *Studies in the Renaissance*, xv, 1968, 70–91 (see esp. p. 90), which contains other useful information on Linacre and his contemporaries.

[2] Angelo Poliziano, *Le Selve e la Strega. Prolusioni nello Studio Fiorentino (1482–1492)*, ed. I. del Lungo, Florence, 1925, esp. pp. 232–41, where del Lungo's article 'Angelo Poliziano, il "greco" dello Studio Fiorentino' is reprinted. This briefly outlines Poliziano's teaching activities in the *Studio*. New information is contained in V. Branca, 'Il Poliziano nello Studio Fiorentino, nuove notizie e nuovi dati', *Humanisme actif. Mélanges d'art et de littérature offerts à Julien Cain*, Paris, 1968, ii. 181–6. Now see also A. F. Verde, *Lo Studio fiorentino, 1473–1503: ricerche e documenti*, i–ii, Florence, 1973, i. 26–9, which collects information on Poliziano's connection with the *Studio Fiorentino* and provides additional bibliography on the subject.

[3] M. Burrows, 'Memoir of William Grocyn', in *Collectanea*, ii, Oxford Historical Society xvi, 1890, p. 346.

[4] Del Lungo (p. 38 n. 2), pp. 236–8.

[5] This is clear from Poliziano's annotations to a copy of C. *Plinii Secundi Historia naturalis*, Rome, 1473; H 13,090, now in the Bodleian Library (shelf-

his Florentine stay, Linacre was a fellow student in Poliziano's class-room with Giovanni de' Medici (1475–1521), the future Pope Leo X, to whom Linacre was later to dedicate a translation of Galen.[1] Of Linacre's period of study with Chalcondylas we know even less. Early reliable witnesses[2] agree that the young Englishman studied with the eminent Greek scholar while in Florence, but all details of the association seem to have vanished. In any case it seems clear that Thomas Linacre's mastery of the Greek language dates from his study with Poliziano and Chalcondylas, who rank among the most distinguished Hellenists of the late Quattrocento. It was during his years in Florence that Linacre gained the complete control of Greek which was later attested to, not only by the unreserved praise of Erasmus and others of high philological standards, but also by the excellence of his translations of Galen.[3] Whatever Greek he might have had when he left England for Italy[4] was perfected in his stay in that seed-bed of learning in the classical languages.

II. *Linacre in Rome*

The precise date of Linacre's move from Florence to Rome is indeterminable. We do, however, have two firm dates connected

mark Inc. Auct. Q.1.2). The relevant text is printed in J. M. S. Cotton, 'Ex libris Politiani II. Incunabula Bodleiana', *Modern Language Review*, xxxii, 1937, 394–9 (with a discussion of its significance), and in I. Maïer, *Les manuscrits d'Ange Politien*, Geneva, 1965, pp. 351–2.

[1] Linacre recalls his former association with Leo in his dedication letter to Galen, *De temperamentis* . . ., Cambridge, 1521; reprint with introduction by J. F. Payne, Cambridge, 1881. The letter is also printed in J. N. Johnson, *The Life of Thomas Linacre*, ed. R. Graves, London, 1835, pp. 324–5. For Poliziano's relation to Giovanni de' Medici see G. B. Picotti, *La giovinezza di Leone X*, Milan, 1928. Some scholars may have overestimated the amount of contact between Linacre and the future Pontiff. The latter was Poliziano's pupil for only a few months (Picotti, pp. 10–11) and then went from Florence to Pisa, where he had begun university studies by November 1489 (ibid., pp. 238–9).

[2] These include Aldus Manutius (in the prefatory letter to Marcus Musurus printed in *Statii Sylvarum libri quinque*, Venice, 1502, sig. aiv–aiir) and William Latimer (in his letter to Erasmus, dated 30 January 1517, in Allen, ii. 441–2). For information on Chalcondylas's teaching at Florence see Verde, op. cit. ii. 178–9.

[3] For Linacre's translations of Galen, see R. J. Durling, 'Linacre and Medical Humanism', below, pp. 76–106.

[4] See C. H. Clough, 'Thomas Linacre, Cornelio Vitelli, and Humanistic Studies at Oxford', above, pp. 1–23.

with his stay in Rome, the first of which is probably fairly close to his time of arrival. On 4 November 1490[1] Thomas Linacre was admitted to the English Hospice of Saint Thomas of Canterbury in Rome and on 3 May 1491[2] he was named a *custos* of that institution. Presumably Linacre maintained an association with the Hospice as long as he remained in Rome,[3] for it would supply his practical needs and provide him with the intellectual companionship which life in a foreign country necessitated. The Hospice of Saint Thomas[4] has been a centre for visiting Englishmen in Rome from the date of its foundation in 1362 until the twentieth century, and those listed on its registers during the years immediately after Linacre's arrival include William Lily (who entered the same day as did Linacre), Cardinal Bainbridge, John Colet, William Latimer, Richard Pace, Cardinal Pole, and John Fisher.[5] Other than his clear connection with the Hospice, we know very little indeed about Linacre's stay in Rome, which must have lasted for two or three years. There is, it is true, an anecdote going back to the sixteenth century, which asserts a connection with the distinguished Venetian humanist Ermolao Barbaro (1453–93), who was in Rome at the time, but the

[1] Rome, Venerabile Collegio Inglese, MS. 17, fol. 18ᵛ. This document is clearly dated 4 November 1490, as verified from a photostat of the manuscript. I am grateful to Mr. Kevin McGinnell, the Archivist of the Collegio Inglese, for supplying photostats. The correct date of Linacre's admission to the Hospice is given by V. J. Flynn, 'Englishmen in Rome during the Renaissance', *Modern Philology*, xxxvi, 1938, 137. Two other publications, which claim to be based on an examination of MS. 17, are mistaken as to the precise date. G. B. Parks, *The English Traveler to Italy*, i, *The Middle Ages (to 1525)*, Rome, 1954, pp. 362, 457, gives 'November 1489' as the date. B. Newns, 'The Hospice of St. Thomas and the English Crown, 1474–1538', *The Venerabile* [Sexcentenary Issue: *The English Hospice in Rome*, Exeter, 1962], xxi, 1962, 190, gives the date as 3 May 1490. It is important to establish a clear date *ante quem non* for Linacre's arrival in Rome, for this increases the probability of his being present at Florence for Poliziano's lectures on Pliny earlier in the year. Cf. the publications of Cotton and Maïer cited above, p. 38 n. 5.

[2] MS. cit., fol. 19ʳ. Flynn (p. 137), Parks (p. 457), and *The Venerabile* (p. 267), all cited in the previous note, give 1491 for the date, only Parks specifying it to be May.

[3] There is no evidence for Linacre's reception into the Hospice before 1490, which further supports the hypothesis that he did not reach Rome with Sellyng.

[4] For further information see especially the publications listed above, p. 40 n. 1.

[5] see e.g. the list in Parks, op. cit., pp. 374–6.

story has no firm foundation.[1] We have no contemporary evidence whatever that Linacre ever met Barbaro, let alone entered into an extended and fruitful friendship with him as various later historians suggest. The alleged encounter between them, said to have taken place in the Vatican Library, suggests that Linacre may have frequented that institution, which was already in 1490 an important centre for scholarly study and at the time was directed by another Venetian humanist, Giovanni Lorenzi.[2] An extant register of books borrowed from the Vatican indicates that Barbaro did sign out for a number of books during the period June 1490 to May 1491.[3] What the register fails to reveal is any entry under Linacre's name, though

[1] It seems to originate with Paolo Giovio (1483–1552): 'Inde vero multis variae doctrinae ornamentis adauctus [sc. Linacre], quum Romana quoque ingenia certius agnoscenda, ac opulentiores bibliothecas inspiciendas existimaret, ad Urbem contendit. In primo autem appulsu forte accidit, ut Hermolao Barbaro amicitia iungeretur. Nam ingresso Vaticanam Bibliothecam & Graecos codices evoluenti, supervenit Hermolaus, ad pluteumque humaniter accedens. "Non tu hercle", inquit, "studiose hospes, uti ego plane sum, Barbarus, esse potes, quod lectissimum Platonis librum (is erat Phaedrus) diligenter evoluas." At id Linacrus laeto ore respondit, "Nec tu, sacrate heros, alius esse iam potes, quam ille fama notus Patriarcha Italorum Latinissimus." Ab hac amicitia (uti casu evenit, feliciter conflata) egregiis demum voluminibus ditatus in Britanniam rediit.' *Pauli Jovii* . . . *Elogia virorum literis illustrium* . . ., Basle, 1577, p. 119. This is repeated by George Lily in *Descriptio Britanniae, Scotiae, Hyberniae, et Orchadum ex libro Pauli Jovii* . . ., Venice, 1548, fol. 49ʳ. There is no evidence for the connection of Linacre with Barbaro other than Giovio's statement. Giovio himself came to Rome about 1514 and could not himself have been a witness to a meeting of Barbaro and Linacre. I have been unable to discover anything in Barbaro's writings or in the secondary literature about him to suggest a meeting. Barbaro was in Rome while Linacre was there, though he died in 1493 (probably in July). For further information and bibliography see the article by E. Bigi in *Dizionario biografico degli italiani*, vi, 1964, 96–9. The unreliable book by A. Ferriguto, *Almorò Barbaro* . . ., Venice, 1919, pp. 375–6, claims a connection between Linacre and Barbaro, but cites only Giovio as evidence.

[2] On Lorenzi as Papal Librarian see esp. P. de Nolhac, 'Giovanni Lorenzi, bibliothécaire d'Innocent VIII', *Mélanges d'archéologie et d'histoire*, viii, 1888, 3–18; P. Paschini, 'Un ellenista veneziano del Quattrocento: Giovanni Lorenzi', *Archivio veneto*, 5th ser., xxxii–xxxiii, 1943, 114–46. For further information and bibliography on Lorenzi see my forthcoming 'An Unstudied Fifteenth-Century Latin Translation of Sextus Empiricus by Giovanni Lorenzi (Vat. Lat. 2990)', *Cultural Aspects of the Italian Renaissance: Essays in Honour of P. O. Kristeller*, ed. C. H. Clough, Manchester, 1975, pp. 244–61.

[3] M. Bertòla (ed.), *I Due Primi Registri di prestito della Biblioteca Apostolica Vaticana*, Vatican City, 1942, pp. 50, 51, 76, 77, 114.

this cannot be taken to mean that he did not frequent the Vatican Library. Linacre may well have had all sorts of encounters and important relationships while in Rome, but so far firm evidence for them is singularly lacking. He may well have benefited enormously from the intellectual circle of the Papal Court of Innocent VIII, and have studied with the noted Pomponio Leto, as some suggest, but as yet we possess no documents to compel belief in such things.

III. *Linacre in Padua*

The precise date of Linacre's arrival in Padua to begin his medical studies is not clear and, indeed, no specific information whatever has come to light thus far to fix precisely the years he spent there as a student. We do have evidence that he took his degree in medicine at the end of summer, 1496,[1] but the bare documents which indicate this fact, along with the later statements of several contemporaries who mention that he studied at Padua,[2] seem to be all we have to connect him with that famous university city. While Linacre maintained contacts with quite a number of Italians, long after he had left the peninsula forever, few if any of these lasting friendships seem to derive from his years as a student at Padua. The precise details of his studies, his friendships, his associations with fellow students, his intellectual development while pursuing the medical art seem to be irretrievably lost to us.

However, one can offer at least a brief, impressionistic picture of the intellectual life in the university during Linacre's stay, and give an indication of the sort of learning he imbibed there. What is needed, of course, is a full-scale study of the instruction in medicine —and indeed, in the arts subjects in general—at *dotta Padova* during the late fifteenth and early sixteenth centuries, when so many changes and new developments were taking place there, establishing the foundation for the world-famous medical school which was to train William Harvey a century later. I propose to sketch in some information concerning the Faculty of Arts—and of other faculties as well, where relevant—during the 1490s and try to relate this to Linacre where possible.

[1] R. J. Mitchell, 'Thomas Linacre in Italy', *English Historical Review*, l, 1935, 696–8.

[2] The best witness is perhaps Richard Pace (1483–1536), who studied at Padua just after Linacre. See his *De fructu qui ex doctrina percipiatur* (first edn. 1517), ed. F. Manley and R. S. Silvester, New York, 1967, pp. 96–7 and *passim*.

Before coming to Padua,[1] Linacre certainly was much better prepared, as well as being significantly older—he was over 30—than
most of his fellow students. Though the level of the education he
had received at Canterbury and Oxford was, one suspects, significantly lower than he might have attained in Italy at the same time,
it was nevertheless sufficient to obtain for him an All Souls fellowship in 1484.[2] The fact that he had studied with Poliziano and
Chalcondylas for several years at Florence, as well as the esteem in
which he was held by men of severe standards such as Aldus Manutius and Erasmus,[3] amply indicate that his preparation in Greek
upon reaching Padua was of an unusually high level. Indeed one
might wonder why he decided to undertake medical studies at such
an advanced age, though it was not unusual for older students to
seek a degree, and we have more than one instance of university
teachers taking degrees quite late in their careers when their reputa-

[1] For Linacre and Padua we must still rely, to a large degree, upon such
older works as G. F. Tomasini, *Gymnasium Patavinum*, Udine, 1654; A. Ricco-
boni, *De Gymnasio Patavino*, Padua, 1598; and I. Facciolati, *Fasti Gymnasii
Patavii*, Padua, 1757. Also useful but outdated is F. M. Colle, *Storia scientifico-
letteraria dello Studio di Padova*, 4 vols., Padua, 1824–5. For a bibliography of
writings on the history of the university see A. Favaro, *Saggio di bibliografia
dello Studio di Padova*, 2 vols., Venice, 1922, which is being supplemented and
brought up to date periodically by the *Quaderni per la storia dell'Università di
Padova*, 1968– . Though a list of graduates from 1406 onwards based on all
known extant records was begun in 1922 with C. Zonta and I. Brotto (eds.),
*Acta gradum academicorum Gymnasii Patavini ab anno MCCCCVI ad annum
MCCCCL*, Padua, 1922, the work was resumed only in 1969 with E. Martel-
lozzo Forin (ed.), *Acta graduum academicorum ab anno 1501 ad annum 1525*,
Padua, 1969. The publication of the volumes of this series dealing with the
period after 1501 is continuing, but the section for the years 1451–1500 (when
Linacre was a student) has not yet appeared. Gloria published the lists of
professors (*rotuli*) for the period before 1405, but there is as yet no publication
concerning the later period. B. Bertolaso, 'Ricerche d'archivio su alcuni
aspetti dell'insegnamento medico presso l'Università di Padova nel Cinque-
e Seicento', *Acta medicae historiae patavina*, vi, 1959–60, 17–18, claims that
51 per cent of the fifteenth-century *rotuli* are lost.

[2] Emden, ii. 1147. In the present volume, Clough, op. cit., and J. M.
Fletcher, 'Linacre's Lands and Lectureships', below pp. 107–97, give further
information on education at Oxford.

[3] Aldus seems to have taken him into his circle rather early, not only
praising him in the prefatory letter to the famous *editio princeps* of Aristotle
(1495–8) but also printing Linacre's translation of (pseudo-)Proclus' *Sphaera*.
See below (pp. 74–5) for further information on the attitude of Aldus and
Erasmus towards Linacre.

tions were already well established.[1] The decision must have come relatively late, for he had already spent at least five years in Italy before he left Rome for his Paduan studies. Though Padua could perhaps teach him little as far as Greek and classical literature were concerned, it must have held forth a desirable prize in the form of a more traditional sort of medical learning. Benedetti's teaching of anatomy, Bagellardo's work on children's diseases, and, indeed, the normal curriculum of theoretical and practical medicine being taught by dell'Aquila, Zerbi, and others may have appealed to him and must have been new to his experience, which from all indications had previously been largely confined to the study of classical texts.[2] It was at this time that Padua was beginning to achieve the position of eminence in medical and scientific studies which it was to hold until the middle of the seventeenth century through the attainments of teachers such as Pomponazzi, Vesalius, Falloppia, Zabarella, Barozzi, Galileo, Fabricius, Cremonini, Rhode, and Liceto. The strong orientation towards medical studies at Padua in Linacre's time stood in bold contrast to northern universities such as Paris and Oxford—where even a moderate level of prestige in this field would not be attained until later—institutions at which theology of a traditional scholastic variety held sway and little attention was being devoted to more empirical studies. This is not to say that theology was absent from Italian universities. Indeed, one must not fall into the trap, as has a whole historiographical tradition, of over-emphasizing the lay and secular aspects of Padua. Theology was indeed being taught at the *Studio* in Linacre's time and, as we shall see, it was not weak, nor was it subjugated to a radical 'naturalism' as has sometimes been supposed. The teaching of theology goes back to 1363[3]—not to the founding of the univer-

[1] Several instances from the Padua of Linacre's time can be cited. Lorenzo da Molino (Amolinus, Amolendinus) took a degree *in artibus* some years after he had begun lecturing in logic. See B. Nardi, *Studi su Pietro Pomponazzi*, Florence, 1965, p. 62 (hereafter cited as *Pietro Pomponazzi*). Nicoleto Vernia, who was named *ordinarius* in natural philosophy in 1468, and was one of the mainstays of the teaching staff by the time Linacre appeared on the scene, took a medical degree in 1496, the same year as did Linacre. See B. Nardi, *Saggi sull'aristotelismo padovano dal secolo XIV al XVI*, Florence, 1958, pp. 98–9 (hereafter cited as *Aristotelismo padovano*).

[2] Information on Linacre's life before he went to Padua—though slight—shows no evidence whatsoever that he had then any interest in medical studies.

[3] The Papal Bull of Urban V for founding a faculty of theology is printed in A. Gloria, *Monumenti della Università di Padova (1318–1405)*, p. 55. For

sity in 1222, it is true—and it seems to have been quite flourishing by the last decade of the fifteenth century.

Linacre came to Northern Italy some time after 1491; there is no evidence of his activities between the time of his election to a wardenship in the English Hospice at Rome in May, 1491, and his graduation at Padua in August, 1496. It is possible that during the interval he returned to England, since his name appears in the Bursar's Book of All Souls College for 1495.[1] The evidence for a return to England is very shaky, however, and it seems more probable that his stay in Italy was continuous and that he moved to Padua some time about 1492 or 1493. Such a supposition would allow him adequate time to pursue medical studies and to procure a degree by 1496. Though the normal Italian *laurea* required four

further details on theological studies at Padua see G. Brotto and G. Zonta, *La facoltà teologica dell' Università di Padova. Parte I (secoli XIV e XV)*, Padua, 1922; the papers contained in *Problemi e figure della Scuola Scotista del Santo*, Pubblicazioni della Provincia Patavina dei Frati Minori Conventuali, 5, Padua, 1966; A. Poppi, 'Per una storia della cultura nel Convento del Santo dal XIII al XIX secolo', *Quaderni per la storia dell' Università di Padova*, iii, 1970, 1–29; and L. Gargan, *Lo studio teologico e la biblioteca dei domenicani a Padova nel Tre e Quattrocento*, Padua, 1971.

[1] Oxford, MS. All Souls College b. 29 (Bursars' Books, 1450–1520). The Book for 1495, which is a weekly list of battels for each member of the College, names Linacre throughout the year. Though the debts of each member of the College are listed week by week, there is no entry for debt after Linacre's name at any time during the year. The same is the case with several other members of the College, including William Latimer. I think that this information is to be interpreted to mean that Linacre, Latimer, and several other members of the College were retained on the books during the year 1495, even though they were not in residence and hence incurred no debts throughout the year. Emden, ii. 1147, has the year of this Bursar's Book as 1493, but he gives 1495 in his article on Latimer (ii. 1106). There is no extant Bursar's Book for 1493. The case for Linacre's return to Oxford during his years in Italy has been made by various scholars including Allen, 'Linacre and Latimer'; Emden is ambiguous on the point. The passage of Thomas Stapleton's life of More (*Tres Thomae*, Cologne, 1612), p. 155, referred to by Allen (p. 514), which asserts that More learned Greek from Linacre at Oxford, seems to be mistaken. Its author seems to have confused More's Oxford studies with his studying Greek with Linacre in London about 1500. More recalls having read Aristotle's *Meteorology* with Linacre in a letter of 21 October 1515 to Martin Dorp. See *The Correspondence of Sir Thomas More*, ed. E. F. Rogers, Princeton, 1947, p. 65. There is general agreement that this refers to his London period rather than to his Oxford studies; see R. W. Chambers, *Thomas More*, London, 1935, pp. 83–4.

or five years of study, there was then a greater degree of flexibility and the whole degree-granting procedure was less standardized than it later became.

The fifteenth-century statutes of the Faculty of Arts of Padua specifically state that a student could not be admitted to an examination for a degree *in artibus* unless he had studied for five years. For a degree *in medicina* it was necessary to study at least three years, during the course of which the student was required to have heard all of the *lectiones ordinariae*, as well as having practised a year with a well-known doctor.[1] We know, however, that such regulations were not always followed *ad litteram* and that 'graces'—to use the term which became common at Oxford—were often given. Given Linacre's unusual background and his extensive earlier training there is good reason to believe that he might have been granted certain exemptions not given to the ordinary student. Moreover, Linacre's Padua degree was *in medicinis*[2] alone rather than *in artibus et medicina*, as was apparently more common, perhaps indicating that in view of his earlier training it was not necessary for him to go through the normal preliminaries such as logic and philosophy.

Whatever courses of lectures Linacre actually followed at Padua, he lived in the atmosphere of the *Studio* for several years and must have come into contact with a variety of students and professors. Consequently, it should not be out of place to devote some attention to the intellectual life of the University during the years immediately before 1496. One finds, first of all, that there were three separate faculties at Padua: Law, Theology, and Arts. The first of

---

[1] There is a printed edition of the Statutes from about 1496 [H–C 15,015; cf. F. R. Goff, *Incunabula in American Libraries*, New York, 1964, p. 572 (S 720)] which is very rare: *Statuta Dominorum Artistarum Achademiae Patavinae*, Venice, c. 1496 (hereafter cited as *Statuta* (1496)). I have used a microfilm of the Marciana copy (shelfmark 12.c.141) now in the Wellcome Library (microfilm 89). The text seems to be essentially the same as the sections printed from MS. 776 of the Biblioteca Universitaria di Padova in A. Favaro, 'Lo Studio di Padova al tempo di Niccolò Copernico', *Atti del Reale Istituto Veneto di Scienze, Lettere ed Arti*, 5th ser. vi, 1880, 349–56. There is also little difference, at least in the sections with which we are here concerned, between these and the later (and more easily accessible) edition of 1589. The relevant section (fol. 28ᵛ) reads as follows: 'Nullus ad examen liberalium artium admitti possit nisi in artibus per annos 5 studuerit. In medicina vero promovendus studuerit ad minus per annos 3 et lectiones omnes ordinarias audierit, et cum aliquo famoso doctore per annum ad minus practicasse, et infirmos visitasse constet.'

[2] Mitchell (p. 42 n. 1), p. 697.

these, as at most other Italian universities of the period, was by far the most important, both in terms of size and of prestige. This fact should not be lost sight of, even though the attention of many historians has been directed towards arts teaching.[1] Since Linacre himself was enrolled in the arts faculty one must concern oneself primarily with that faculty, though some consideration will also be given to the theology faculty, especially as there was a considerable interchange between arts and theology at Padua during his time.[2]

With regard to the teaching of theology at Padua there was a rather unusual division in the allotment of chairs. Both metaphysics and theology had two chairs each,[3] one *in via Thomae* and the other *in via Scoti*. The Thomist chairs were invariably held by Dominicans and the Scotist chairs by Franciscans. Moreover, the teaching of these subjects was partly carried on in the local convents of the two orders.[4] This tradition, which was unusual, though not unique to Padua,[5] continued for at least two centuries.

During Linacre's time the Thomist chair of theology was held by Gerolamo da Monopoli,[6] and the Scotist chair first by a certain

---

[1] There is an extensive literature on the faculty of law. More foreign students came to Italian universities in the fifteenth century to study law than any other subject. See R. J. Mitchell, 'English Students at Padua, 1460–1475', *Royal Historical Society Transactions*, 4th ser. xix, 1936, 101–17. Of the 18 students listed by Miss Mitchell as taking degrees at Padua in the fifteenth century, 5 were in arts (1 in philosophy and 4 in medicine), 4 in theology, and 9 in law (5 in canon law, 3 in civil law, and 1 in canon and civil law combined). See idem, 'English Law Students at Bologna in the Fifteenth Century', *English Historical Review*, li, 1936, 270–87.

[2] See below for the late fifteenth- and early sixteenth-century discussion of immortality.

[3] This arrangement began in the fifteenth century, first with separate chairs of metaphysics; then in about 1490 separate chairs of theology were added. See esp. Brotto and Zonta (p. 44 n. 3). Facciolati (p. 43 n. 1) has a list of the incumbents of the chairs during this period.

[4] For details see the literature cited above in p. 44 n. 3.

[5] When the University of Alcalá was founded in the early sixteenth century by Cardinal Cisneros, the faculty of theology had chairs not only of Thomism and Scotism, but also of Nominalism. See M. Bataillon, *Érasme et l'Espagne*, Paris, 1937, p. 17.

[6] After taking a degree at Ferrara in 1493, Gerolamo held the Thomist chair at Padua from 1495 until 1502, when he moved to the chair of metaphysics. He later held various administrative posts in the Dominican order and taught metaphysics at Naples before his death in 1528. He wrote several philosophical and theological works including one against the Reformer Huldrych Zwingli, and edited the *editio princeps* of Pseudo-Thomas, *Summa*

Magister Gratia da Brescia (for the years 1490–5)[1] and then by Maurice O'Fihely (Mauritius de Portu, Mauritius Hibernicus, etc.),[2] an Irish Franciscan. The latter, who was a prominent figure in Scotist studies, editing several works of Duns Scotus and of later writers in the same tradition, was one of those present at Linacre's degree examination in 1496. The metaphysics chairs were held by two of the most prominent spokesmen for their respective traditions in the later Middle Ages: the Franciscan Antonio Trombetta[3] and the Dominican Tommaso de Vio.[4] Were we to look deeper into the

totius logicae, Venice, 1496. For further details and bibliography see Gargan (p. 44 n. 3), pp. 154–5.

[1] Little is known about this figure; see Facciolati (p. 43 n. 1), ii. 97; *Problemi e figure* (p. 44 n. 3), pp. 69, 125, 663, 664, 666.

[2] Maurice was born about 1460 in Baltimore or Clonfert, Ireland, and died at Galway, 25 May 1513. After holding minor teaching posts at Milan, Padua, and Siena, he was promoted to the theology chair *in via Scoti* at Padua in 1495. In 1506 he was named Archbishop of Tuam. For further details and bibliography see C. H. Lohr, 'Medieval Latin Aristotle Commentaries, Authors: Johannes de Kanthi—Myngodus', *Traditio*, xxvii, 1971, 344–5, as well as Poppi's paper cited in the next note.

[3] Trombetta (1436–1517) was the outstanding Scotist spokesman at Padua for half a century. He was professor of metaphysics there from 1469 until 1511, moving to the Scotist chair in the *Studio* in 1476. He published various works, including several on metaphysics and the anti-Averroist *Tractatus de humanarum animarum plurificatione*, 1498. See especially A. Poppi, 'Lo scotista patavino Antonio Trombetta (1436–1517)', *Il Santo*, ii, 1962, 349–67, and Lohr in *Traditio*, xxiii, 1967, 366–7.

[4] Tommaso de Vio (Cardinal Caietanus) was born at Gaeta in 1468. He studied at Naples (1484) and Bologna (1488) before coming to Padua in 1491. After several years of study he became *magister* in theology and then held the Thomistic chair of metaphysics from 1494 to 1497. After teaching at Pavia (1497–9) and Rome (1501–8) he moved increasingly into administrative and diplomatic posts, though he continued to write many doctrinal and polemical works in philosophy and theology. He was General of the Dominican Order from 1508 to 1518 and, as such, played an important role in the Fifth Lateran Council (1512–17). In 1517 he was created Cardinal by Leo X and was named bishop of his native Gaeta two years later. He died in Rome in 1534. Of de Vio's numerous philosophical and theological works, of particular importance and influence are his interpretative works on Thomas Aquinas, and he was without doubt one of the most significant continuators of the Thomistic tradition during the Renaissance. While at Padua he wrote a commentary on the *Sentences* of Peter Lombard (MS. Paris, BN lat. 3076) and a commentary on Aquinas's *De ente et essentia* (1st edn., Venice, 1496). For his period at Padua see especially A. Poppi, *Causalità e infinità nella scuola padovana dal 1480 al 1513*, Padua, 1966, pp. 170–85 and *passim*; Gargan (p. 44 n. 3), pp. 156–8 (further

theological and metaphysical disputes taking place at Padua at the time we would see that, far from being the secularized haven for anti-religious sentiment which certain historians have tried to make of it, a high level of interest in theological and religious matters was maintained during the Quattrocento. Not only were some of the leading theologians of the time present at Padua, but the twofold orientation of the faculty allowed fruitful discussions and disputations to take place with full University and communal approval.

The Faculty of Arts was oriented primarily towards the preparation of trained physicians. Though subjects such as moral philosophy, Greek, Latin, and mathematics were taught, the principal emphasis was on medical studies and those topics, such as logic and natural philosophy, which were considered important prerequisites for the study of medicine. The central position of medicine at Padua —and indeed in Italian universities in general—needs to be underlined. Many recent scholars who have worked on the intellectual history of the *Studio* during the late fifteenth and sixteenth centuries have apparently lost sight of this and they deal with the philosophical teaching of the time as though it were primarily a self-contained discipline. Medical training in the Faculty of Arts at Padua—and the situation there does not appear to be very different from that obtaining in other Italian universities at the time—consisted of a sort of two-tier education. Preliminary studies involved work in logic and natural philosophy. After such preparation the student then advanced to the study of medical subjects. The normal procedure was apparently for a student first to take a degree *in artibus* and then, after spending several more years in the study of medical subjects, to take a further degree in medicine.[1] Moreover, the medical degree had, as did lectureships in medical studies, greater prestige attached to it than did an arts degree. The value of a medical degree is perhaps attested by the fact that Nicoleto Vernia sought and obtained one very late in his career, nearly forty years after taking a first degree in philosophy.[2]

As far as teaching in the Faculty of Arts was concerned a common progression was from teaching logic to teaching natural philosophy

bibliography); and A. Maurer, 'Cajetan's Notion of Being in his Commentary on the *Sentences*', *Mediaeval Studies*, 28, 1966, 268–78.

[1] Bruno Nardi cited a number of examples of this; see especially *Saggi sulla cultura veneta del Quattro e Cinquecento*, Padua, 1971, pp. 103–4 (hereafter cited as *Cultura veneta*).   [2] Nardi, *Aristotelismo padovano*, pp. 161–2.

and then finally to medicine, a position which was not only more remunerative than the others, but was also considered to carry with it a higher social status. Consequently, even though modern interpreters have emphasized the importance of logic and methodology in Renaissance curricula, the teaching of these subjects was largely in the hands of beginning teachers who after two or three years passed to more lucrative and prestigious positions.[1] Thus even a Zabarella, whose posthumous fame is largely based on his work in logic, actually taught that subject for only a few years at the beginning of his career.[2] The move from teaching positions in natural philosophy to those in medicine was a relatively common occurrence at Padua during the second half of the fifteenth century. During Linacre's time, for instance, it was made by Paolo Bagellardi, Gerolamo de Polcastris, Pietro Trapolin, and Gabriele Zerbi.[3]

Having made these general points about the Faculty of Arts, one can look more closely at its actual make-up during Linacre's years there. First, it is necessary to examine the status of philosophy at Padua. As already noted, this topic has been far more studied in recent times than has the equivalent area in the history of medicine. As at other universities the curriculum was clearly set out in the statutes. At Padua, as elsewhere in Italy, the basic texts were several writings of Aristotle on logic and natural philosophy. Teachers of logic lectured on the *Posterior Analytics*,[4] presumably lecturing on the same text every year. In natural philosophy[5] the *Physics* (Books 1, 2, and 8), *De generatione et corruptione*, *De anima*, and *De coelo* were read. The teaching of philosophy, as with most other subjects, was generally expected to be an actual 'reading' of the assigned books with commentary and explication. To what extent outside material was introduced into the lectures is difficult to determine, though in certain specific cases, where appropriate manuscript or other sources remain, this can be partly established. In addition to the required teaching, the tone and emphasis of the lectures certainly must have

[1] This was not always the case, however. See below for the case of Lorenzo dal Molino who continued to teach logic for many years.

[2] See W. F. Edwards, 'The Logic of Iacopo Zabarella (1533–1589)' (Columbia University dissertation), 1960, pp. 28–30, from which we learn that Zabarella taught logic only for the period 1563 (or 1564) to 1568 before moving on to the teaching of natural philosophy.

[3] Nardi, *Aristotelismo padovano*, pp. 157–8.

[4] Facciolati (p. 43 n. 1), ii. 113, which cites the appropriate text from the statutes.   [5] Ibid. ii. 100.

been determined by current fashions and tendencies. For example, we know that certain repercussions of the immortality controversy found their way into courses of lectures given by Pomponazzi during his career.[1]

Linacre was at Padua during a crucial period in the development of philosophical thought there, one marked by a number of significant developments as well as numerous internal disputes. Renan, Ragnisco, and Fiorentino, and more recently Randall, Nardi, Kristeller, Gilson, Di Napoli, Poppi, and Mahoney, among others, have done much to illuminate philosophical life at Padua in the closing years of the fifteenth century and the early years of the sixteenth. This was the period during which the immortality controversy, which split the Fifth Lateran Council and forced that august gathering into a much-discussed decision on personal immortality, was taking shape. After the Averroist controversy, which had rocked Paris and Oxford in the thirteenth century and then spread to other centres including Bologna, Pavia, and Padua, had died down, it erupted again at Padua during the closing quarter of the fifteenth century.[2] The refocusing of interest on the psychological problem of individual immortality seems to have been initiated by Nicoleto Vernia (*c.* 1420–99).[3] During the 1480s

[1] In addition to the texts published by Nardi, *Pietro Pomponazzi*, and Poppi (cited below, p. 53 n. 1) see also the other published by F. Fiorentino, *Pietro Pomponazzi. Studi storici sulla scuola bolognese e padovana del secolo XVI con molti documenti inediti*, Florence, 1868; L. Ferri, 'La psicologia di Pietro Pomponazzi secondo un manoscritto inedito dell'Angelica di Roma', *Atti della R. Accademia dei Lincei*, 2nd ser., part iii, 1875–6, 333–548; P. O. Kristeller, 'A New Manuscript Source for Pomponazzi's Theory of the Soul from his Paduan Period', *Revue internationale de philosophie*, xvi, 1951, 144–57; idem, 'Two Unpublished Questions on the Soul of Pietro Pomponazzi', *Medievalia et humanistica*, ix, 1955, 76–101. See also C. Oliva, 'Note sull'insegnamento di Pietro Pomponazzi', *Giornale critico della filosofia italiana*, vii, 1926, 83–103, 179–90, 254–75.

[2] Among recent studies of late fifteenth-century Padua are: G. di Napoli, *L'immortalità dell'anima nel Rinascimento*, Turin, 1963; E. P. Mahoney, 'The Early Psychology of Agostino Nifo' (Columbia University dissertation), 1966; idem, 'Nicoletto Vernia and Agostino Nifo on Alexander of Aphrodisias: an Unnoticed Dispute', *Rivista critica di storia della filosofia*, xxiii, 1968, 268–96; B. Nardi, *Aristotelismo padovano* and *Pietro Pomponazzi*; A. Poppi, 'Lo scotista . . .' (p. 48 n. 3); and idem, 'L'anti-averroismo della scolastica padovana alla fine del secolo XV', *Studia patavina*, xi, 1964, 102–24.

[3] Vernia took a degree in philosophy at Padua in 1458 and, as mentioned above (p. 49), in medicine in 1496. From 1468 until his death he was

Vernia began putting forth ideas in his psychological teaching which were considered to be dangerously tinged with what has been called 'Averroism'. This led to a condemnation by doctrine, if not by name, by Pietro Barozzi, Bishop of Padua, in 1489.[1] This, in turn, provoked a protracted discussion of the problem at Padua and elsewhere. At Padua, during the first few years after Barozzi's condemnation, the discussions involved, in addition to Vernia himself, a number of other lecturers, including Trombetta,[2] Agostino Nifo,[3]

ordinarius of natural philosophy at Padua. He apparently held to the 'one intellect' (Averroistic) interpretation of Aristotelian psychology for many years before rejecting it in a work entitled *Contra perversam Averrois opinionem de unitate intellectus et animae felicitate quaestiones divinae*, completed in 1499, but not published until 1504. A number of other brief works, principally on natural philosophy, also survive. Currently in the press is E. P. Mahoney, *Nicoletto Vernia's Early Treatise on the Intellective Soul: Introduction and Critical Text*, Saggi e Testi, 14, Padua, ?1975. For further information on Vernia see P. Ragnisco, 'Nicoletto Vernia. Studi storici sulla filosofia padovana nella 2ª metà del secolo decimoquinto', *Atti del R. Istituto Veneto di scienze, lettere ed arti*, 7th Ser. ii, 1890–1, 241–66, 617–64; idem, 'Documenti inediti e rari intorno alla vita ed agli scritti di Nicoleto Vernia e di Elia di Medigo', *Atti e memorie della R. Accademia di scienze, lettere ed arti in Padova*, N.S. vii (1890–1), 275–302; Nardi, *Aristotelismo padovano*, esp. pp. 95–126; Mahoney (p. 51 n. 2); C. Vasoli, 'La scienza della natura in Nicoleto Vernia', in his *Studi sulla cultura del Rinascimento*, Manduria, 1968, pp. 241–56, and Verde, ii. 510–11, who also announces (i. 166) that a 'complete' study on Vernia by E. P. Mahoney will soon be published besides the edition of one of Vernia's works by him cited above.

[1] For the text of the decree see Ragnisco, 'Documenti inediti . . .', pp. 278–9. For further information on Barozzi see F. Gaeta, *Il vescovo Pietro Barozzi e il trattato 'De factionibus extinguendis'*, Venice/Rome, 1958, and Mahoney, 'Nicoletto Vernia . . .' (p. 51 n. 2), especially p. 271 n. 11, for a summary of relevant literature.

[2] See above, p. 48 no. 3, for further information.

[3] Nifo (1470–1538), from Sessa Arunca in Southern Italy, took a degree at Padua *c.* 1492, in which year he was named *extraordinarius* in natural philosophy. In 1495 he became *ordinarius in secundo loco* and a year later was promoted to first place. He left Padua in 1499 and spent the remainder of his life teaching in various Italian universities. After leaving Padua, Nifo learned Greek; he marks a transition from the medieval approach to the teaching of Aristotle to the more humanistic and more broadly based sixteenth-century conception. For Nifo and his prolific writings see P. Tuozzi, 'Agostino Nifo e le sue opere', *Atti e memorie della R. Accademia di scienze, lettere ed arti in Padova*, N.S. xx, 1903–4, 63–86; B. Nardi, *Sigieri di Brabante nel pensiero del Rinascimento italiano*, Rome, 1945; idem, *Aristotelismo padovano, passim*; and the following works of E. P. Mahoney, which have additional bibliography:

and Pietro Pomponazzi.[1] This is one of the currents of thought
—the modish philosophical debate—which was still in full swing
when Linacre was a student at Padua. While it is probable that the
mature Englishman was more inclined towards medical studies than
those in natural philosophy or metaphysics, he must have been
aware of the philosophical disputes which played so prominent a
role in university life at the time.

One further aspect of natural philosophy which was being discussed with verve by various thinkers about the time Linacre was
at Padua, involved the question of how celestial bodies are moved.
As Fr. Poppi has shown, much attention was being devoted to this
traditional problem and several related ones by Paduan philosophers
and theologians of various orientations.[2]

Among the other philosophers teaching at Padua during the
1490s were Pietro Trapolin (1451–1509),[3] who moved from a philosophy lectureship to one in medicine during Linacre's stay, and
Girolamo Avanzi (d. 1534).[4] Particularly interesting is the latter, for

'Early Psychology . . .' (p. 51 n. 2); 'Nicoletto Vernia . . .' (p. 51 n. 2);
'Agostino Nifo's Early views on Immortality', *Journal of the History of
Philosophy*, viii, 1970, 451–60; 'Pier Nicola Castellani and Agostino Nifo on
Averroes' Doctrine of the Agent Intellect', *Rivista critica di storia della filosofia*,
xxv, 1970, 387–409; 'A Note on Agostino Nifo', *Philological Quarterly*, l, 1971,
125–32; 'Agostino Nifo's *De sensu*', *Archiv für Geschichte der Philosophie*, liii,
1971, 119–42.

[1] See P. O. Kristeller, *Eight Philosophers of the Italian Renaissance*, Stanford,
1964, pp. 72–90; Nardi, *Pietro Pomponazzi*; A. Poppi (ed.), *Pietro Pomponazzi:
corsi dell'insegnamento padovano*, i–ii, Padua, 1966–70; idem, *Saggi sul pensiero
inedito di Pietro Pomponazzi*, Padua, 1970, and the publications cited on p. 51
n. 1.

[2] Poppi, *Causalità e infinità* (p. 48 n. 4). Among the thinkers discussed—
to single out only those who were teaching at Padua while Linacre was a
student—are Gabriele Zerbi, Tommaso de Vio, Pietro Pomponazzi, Agostino
Nifo, and Antonio Trombetta.

[3] For information on Trapolin see below, p. 60 n. 4. Besides his interest
in philosophy and medicine, he was apparently also a renowned mathematician. See A. Favaro, *Galileo Galilei e lo studio di Padova*, Florence, 1883, i. 122.

[4] Avanzi was born in Verona and began teaching philosophy at Padua in
1493 (according to Facciolati (p. 43 n. 1), ii. 110). His degree *in artibus*
dates from 1494 (Nardi, *Aristotelismo padovano*, p. 159). He apparently also
taught moral philosophy and had close connections with Venice and Aldus's
Neakademia. Avanzi's emendations of classical Latin poets (e.g. Catullus and
Lucretius) were incorporated into the Aldine editions and won him recognition as a Latin scholar. I know of no major study on Avanzi, but for some
information see G. M. Mazzucchelli, *Scrittori d'Italia*, Brescia, 1753–63,

he seems to form a bridge between the scholasticism at Padua and the humanism of the Aldine circle in Venice. This, however, is a topic to which we must return later.

Padua at the end of the Quattrocento could scarcely be considered one of the great centres of humanistic culture in Italy, but classical languages and literature were cultivated there to some extent. A chair of Greek had been instituted in 1463 and the first incumbent was Demetrios Chalcondylas,[1] with whom Linacre was later to come into contact in Florence. During Linacre's own stay at Padua the chair seems to have been held by a certain Laurentius Camertus, also called 'Creticus' from his place of origin. Of him little is known and the sources are somewhat vague as to precisely when he was teaching at Padua.[2]

There was also a chair of rhetoric, which from 1486 until 1503 was held by Giovanni Calfurnio of Bergamo (1443–1503).[3] While we know very little indeed about the teaching of humanistic subjects at the *Studio* during Linacre's time, it can be at least stated that Padua possessed a certain humanistic tradition. This is evident from the reputation established by Chalcondylas and from the distinction Padua regained in the early years of the sixteenth century by the presence of Marino Becichemo, Marcus Musurus, and others.

In 1497, a year after Linacre left Padua degree in hand, there was instituted a special chair for the teaching of Aristotle in Greek. The first incumbent was Niccolò Leonico Tomeo (1456–1531),[4] with

i. 1226–7; S. Maffei, *Verona illustrata*, Venice, 1792–3, iv. 16–17; A. Firmin-Didot, *Alde Manuce et l'hellénisme à Venise*, Paris, 1875, pp. 145–6, 150, 239–40, 444; Nardi, *Aristotelismo padovano*, pp. 159–61, 167; M. E. Cosenza, *Biographical and Bibliographical Dictionary of the Italian Humanists*, Boston, 1962, i. 349–50.

[1] Chalcondylas left Padua for Florence about 1475. For his years in Padua see G. Cammelli, *I dotti bizantini e le origini dell'Umanesimo*, iii, *Demetrio Calcondila*, Florence, 1954, pp. 27–51.

[2] See Facciolati (p. 43 n. 1), i, p. lv. Cf. D. J. Geanakoplos, *Greek Scholars in Venice*, Cambridge, Mass., 1962, p. 39 n. 85. No additional information is brought to light concerning the teaching of Greek at Padua during this period by E. Ferrai, *L'ellenismo nello Studio di Padova*, Padua, 1876, which seems to be the fullest treatment of the subject.

[3] For further details see V. Cian, *Un umanista bergamesco del Rinascimento: Giovanni Calfurnio*, Milan, 1910 (also published in *Archivio storico lombardo*, xxxvii [1910]). We have an inventory of the books left by Calfurnio on his death which indicates the range of his interests (published by Cian, pp. 22–32).

[4] For the document telling of his appointment see J. L. Heiberg, *Beiträge zur Geschichte Georg Valla's und seiner Bibliothek*, Leipzig, 1896, p. 19. Cf.

whom Linacre apparently came into contact while in Padua or Venice. This distinguished Albanian Hellenist may have assisted with Linacre's education in some way.[1] What is certain is that, until his death, Linacre remained on good terms with Tomeo.[2] The importance of the new chair, perhaps the first specifically to require that the Philosopher be taught in Greek,[3] would be difficult to exaggerate. It indicates perhaps more clearly than any other single event the extent to which humanism was beginning to transform—at least in some centres—the teaching of traditional philosophy. It shows, furthermore, a progressive tendency at Padua, and one which certainly would have earned Linacre's approval. But it was for its celebrated medical studies that Linacre was attracted to Padua.

Medical teaching, as well as that of humanistic subjects and philosophy, took place in the Faculty of Arts and was generally considered to be the more advanced stage of study. After a student had a thorough grounding in the propaedeutic studies—logic and natural philosophy—he normally moved on to medical studies proper. As a rule medical teaching at the universities of Linacre's time was divided into two major areas of study: theoretical medicine and practical medicine. Such was the case at Padua. Beyond these two major categories, there were sometimes established teaching positions in anatomy and surgery, and later, towards the middle of the sixteenth century, in botany.[4] The teaching texts for

Facciolati (p. 43 n. 1), i, pp. lv–lvi. There is too little literature on Leonico Tomeo, but see A. Serena, *Appunti letterari*, Rome, 1903, pp. 3–32; F. A. Gasquet, *Cardinal Pole and His Early Friends*, London, 1927; Allen, v. 520–1; and Cosenza, op. cit., p. 53 n. 4), iv. 3394–7; v. 1749–51.

[1] Linacre is said to have been among Leonico Tomeo's pupils, in a diplomatic dispatch to Henry VIII, dated 25 May 1530. See *Letters and State Papers, Foreign and Domestic, of the Reign of Henry VIII . . .*, 2nd edn., rev'd and enlgd., by R. H. Brodie, London, 1920, iv. 2873–4 (doc. 6403). There seems to be no other extant source indicating such a relationship.

[2] There is a letter of Tomeo to Linacre dated 19 January 1524, with which Tomeo sent a copy of his translation of Aristotle's *Parva naturalia*, Venice, 1523; Index Aureliensis 107,886. This letter is contained in MS. Vat. Ross. 997 (see P. O. Kristeller, *Iter Italicum*, London/Leyden, 1967, ii. 471). An edition of Tomeo's correspondence is being prepared by Mr. C. H. Talbot, who has kindly made this letter available to me. An English translation is published in Gasquet, op. cit. (p. 54 n. 4).

[3] But see below, p. 61 n. 1.

[4] Mathematics was often taught in the faculty of arts of Renaissance universities. Some aspects of mathematics, especially astrology, were relevant

both branches of medical studies were clearly set out by statute and reflect the medieval tradition of medical education rather than any novel or humanistic tendency. The statutory requirements in medicine, as in philosophy, during Linacre's time show little change from what they were a century or two previously. In medicine, as in philosophy, the teaching staff was divided into *ordinarii* and *extraordinarii*.[1] At Linacre's time there were four basic chairs of

to medical teaching. For some details, taken from Pisa in the sixteenth century, see my 'The Faculty of Arts at Pisa at the Time of Galileo', *Physis*, xiv, 1972, 243–72. At Padua about 1480 Paul of Middleburg, a well-known practitioner of the occult side of mathematical arts, was the lecturer in astronomy (i.e. mathematics). However, he had left by the time of Linacre's arrival.

During the student days of Linacre, several mathematicians apparently taught the subject for short periods. Giacomo Filippo Aristofilo de' Fiorenzuoli da Viterbo held the chair in 1492 and in the next year it was occupied by Clementino de' Clementini. Also about the same time the important mathematician Luca Pacioli gave some public lectures in Padua. During the year 1494–5 Francesco Capuano lectured on astronomy in the *Studio*. From 1495 to 1498 mathematics was taught by Federico Crisogono.

Little, however, is known about the nature of the mathematics being taught at Padua while Linacre was there. It is possible that while still in Padua—or immediately afterwards, in Venice—he decided to undertake his translation of (pseudo-)Proclus' *Sphaera*. For further information on mathematics at Padua during Linacre's time see Favaro, *Galileo Galilei* (p. 53 n. 3) and especially idem, 'I lettori di matematiche nella Università di Padova dal principio del secolo XIV alla fine del XVI', *Memorie e documenti per la storia della Università di Padova*, i, 1922, 1–70, especially pp. 40–57. Facciolati (p. 43 n. 1), ii. 116–18 is very vague on these matters.

A mathematician with whom Linacre may have come into contact while at Padua is Benedetto del Triaca (or Tiriaca), a student of Pomponazzi, who took an arts degree in 1494, taught logic in 1495 and 1496, and held the chair of mathematics from 1498 to 1506. Triaca was the lecturer in mathematics during the years when Nicolaus Copernicus was a student in Padua. For further information see Favaro, *Galileo Galilei* (p. 53 n. 3), i. 125–8; idem, 'Lo studio di Padova . . .' (p. 46 n. 1); Nardi, *Pietro Pomponazzi*, index; idem, *Cultura veneta*, pp. 107–8, 114–17 (further bibliography); and especially Jo. Brunatius, 'De Ben. Tyriaco Mantuano', in A. Calogierà (ed.), *Raccolta d'opuscoli scientifici e filologici*, xliii (1750), i–xlvi.

[1] For the origin and development of this distinction see H. Rashdall, *The Universities of Europe in the Middle Ages*, ed. F. M. Powicke and A. B. Emden, 3 vols., London, 1936, i. 206–7. It should be noted that the former position was the more prestigious and better-paying one. In some universities and in certain fields of study the two types of teacher lectured on different materials. The medical professors at Padua during the period under consideration apparently taught the same materials whether *ordinarii* or *extraordinarii*. See

medical studies at Padua—in addition to the *extraordinarii*, who repeated the same material. The professor of theoretical medicine taught in a three-year cycle:[1] (1) The First Book of Avicenna's *Canon medicinae*; (2) Hippocrates' *Aphorisms* with Galen's commentary and, if time permitted, Hippocrates' *Liber prognosticorum*; (3) Galen's *Ars parva* and, again time permitting, something from the Fourth Fen of Avicenna's *Canon*.

As one can see, this aspect of the medical curriculum was highly theoretical and covered the basic outline of late medieval medical theory. The First Book of Avicenna's *Canon*, which initiated the young student into medical thought, begins with a discussion of elements, temperaments, and humours, before passing on to more practical matters including anatomy. The works of Galen and Hippocrates listed here are also highly theoretical, the *Ars parva*, of course, being one of the most discussed works of scientific and medical methodology of the period.[2] According to the Padua statutes, it was recommended that this work should be read along

Favaro, 'Lo studio di Padova . . .' (p. 46 n. 1), pp. 351–2, for extracts from the relevant statutes.

[1] *Statuta* [1496], fol. 24ᵛ, reads as follows (liber II, cap. 16): 'Quae teneantur legere doctores. Ordinarii Theorici primo anno legere teneantur primum *Canonis*; secundo anno legere teneantur totum primum librum *Aphorismorum* Hipocratis, cum commento Galieni, quem si compleverint ante finem anni continuare debent librum *Pronosticorum* Hipocratis; tertio anno legant librum *Microtegmi* [sic] Galieni cum expositione Trusiani seu expositione Jacobi cum questionibus ad libitum audire volentium, quem si compleverint ante finem anni, continuent quartum phen primi *Canonis*. Extraordinarii Theoricae similiter alternatim legant ut quod ordinarii in praecedenti anno legerunt, ipsi in sequenti legant, nisi fuerit concurrens eius, legere audeat ullo modo sub poena periurii et lib. l [i.e. 50 lire]. Nec rectori et consiliariis hoc alicui concedere liceat. Si quis vero doctor aliquam lectionem ultra sibi deputatam legere voluerit, nunquam legere possit materiam ab alio doctore incaeptam vel publicatam, vel ut supra alteri deputatam.'

[2] See especially J. H. Randall, *The Development of Scientific Method in the School of Padua*, Padua, 1961, pp. 13–68; D. P. Lockwood, *Ugo Benzi, Medieval Philosopher and Physician*, Chicago, 1951, pp. 222–7; N. W. Gilbert, *Renaissance Concepts of Method*, New York, 1960; W. P. D. Wightman, 'Quid sit Methodus? "Method" in Sixteenth-Century Medical Teaching and "Discovery"', *Journal of the History of Medicine*, xix, 1964, 360–76; W. F. Edwards, 'Randall on the Development of Scientific Method in the School of Padua—a Continuing Reappraisal', in J. P. Anton (ed.), *Naturalism and Historical Understanding*, State University of New York Press, 1967, pp. 53–68; C. Vasoli, *Studi sulla cultura del Rinascimento*, Manduria, 1968, pp. 257–344 ('Su alcuni problemi e discussioni logiche del Cinquecento').

with an accompanying commentary by one of its two principal late medieval interpreters, Pietro Torrigiano de' Torrigiani (*c.* 1270–*c.* 1350)[1] or Jacopo da Forlì (d. 1413/14).[2] These commentaries are thus the two most recent works listed in the statutes to be used for the instruction of students in theoretical medicine.

Practical medicine was likewise closely tied to traditional teaching texts. Again, it was arranged in a three-year cycle of teaching, this time largely based upon Avicenna's *Canon.*[3] In the first year the section on fevers taken from the Fourth Book was taught and in the two succeeding years the Third Book of the same work was covered. This important book, which systematically deals with the symptoms, diagnosis, and treatment of specific diseases, was divided into two parts as convenient year-long teaching units. These are usually designated as 'De morbis particularibus a capite ad cor' and 'de corde et infra'. In the second and third years the teaching was apparently supplemented by some lectures on Rhazes's *Liber nonus ad Almansorem,*[4] which covers largely the same ground as the Fourth Book of the *Canon.*[5]

The importance of practical medicine was such that there was an additional chair in the subject specifically instituted to repeat the Third Book of Avicenna. The teaching presumably took place out of phase with what was being lectured on in *practica.*[6] Anatomy and surgery were also taught and there is evidence for a single chair combining these subjects as far back as 1387.[7] For the period of the

[1] See G. Sarton, *Introduction to the History of Science*, Baltimore, 1927–48, iii. 839–40.

[2] Ibid., iii. 1195.

[3] Facciolati (p. 43 n. 1), ii. 122; Bertolaso (p. 43 n. 1), pp. 24–5.

[4] This is part of Rhazes's larger *Kitāb al-Manṣūrī* in ten books, which was one of the mainstays of medieval and early modern medical education. There are several Latin editions of the *Liber nonus* alone (accompanied by various commentaries) including at least nine printed at Padua and Venice between 1476 and 1500. See *Indice generale degli incunaboli delle biblioteche d'Italia*, Rome, 1943 ff., iv. 362–4 (nos. 8343–8352, except 8345 which was printed at Milan). See also M. B. Stillwell, *The Awakening Interest in Science during the First Century of Printing, 1450–1550*, New York, 1970, pp. 156–7.

[5] Bertolaso (p. 43 n. 1), p. 24.

[6] Ibid., pp. 32–4. I am not entirely satisfied with this explanation of the relationship of the chair of practical medicine and that *ad lecturam tertii Avicennae*. There must have been a somewhat greater distinction between them than Bertolaso indicates. See also Favaro, 'Lo studio di Padova . . .' (p. 46 n. 1), pp. 320–1.

[7] Bertolaso (p. 43 n. 1), pp. 29–31.

1490s it is not yet wholly clear just how the teaching in this field was divided up and the information on who was teaching these subjects at the time is quite scanty.[1] None the less, as we shall see below, anatomy teaching in particular was undergoing a crucial transformation during the 1490s at Padua.

Surgery, like other subjects, was divided into a three-year cycle of lectures. According to Tomasini,[2] the scheme was as follows: First year, surgery of tumours; second year, surgery of wounds and ulcers; third year, surgery of dislocations and fractures. During Linacre's time the subject was taught by a certain Marcus Doctus, who lectured on surgery from 1477 to 1496, after having lectured on medicine for the previous thirty years.[3]

The bulk of medical teaching at Padua was carried out in the morning, when the *ordinarii* lectured.[4] There was first 'at least' two hours of theoretical medicine, followed by 'at least' an hour of practical medicine. The afternoons were given over to private teaching, as well as to the lectures of the extraordinary professors, who lectured on the same material as had the *ordinarii*, but usually a year out of phase and in more summary fashion. In January anatomy lessons were added and public dissections performed (see below). To the formal requirements of the course was added a year's practical study with a 'famous physician', as has been noted above.[5] Precisely what the last requirement meant in practice is difficult to say. Perhaps a student had the opportunity of working alongside a mature and experienced physician, gaining a broad working knowledge of the practical aspects of what was to be his life's profession. However, the amount of practical training a student received probably varied a great deal.

In both fields, theoretical and practical medicine, Padua boasted several men of more than routine accomplishment.[6] In the former

[1] For example, the standard histories of the university do not mention the anatomical teaching of Alessandro Benedetti (see below).

[2] Op. cit. (p. 43 n. 1), p. 71. Cf. Bertolaso, p. 30. This was the scheme in practice in Tomasini's time and may possibly have been instituted after Linacre's stay.

[3] Facciolati (p. 43 n. 1), ii. 140.

[4] This paragraph is largely based on Bertolaso, and the Statutes of 1496 (p. 46 n. 1).

[5] See above, p. 46 n. 1.

[6] In addition to those mentioned below, Facciolati, ii. 134, also lists Philippus Rambertus Venetus, who began teaching medicine in 1490, and

field are to be included Giovanni da Schio,[1] Gabriele Zerbi,[2] Girolamo Polcastro,[3] and Pietro Trapolin.[4] Teachers of practical medicine included Girolamo della Torre,[5] Giovanni dell'Aquila,[6] and
Onofrius Fontana, who began in 1492. Victor Maripetrus began teaching
practical medicine in 1484 (Facciolati, ii. 133), but I have been unable to
determine whether he was still active in Linacre's time.

[1] Giovanni da Schio (Joannes de Scledo) began teaching at Padua in 1491,
according to Facciolati (ii. 134). See also Nardi, *Aristotelismo padovano*, pp. 152,
165.　　　　　　　　　　　　　　　　　　　　　　　　　[2] For Zerbi see below.

[3] Girolamo da Polcastro (Hieronymus de Polcastris) began teaching
theoretical medicine in 1492 (see Facciolati, ii. 135). See also Nardi, *Aristotelismo padovano*, pp. 152–3.

[4] Pietro Trapolin (1451–1509) took a degree at Padua in arts in 1483 and
in medicine three years later. He taught philosophy from 1481 until 1494,
when he began teaching practical medicine. A year later he moved again, to
a chair of theoretical medicine. Trapolin was one of the philosophy teachers
of Pietro Pomponazzi. He published nothing, but left behind MSS., including
lectures on Aristotle's *De anima*, and 'quaestiones' on Hippocrates' *Aphorisms*
and Avicenna's *Canon*. See Nardi, 'Appunti intorno al medico e filosofo
padovano Pietro Trapolin' (*Aristotelismo padovano*, pp. 147–78) and idem, 'Il
frammento marciano del commento al *De anima* e il maestro del Pomponazzi,
Pietro Trapolin' (*Pietro Pomponazzi*, pp. 104–21).

[5] Girolamo della Torre (Hieronymus a Turre, Turrianus, d. 1506) of
Verona began teaching practical medicine at Padua in 1487. He published
nothing, but left MSS., including a treatise *De venenis* (Vatican, Barb. lat. 229;
cf. Kristeller, *Iter Italicum*, i. 443). He edited Joannes Arculanus, *Practica*,
Venice, 1493; H 13,899; BMC v. 367 (IB 22178). His four sons, Giulio,
Giambattista, Marcantonio, and Raimondo surpassed their father. Marcantonio in particular achieved lasting importance as an anatomist, and teacher
of Leonardo da Vinci. See Facciolati (p. 43 n. 1), ii. 131; Maffei, *Verona illustrata*, iv. 12–16; Nardi, *Aristotelismo padovano*, index s.v. Torre; G. Favaro,
Leonardo da Vinci, i medici e la medicina (Rome, 1923).

[6] Giovanni dell'Aquila (Joannes de Aquila, Aquilanus, d. 1510), b. Lan-
ciano (near Naples), held various posts at Padua and Pisa. In 1491 he
became the first professor of practical medicine at Padua, a post held until his
retirement in 1506. He published nothing, but see his medical poem *De
phlebotomis* in *Collectio Salernitana*, ed. S. de Renzi, Naples, 1852–9, iii. 255–70.
He is also credited with *De sanguinis missione in pleuritide*, Venice, 1520, but as
yet no copy of it has been discovered. With Alessandro Sermoneta (a Paduan
colleague who had gone by Linacre's time), he edited Michele Savonarola's
Practica de aegritudinibus, Padua, 1479; H 14,480; *BMC* vii. 1079. The colophon
(fol. 323vb) reads in part as follows: 'Michael Savonarola . . . hoc divinum opus
edidit. Alexander Sermoneta et Johannes Aquilanus, phisici et medici nostra
etate omnium praestantissimi collatis exemplaribus hoc opus sive divinam
practicam diligentissime recognoverunt . . .' He also worked on Pietro
d'Abano's *Conciliator* and some of the materials from his own copy of the work
were incorporated into the Venice, 1521, and several later editions of the

Francesco Cavalli.[1] In all probability Linacre obtained as good a medical education from these men as could be provided anywhere work. The title-page of the 1521 edition reads in part as follows: '*Conciliator Petri Aponensis . . . noviter castigatissime impressus collatusque cum exemplari quod fuerat manu propria castigatum senis illius nostra tempestate celeberrimi Joannis Aquilani, qui summa cum laude diu practicam medicine ordinarie Patavii est professus . . .*' Dell'Aquila is also praised by Amadeus Scotus in the prefatory letter to the same edition (fol. 1ᵛ). MS. Bergamo, Biblioteca civica, λ 117, contains some notes taken down from dell'Aquila's lectures (Kristeller, *Iter Italicum*, i. 13) and several letters of his are extant (ibid., ii. 100, 268). See also Mazzuchelli (p. 53 n. 4), ii. 900; A. Fabroni, *Historia Academiae Pisanae . . .* (Pisa, 1791–5), i. 345–6, 396; P. Verrua, 'Giovanni dell'Aquila e lo studio di Padova (1480–1506)', *Annuario 1927–1929 del R. Istituto Magistrale di Padova*, 1929, pp. 5–52; Nardi, *Aristotelismo padovano*, index s.v. Aquilano; G. de Sandre, 'Chiose all'inedito testamento di Giovanni dell'Aquila', *Quaderni per la storia dell'Università di Padova*, i, 1968, 167–71; Verde, op. cit., ii. 314–17.

[1] Francesco Cavalli (Franciscus de Caballis, d. 1540) of Brescia was named professor of practical medicine in 1492. He published *De numero partium ac librorum physicae doctrinae Aristotelis* (Venice, c. 1490; GKW 5832) as well as a treatise *De animali theria*, which was published several times in various collections of medical works (e.g. in Antonius Cermisonus, *Consilia medica* (Venice, c. 1498; GKW 6515)). Some poems are in MS. Parma, Biblioteca Palatina 555, fols. 157–60 (Kristeller, *Iter Italicum*, ii. 36). According to Peroni (cited below) there were letters of his, as well as a MS. work, 'Del numero e dell'ordine delle parti', extant in the library of S. Pietro in Oliveto in the early nineteenth century. Cavalli's knowledge of Aristotle was highly regarded and he was praised in one of Aldus Manutius's prefatory letters to the *editio princeps* of Aristotle (to vol. ii, printed in B. Botfield (ed.), *Praefationes et epistolae*, Cambridge, 1861, p. 201). On this see L. Minio-Paluello, 'Attività filosofico-editoriale aristotelica dell'umanesimo', *Umanesimo europeo e umanesimo veneziano*, Florence, 1964, pp. 253–4. According to Francesco Patrizi da Cherso and others, Cavalli began teaching Aristotle from the Greek text at Padua even before Niccolò Leonico Tomeo (see above, p. 55), and also began making use of the Greek commentators in his interpretation at an early date: 'Franciscus autem Caballus, qui inter primos Aristotelicae philosophiae professores, Graecos interpretes in Scholis nominavit, et est secutus, duos libros de ordine Physicorum Aristotelis librorum conscripsit' (*Francisci Patricii Discussionum Peripateticarum tomi IV . . .*, Basle, 1581, p. 112 (liber I, cap. 9)). Later Patrizi is even more explicit: 'Primus in Galliis Joan. Faber Stapulensis, in Italia vero Patavii Franciscus Caballus, et post eum Nicolaus Leonicus eiusmodi philosophandi rationem neglexerunt, Aristotelem Graece, Graecosque Aristotelis interpretes in scholas induxerunt, inde coeptum aliud mixtionis in philosopando genus; uti Aven Rois et Latinis Graecos interpretes admiscerent' (ibid., p. 163 (liber I, cap. 12)). The secondary literature on Cavalli is remarkably meagre, but see V. Peroni, *Biblioteca Bresciana*, Brescia, 1818–23; reprint Bologna, 1968, i. 246–7.

in Europe at the time. Of the medical men there during the final decade of the fifteenth century Gabriele Zerbi,[1] a man who served on Linacre's committee of examiners when he obtained his degree, was undoubtedly the most famous. Though his posthumous reputation has largely been eclipsed, he left behind several quite substantial works, both philosophical and medical. In addition to his treatise on metaphysics, which has recently attracted interest,[2] he is also known for several important medical works which must have been at the centre of discussion at Padua around 1500. His published *Anatomia*, which took form during his later years at Padua,[3] is a substantial and detailed treatise on the subject, meant apparently to be a self-subsistent treatment of anatomy, rather than a brief outline to be used along with practical demonstration.[4] It was, however, severely criticized later by Berengario da Carpi, though recent scholarship tends to show that Zerbi was not as incompetent as Berengario thought.[5] Zerbi was also responsible for a treatise on

[1] On Zerbi (Zerbus, Zerbo, de Zerbis, etc.), see especially F. W. O. Bandtlow, *Die Schrift des Gabriel de Zerbis: De cautelis medicorum* (inaugural dissertation), Leipzig, 1925; G. Romagnoli, 'Contributi alla biografia di Gabriele Zerbi desunti dal suo testamento del 1504', *Pagine di storia della medicina*, xi, no. 6, 1967, 82–98; L. Münster, 'Studi e ricerche su Gabriele Zerbi. Nota 1: nuovi contributi biografici—la sua figura morale', *Rivista di storia delle scienze mediche e naturali*, xli, Supplemento, 1950, 64–83; J. Riesco, 'Gabriel de Zerbis médico y filósofo humanista', *Giornale di metafisica*, xix, 1964, 90–7, which contains new archival material; A. Poppi, *Causalità e infinità* (p. 48 n. 4), pp. 151–69.

A probable account of Zerbi's life is that he was born at Verona in 1445 and took a medical degree at Padua in 1466. After teaching medicine at Padua until 1475, he lectured on logic, philosophy, and medicine at Bologna from 1475 until 1482. He then went to the Sapienza in Rome, where he held the Chair of Theoretical Medicine. He returned to Padua in May 1494 to accept the offer of the Chair of Theoretical Medicine, a position he held until his death in 1504.

[2] *Questiones metaphysice*, Bologna, 1482. On this see especially Poppi and Riesco cited in the previous note.

[3] *Liber anathomice corporis humani et singulorum membrorum illius . . .*, Venice, 1502. Particularly noteworthy is the section on the anatomy of infants, which was reprinted in 1537. See Stillwell (p. 58 n. 4), p. 230.

[4] As was Benedetti's work, on which see below.

[5] See E. dall'Osso, 'Gabriele Zerbi visto attraverso le pungenti postille di Berengario da Carpi', *Pagine di storia della medicina*, i, no. 4, 1957, 12–23, and M. C. Nannini, 'Processo storico a Jacopo Berengario ed a Gabriello Zerbi', ibid., xi, no. 2, 1967, 78–85.

medical ethics and medical practice, *De cautelis medicorum*,[1] published in 1495 at Venice while Linacre was among his students. Before returning to Padua from Rome he also published what seems to be the first printed work on geriatrics, *Gerontocomia scilicet de senum cura atque victu*, which appeared at Rome in 1489, dedicated to Pope Innocent VIII.[2] Zerbi was drawn to Padua by a substantial increase in pay above his earnings in Rome.[3]

One further person who contributed to the intellectual *ambiente* of late Quattrocento Paduan medicine was Paolo Bagellardo. Bagellardo (d. 1492/4)[4] was an old man when Linacre arrived in Padua and he died before the English student took his degree. He was probably no longer teaching, but undoubtedly one of the eminent medical figures of the Veneto region. Perhaps Linacre came into contact with him or at least read his *Libellus de aegritudinibus et remediis infantium*, Padua, 1472, the first printed book to deal

[1] A good description of the work is in *BMC*, v. 470. On it see, in addition to the work of Bandtlow (p. 62 n. 1), L. Münster, 'Il tema di deontologia medica. Il *De cautelis medicorum* di Gabriele Zerbi', *Rivista di storia delle scienze mediche e naturali*, xlvi, 1956, 60–83, and C. Mancini, *Un codice deontologico del secolo XV. Il De cautelis medicorum di Gabriele de Zerbi*, Scientia veterum, no. 44, Pisa, 1963.

[2] See *BMC*, iv. 110 and Bandtlow (p. 62 n. 1), p. 7. It is apparently the first printed treatise on geriatrics, though it has received little attention from writers on the history of the subject. P. Lüth, *Geschichte der Geriatrie*, Stuttgart, 1965, p. 125, is derivative.

[3] In 1490 his salary at Rome was raised from 150 to 250 florins. In 1492 he refused an offer of 400 florins to come to Padua, but was attracted there two years later by an increased salary of 600 florins. For details see Riesco (p. 62 n. 1), p. 94.

[4] Bagellardo (also called Paulus a Flumine or Paolo da Fiume), probably b. Padua in the early fifteenth century. After taking degrees in arts and medicine, he taught philosophy for three years from 1441, and then medicine for the next twenty-eight years. In 1472 he finally obtained a chair and retired to Venice eight years later, returning to Padua some time before his death in 1492 or 1494. His *Libellus de aegritudinibus et remediis infantium* was first published in Padua in 1472 and at least four times later, besides appearing in Italian translation at Brescia in 1486. On it see K. Sudhoff, *Erstlinge der pädiatrischen Literatur*, Munich, 1925, pp. vii–xxii and the first section of the reprints, which reproduces the first edition of the work in facsimile. On Bagellardo see also Mazzuchelli (p. 53 n. 4), ii. 42–3, and the article by E. Carone in *Dizionario biografico degli italiani*, v, 1963, 179–81. For his significance in the history of medicine see G. F. Still, *History of Paediatrics*, London, 1931, pp. 59–66, and A. Pieper, *Quellen zur Geschichte der Kinderheilkunde*, Berne/Stuttgart, 1966, pp. 45–7.

specifically with the subject of pediatrics. While the book was not an epoch-making work as were the works of Vesalius or Harvey, it was a significant milestone in the history of medicine, again indicating the vitality and importance of Padua at the time.

Though the authors of the first printed books on both pediatrics and geriatrics were at Padua in the years around 1490, the medical subject in which the most significant advances were being made was probably anatomy. Linacre was at Padua a half-century before Vesalius arrived to revitalize anatomical instruction, but students of the subject[1] agree that some important changes began to take place at Padua during the last decades of the fifteenth century, which persisted until the time of Fabrizio d'Acquapendente a century later. A key figure here whom one might suppose—at least in the absence of firm evidence to the contrary—to have been Linacre's instructor in the subject, was Alessandro Benedetti of Legnago (c. 1450–1512).[2] Benedetti, if not the first to give public demonstrations at Padua, was among the earliest and he utilized the anatomical theatre, which was later to play such an important role in medical education.[3] Benedetti's use of this pedagogical device, as well as his

[1] See, for example, G. de Bertolis, 'Alessandro Benedetti: il primo teatro anatomico padovano', *Acta medicae historiae Patavina*, iii, 1956–7, 1–13, especially pp. 4–9; E. A. Underwood, 'The Early Teaching of Anatomy at Padua with Special Reference to a Model of the Padua Anatomical Theatre', *Annals of Science*, xix, 1963, 1–26, esp. pp. 5–6; C. D. O'Malley, *Andreas Vesalius of Brussels, 1514–1564*, Berkeley/Los Angeles, 1964, esp. pp. 17–20.

[2] Benedetti, with his teacher Antonio Benivieni, represents the humanistic tendency in Italian medicine of the late fifteenth century. After training in both classical subjects and in medicine, Benedetti held a chair of anatomy at Padua from about 1490. For his experiences during Charles VIII's invasion of Italy, 1495–6, see *Diaria de Bello Carolino*, Venice, 1496. His medical publications include works on anatomy, and commentaries on Pliny. For further information, with bibliography, see especially the article by M. Crespi in *Dizionario biografico degli italiani*, viii, 1966, 244–7, and his *Diaria de Bello Carolino*, ed. Dorothy Schullian, New York, 1967. I have not been able to see H. D. Kickartz, *Die Anatomie des Zahn-, Mund-, und Kieferbereiches in dem Werk 'Historia corporis humani sive anatomice' von Alessandro Benedetti*, Institut für Geschichte der Medizin der Medizinischen Akademie, Düsseldorf, 1964.

[3] For details see the articles by de Bertolis and Underwood cited on p. 64 n. 1. Cf. Gottfried Richter, *Das anatomische Theater*, Abhandlungen zur Geschichte der Medizin und der Naturwissenschaften, Heft 16, Berlin, 1936. Private anatomical dissections were already being carried on at Padua in the late thirteenth and early fourteenth centuries; see L. Premuda and G. Ongaro, 'I primordi della dissezione anatomica in Padova', *Acta medicae historiae Patavina*, xii, 1965–6, 117–42.

clear understanding of the subject-matter of anatomy, are clearly brought out in his *Historia corporis humani sive Anatomice libri quinque*, first published at Venice in 1502 and reprinted at least eight times by 1549.[1] Benedetti's book shows in an unequivocal fashion that public dissection was the basis of his teaching method[2] and, to some degree at least, he was moving away from a complete dependence on the textbook of Mondino de' Luizzi, which had been the standard teaching manual for two centuries.[3] What is more, the strong language of the statutes of 1496 seems to indicate that in the past the required anatomical demonstrations had not always been carried out, and it is quite precisely stated that the demonstrations must be given or substantial fines would be imposed upon those responsible (i.e. the Rector and other officials of the *Studio*) for the omission.[4] Benedetti's *Anatomice*, though published in 1502, can be said to reflect the state of his teaching at Padua from the time of his arrival in 1494.[5] In a justly famous passage of his work Benedetti sets forth various details of how public anatomies are to be carried out.

[1] For information on the first edition see F. J. Norton, *Italian Printers, 1501–1520*, London, 1958, p. 138. For a list of four later editions and other works of Benedetti see *Index Aureliensis*, iii. 531–2. For books by him printed before 1500 see *GKW*, i. 427–30. Schullian's notes and bibliography (cited on p. 64 n. 2) have further information on various editions of his works.

[2] See the text of Benedetti's work discussed by de Bertolis (p. 64 n. 1), pp. 8–9, and Underwood (p. 64 n. 1), p. 6. Underwood points out that during this period dissections became more 'public', and an increasing number of observers were admitted to them. See below, p. 66 n. 2.

[3] See E. Wickersheimer, *Anatomies de Mondino dei Luzzi et de Guido de Vigevano*, Paris, 1926. Mondino's textbook was in use until the advent of Vesalius. See R. Eriksson, *Andreas Vesalius' First Public Anatomy at Bologna 1540 . . .*, Lychnos-Bibliotek, 18, Uppsala/Stockholm, 1959, pp. 34–41.

[4] *Statuta*, 1496, 27ʳ. Cf. Favaro, 'Lo studio . . .', pp. 354–6, and see also Bertolaso (p. 43 n. 1), pp. 29–31, who gives evidence that the chair of anatomy went back at least to 1387. Anatomy teaching usually began in January when the weather was cold (according to the Statutes cited above, it was required to begin the subject before the end of February). It was normally taught in the morning, but was often continued in the afternoon as well. The instruction lasted for at least twenty-six days concurrently with instruction in other subjects. After a holiday for *carnivale*, anatomy instruction continued during the third hour of the morning.

[5] A letter by Jacobus Antiquarius to Benedetti, prefaced to the edition, is dated March 1494 and Benedetti's dedication to Emperor Maximilian is dated August 1497. See [Alexander Benedictus], *Historia corporis humani sive Anatomice* [Venice, 1502], fol. 4ᵛ and sig. aʳ–aiiʳ.

After discussing how cadavers are to be selected and prepared he continues:

In a spacious and well-aired place, a temporary theatre with seats arranged in an amphitheatre should be constructed, such as those found at Rome and Verona. It should be of adequate size to accommodate the number of onlookers, so that the master surgeons who perform the dissections are not disturbed by the crowd. . . . The cadaver should be placed in the centre of the theatre, on an elevated bench, in a well-lighted place, convenient for the dissectors . . .[1]

In this and other passages of his work Benedetti strongly emphasizes the importance of public anatomies in the education of medical students.[2]

From the brief sketch given above, it can be seen that Padua in the 1490s was a mixture of medieval tradition and Renaissance novelty.[3] If logic and philosophy teaching still followed the basic

[1] *Historia corporis humani*, sigs. aii^v–aiii^r. I have collated this text with the often better one found in the Paris, 1544 ed. (BM, shelfmark 781.b.1). The relevant sections are printed with modern punctuation and an English translation, which I have consulted but have modified in places, in W. S. Heckscher, *Rembrandt's Anatomy of Dr. Nicolaas Tulp*, New York, 1958, pp. 182–3, a book generally useful for its discussion of the development of anatomy during the Renaissance.

[2] The following passage from the final chapter of his book might be quoted as evidence of this: 'Sed iam finem faciam dissectioni, dimittendum tandem theatrum est, quoniam partes omnes humani corporis utiliter magis quam verbose tractatae sunt, atque historiam ipsam breviario quodam percurrisse non fuerit alienum. Hortor omnes tum tyrones tum veteranos medicos vel chirurgos ad frequens huiusmodi theatrum quod singulis saltem annis celebrandum sit, quoniam in eo vera videmus, aperta contemplamur, ut opera naturae tanquam viventia nostris subiaceant oculis, alioqui scriptura est picturae persimilis, quae saepe recordationis negligentiam excitat et animi caliginem discutit, sed qui litterarum confisi dumtaxat monumentis (ut inquit Plato) sine rerum conspectione res ipsas animo non revolvunt expressas saepe falluntur. Et opinionem potius quam veritatem mentibus tradunt, sicut noviter navigare incipientibus in depictis chartis contigit in quibus insulae, sinus, recessus, promontoria, veris quae oculis subiacent ad plenum non respondent, sed huiusmodi picturae res pridem notas commemorant et viventium veluti simulachra referunt. Scientis enim sermonem viventem dicimus et animatum et orationem eius scriptam, non iniuria, imaginem quandam nuncupabimus.' *Historia corporis humani*, sig. hiii^v–hiiii^r (again corrections have been made on the basis of the Paris, 1544 text). Vesalius, in contrast to Benedetti, insisted that the instructor himself carry out dissections and not leave it to his assistants. See *Andreae Vesalii . . . De humani corporis fabrica libri septem*, Basle, 1543, fol. 2^v.

[3] See above, p. 43 n. 1.

medieval pattern, the roots of a humanistic approach to Aristotle were already apparent. Medical training was still largely based on Hippocrates, Galen, Rhazes, and Avicenna, but the beginnings of a new approach to the study of anatomy can be discerned during the final decade of the fifteenth century, and novel subjects such as pediatrics and geriatrics were being seriously studied by Paduan professors.

Thomas Linacre drew what benefit he could from all this, completed the necessary requirements, and passed the examinations for his Paduan degree *in medicinis* at the end of August 1496.[1] One of the three documents concerning his degree commends Linacre specifically for the excellence of his examination performance.[2] Some scholars have taken this to be a mark of his unusual ability; however, while such praise was not given to all students, it was not unusual.[3] His examiners included a number of names already mentioned: Pietro Trapolin, Giovanni dell'Aquila, Lorenzo da Noale,[4] Gabriele Zerbi, and Nicoletto Vernia. Among the witnesses to his examination was the Professor of Rhetoric, Giovanni Calfurnio.

Thus Linacre left Padua having supplemented his earlier training in classical languages and literature with what was probably the best medical education the Continent had to offer. The Paduan

---

[1] The documents are printed in Mitchell (p. 42 n. 1), where the date of his degree is established as being 1496. Previously, it was widely thought that Linacre had received the degree in 1492 or 1493. The precise date, 30 August 1496, had, however, been given by Brunatius (p. 55 n. 4), p. xxv; there is a copy of this important, but little-known work in the BM: shelfmark 247.c.12.   [2] Mitchell, p. 697.

[3] On 17 February 1502 a student was commended for being 'doctissimus': *Acta graduum* (p. 43 n. 1), III. i. 40 (no. 106). On 5 March of the same year another student was commended in terms very similar to those used in the Linacre document (*Acta graduum*, III. i. 43 (no. 114)). Few documents of the type referred to in the preceding note seem to be extant, so it is difficult to establish just how unusual the praise accorded Linacre is. See also Pace (p. 42 n. 2), pp. 96–7, where Linacre's brilliance in the examination is emphasized and the particular praise of dell'Aquila for Linacre is noted. The accuracy of this information is difficult to assess, but the anecdote concerning dell'Aquila told immediately after the Linacre story strikes one as somewhat fanciful.

[4] I have been unable to identify this man precisely. He is called Lorenzo da Noale (da Anovale, da Novali), but the standard sources give little information. He may well have been a very junior member of the teaching staff (a lecturer in logic?). See Nardi, *Aristotelismo padovano*, pp. 124, 151, 153, 159, 162. He is also listed as examiner on other occasions during the early sixteenth century. See *Acta graduum*, III. i. 6 ff.

education completed, he apparently set his sights on yet another great centre of intellectual and cultural activity on the Italian peninsula, Venice.

IV. *Linacre and Venice*

Thomas Linacre himself offers an excellent illustration of the intellectual interchange which was taking place between 'scholastic' Padua and 'humanistic' Venice. Linacre, from all indications, moved easily from the scholastic and scientific atmosphere of Padua to the literary and humanistic circle around Aldus Manutius in late Quattrocento Venice. Nor was he the only one of his contemporaries at Padua to fuse these two interests, for there were at least several of the teachers at Padua during Linacre's time who did just that.[1]

It is possible that Linacre may already have established contacts with the Aldine group during his medical studies. We have no clear evidence on this point. The link between Aldus and Linacre is first precisely recorded in the former's prefatory letter to Alberto Pio in the second part of Volume I of the *editio princeps* of Aristotle. In this letter, prefaced to a volume which appeared in February 1498, Linacre, along with several others, is invoked as a witness present in Venice to the fact that the edition has been carefully done.[2] This

---

[1] e.g. Benedetti (see pp. 64–6), who studied with the eminent historian Giorgio Merula and had many other contacts with equally eminent humanist figures. His library shows the range of his interests. See Schullian (p. 64 n. 2), esp. p. 15.

Somewhat more unexpected is Aldus's praise of the Professor of Practical Medicine, Francesco Cavalli, since Cavalli's medical writings and teaching would seem to indicate conservatism. Aldus says of him: 'Sed consuluit labori nostro Franciscus Caballus, multi homo studii, philosophusque doctissimus, ac excellens Venetiis medicus. Is enim libellum de ordine librorum Aristotelis in philosophia accurate quidem et erudite composuit, quem ipsi brevi excusum formis publicabimus' (Botfield (p. 61 n. 1), p. 201). Also see above, p. 61 n. 1.

Girolamo Avanzi, one of the Padua philosophy teachers (on whom see above, p. 53 n. 4), collaborated on various editions with Aldus, was a member of his Academy and published commentaries on various Latin poets.

[2] The letter is printed in Botfield, pp. 197–200, especially p. 199. Cf. Allen, 'Linacre and Latimer' (p. 37 n. 3), p. 515. For the details of the preparation of this edition see A. Firmin-Didot, *Alde Manuce et l'hellenisme a Venise*, Paris, 1875. Another letter, which seems to name Linacre as being in Venice on 4 November 1498, is that of William Latimer to Aldus, printed in P. de Nolhac, 'Les correspondants d'Alde Manuce. Matériaux nouveaux d'histoire littéraire (1483–1514)', *Studi e documenti di storia e diritto*, viii, 1887, 247–99; ix, 1888,

would seem to indicate that at that time *Thomas Anglicus*, as he is referred to in the letter, was already well known and respected by the Aldine circle.

Linacre was in fact a member of the so-called Aldine Academy,[1] an organization dedicated primarily to the study and propagation of Greek language and literature. This group not only had its constitution written in Greek, but it was agreed by members that that language was to be used at all sessions. Amongst its members were included some of the foremost Greek *émigrés* to Italy, and some of the most distinguished Italian and northern European scholars of the time, including Girolamo Aleandro, Pietro Bembo, Marcus Musurus, and Alberto Pio. The precise role of Linacre in this group is not clear, though his acceptance into it once again indicates the high esteem felt by the scholarly élite of Italy for his learning in the Greek tongue.

It may have been while at Venice that Linacre first met Alberto Pio (*c.* 1475–1531), Prince of Carpi, who had been a pupil of Aldus, and later was to be the dedicatee of the *editio princeps* of Aristotle, perhaps the most ambitious venture of the Aldine Press in the printing of Greek. Many years later Pio, writing a polemical work against Erasmus, recalls having met Linacre in Aldus's home, but since some of the factual information in this work seems clearly to be false, Pio's recollection of events which happened thirty years before may not be reliable.[2] It was, in any case, undoubtedly in

203–48 (cited from the offprint (pp. 1–104), reprinted Turin, 1967, of which see p. 96).

[1] On the Νεακαδημία, as it was officially called, see Firmin-Didot, op. cit., esp. pp. 147–54, 435–78 (where the Greek constitution is printed) and D. J. Geanakoplos, op. cit., esp. pp. 128–30. The next paragraph is based on these works.

[2] It is contained in the polemical work *Alberti Pii Carporum Comitis illustrissimi ad Erasmi Roterodami expostulationem Responsio accurata et paraenica Martini Lutheri et asseclarum eius haeresim vesanam magnis argumentis, et iustis rationibus confutans* [Paris, 1528?], fol. 3ᵛ, which reads in part as follows: 'Aldum nostrum Venetiis divertebaris: tunc enim primum ego adolescens audivi Erasmi nomen ab Aldo commendari, et (ni fallor) etiam te vidi et Thomam Linacrium virum praeclarum itidem Aldi contubernalem, deinde crescente in dies laudis tuae fama, amor etiam augebatur.' My attention was first called to this by M. P. Gilmore, 'Erasmus and Alberto Pio, Prince of Carpi', *Action and Conviction in Early Modern Europe. Essays in Memory of E. H. Harbison*, ed. T. K. Rabb and J. E. Seigel, Princeton, 1969, p. 306. Cf. H. Semper *et al.*, *Carpi: ein Fürstensitz der Renaissance*, Dresden, 1882, p. 28.

Though Pio's memory of having met Erasmus and Linacre together in

Venice that Linacre made a number of contacts with distinguished members of the international humanist community which congregated there.

The date at which Linacre left Venice and returned to England is yet one more fact which is not known with any degree of precision. We do know that he was already back there when the first printed work to appear under his name was published in October 1499.[1] This is a translation of the *Sphaera*, then attributed to Proclus. It was included in a miscellaneous collection published by the Aldine Press under the general title of *Astronomici veteres*.[2] It would seem likely that Linacre had been assigned the task of producing a translation by Aldus before he left Italy, but Aldus's prefatory letter of 15 October 1499 clearly states that Linacre had recently 'sent' him the translation.[3] Back in England Linacre had evidently already been given charge of the education of the young Prince Arthur (1486–1502), to whom he dedicated his translation of the *Sphaera*.[4]

v. *Linacre in England*

On re-entering his native country some time about 1499, Linacre turned his attention to new activities. His long years of study were over and he entered into medical practice, though he did continue his translating work, producing excellent Latin versions of a number of Galen's works. He also wrote several very popular and influential textbooks on grammar. During the twenty-five years remaining to

Aldus's house seems plausible, it proves to be impossible. Linacre left Italy before 1500 and Erasmus did not arrive there until 1506. It is possible that Pio met them there on different occasions, though he did not spend much time (if any) in Venice during Linacre's stay. Aldus taught Alberto as a youth, but this was at Carpi.

[1] In addition Linacre was in England, and had become acquainted with Erasmus there, by 5 November 1499. On that date Erasmus mentions him for the first time. See Allen, i. 273–4. There would have been no earlier opportunity for the two to meet.

[2] See Firmin-Didot (p. 68 n. 2), pp. 124–31. The full title and the prefaces are printed in Botfield (p. 61 n. 1), pp. 234–43.

[3] '. . . visum est illis [sc. Arati *Phaenomena*] adjungere Procli Sphaeram, et eo magis, quod eam Thomas Linacrus Britannus docte et eleganter Latinam nuper fecerit, ad meque nostris excudendam formis miserit' (Botfield, p. 239).

[4] The prefatory letter is printed in Botfield, p. 242. A presentation MS. of the work is still extant in Trinity College, Cambridge, MS. 936. See M. R. James, *The Western Manuscripts in the Library of Trinity College, Cambridge*, Cambridge, 1900–4, ii. 347.

him he continued to cultivate various contacts which he had made in Italy, though the scanty extant correspondence linking him to Italian friends allows us only a very vague glimpse of these friendly interchanges.[1] Moreover, it appears that new Italian friendships were forged, probably largely through his existing links with that country.

Even from the little information we have, a number of important things emerge. First of all Linacre maintained contacts with the Italian book trade and continued to have manuscripts made for him in Florence.[2] It is also clear from several letters that he had more contacts with the Florentine community than one would suppose from the meagre evidence which has come to light regarding his years in the Tuscan capital as a student. One of his letters is to Giampiero Machiavelli,[3] presumably a little-known member of the prominent Florentine family. In that letter is mentioned Giovanni Cavalcanti (1444–1509),[4] of another prominent family of the same city, and a member of the circle of Marsilio Ficino. Linacre's ties with both Cavalcanti and Poliziano may indicate that he was also in close contact with Ficino, Pico, and the Platonic Academy of Florence during his year there, but, as already noted, no document has been uncovered to substantiate this. Moreover, Linacre's own writings (other than translations) being as sparse as they are, one is given little opportunity to uncover 'Platonic' influences and it can only be suggested that he may have benefited from Ficino and his circle.

At, it seems, Giampiero Machiavelli's instigation, Antonio

[1] As R. Weiss, 'Notes on Thomas Linacre', *Miscellanea Giovanni Mercati*, Vatican City, 1956, iv. 373–80, points out (p. 373), we have only three personal letters from the pen of Linacre. Weiss prints two of them, Linacre's letters to John Claymond and Giampiero Machiavelli. The third, to Guillaume Budé, is printed in *Gulielmi Budaei . . . Epistolae*, Basle, 1521, pp. 25–6.

[2] Weiss (p. 71 n. 1, above), p. 377, where are also listed books and MSS. once in the possession of Linacre. Cf. Emden (p. 37 n. 2, above), ii. 1149.

[3] On Machiavelli see Weiss (p. 71 n. 1, above).

[4] Linacre's letter suggests a rather close connection with Cavalcanti, but reference to the secondary literature on the latter reveals nothing further. Cavalcanti was one of the interlocutors in Ficino's widely known *De amore* (or *Commentarium in Convivium Platonis*). See Marsilio Ficino, *Commentaire sur le Banquet de Platon*, ed. R. Marcel, Paris, 1956. For further information on Cavalcanti see A. della Torre, *Storia dell'Accademia platonica di Firenze*, Florence, 1902, pp. 647–54 and *passim*; P. O. Kristeller, *Supplementum Ficinianum*, Florence, 1937, i. 118.

Francino dedicated his edition of Julius Pollux's *Vocabularium*, published by the Giunta Press in Florence in 1521, to Linacre.[1] Obviously such a dedication not only discloses a continuing close bond between Linacre and the Florentine intellectual community, but also indicates the high esteem which his knowledge of Greek still commanded in Italy. In fact, the prefatory letter is very revealing and perhaps not so well known as it might be, especially considering the light it sheds on cultural ties between Florence and England in the early sixteenth century. In it, Linacre is invited not only to prepare his own Latin translation of Pollux for the press, but also to send any other translations he might have of either Galen or Hippocrates to the Giunta for publication.[2]

In addition to continued epistolary exchange with Niccolò Leonico Tomeo, alluded to above,[3] Linacre maintained or established new friendships with several other Italians. While in Venice he came to know Andrea Torresano (1451–1529),[4] whose daughter married Aldus Manutius and who was himself a distinguished printer. Torresano recalled his meeting with the Englishman a year after Linacre's death in the prefatory letter to the first collected edition of Galen's works.[5] Also while in Venice Linacre may have encoun-

---

[1] *Iulii Pollucis Vocabularium*, Florence, 1521. The preface is also printed in A. M. Bandini, *Iuntarum typographiae annales ab anno MCCCCXCVII ad MDL...*, Lucca, 1791, pp. 159–61, and an English translation is given in Johnson, *The Life of Thomas Linacre*, pp. 242–5. The first edition of Pollux's work was produced by Aldus in 1502, on which see Botfield (p. 61 n. 1, above), pp. 259–60.

Antonio Francino of Montevarchi played an important role in the Giunta Press of Florence and was responsible for seeing many editions of classical authors through the press. See A. M. Bandini, *De Florentia Iuntarum typographia . . .*, Lucca, 1791, pp. 86–91. For a list of the editions for which he was responsible see the other work of Bandini cited above.

[2] '. . . ob egregiam tuam utriusque linguae bonarumque disciplinarum peritiam, hortamurque ut si quando ocium nactus eris, Pollucem ea qua soles felicitate, latinum facias, et siquid habes, aut Galeni, aut Hyppocratis translatum, cui ultimam manum imposueris ad nos excudendum mittere non dedigneris, nos autem curabimus ut quaecunque Galeni opera hic inveniuntur tibi transcribantur' (Pollux (p. 72 n. 1, above), fol. 1ᵛ).

[3] See above, pp. 54–5.

[4] On him see D. Bernoni, *Dei Torresani, Blado, e Raggazzoni*, Milan, 1890, pp. 3–89; Firmin-Didot (p. 68 n. 2), *passim*.

[5] '. . . Thomas Linacrus Aldi nostri contubernio ad aliquot annos usus', Torresano's prefatory letter printed in Botfield (p. 61 n. 1), p. 362. Cf. Alberto Pio's statement cited in p. 69 n. 2.

tered Girolamo Aleandro (1480–1542),[1] who was later to take an important part in the Counter-Reformation. In 1512 we find Aleandro writing to Erasmus and asking to be remembered to his fellow member of the Aldine Academy, Thomas Linacre, and to other English humanists of his acquaintance.[2]

Ambrogio Leone of Nola (1459–1525),[3] whose work has not attracted the attention it deserves, is another Italian humanist-physician who can be linked with Linacre. Once again Erasmus provides us with the evidence; in writing to Leone he tells us that Leone knew Linacre through Aldus and through Erasmus himself.

Finally, when Linacre came to be named Canon and Prebend of the church of St. Stephen, Westminster, in 1517, it was an Italian humanist whom he succeeded in the position. This was Andrea Ammonio of Lucca (1477–1517), who had arrived in London in 1506 and apparently remained in close contact with Linacre from then until his death.[4]

VI. *Conclusions*

What Linacre brought back with him from Italy to Britain was a high-level education in both humanistic and medical studies, which was superior to anything he might have obtained in his native land. His endeavours in the field of medicine were quite remarkable and he might be said to have initiated a new approach

[1] Aleandro studied in Venice, off and on, during the years 1493–4 and perhaps met Linacre at that time. He later became a member of the Aldine Academy. See J. Paquier, *L'Humanisme et la Réforme. Jérôme Aléandre de sa naissance à la fin de son séjour à Brindes (1480–1529)* . . ., Paris, 1900, pp. 12–17. See also *Dizionario biografico degli italiani*, ii, 1960, 128–35.

[2] Allen, i. 507.

[3] Leone (Ambrosius Leo) studied medicine at Padua having had Vernia as one of his teachers. He taught medicine in Naples until the time of the French invasions. He then returned to Padua to study Greek with Musurus. In 1507 he joined the household of Aldus Manutius, serving as both physician and editor. See Allen, iii. 352–3; L. Thorndike, *History of Magic and Experimental Science*, New York, 1923–58, v. 143–7; P. de Montera, 'La Béatrice d'Ambroise Leone de Nola. Ce qui reste d'un *Beatricium* consacré à sa gloire', *Mélanges Hauvette*, Paris, 1934, pp. 191–210; *Catalogus translationum et commentariorum*, ed. P. O. Kristeller *et al.*, Washington, 1960 ff., i. 117–18.

[4] We know of the Linacre–Ammonio association largely through Erasmus; see Allen, i. 456, 458–9. For Linacre's succeeding Ammonio at St. Stephen's see *Letters and Papers* (p. 55 n. 1), ii. 1147 (doc. 3624). For further information see Allen, i. 646, and C. Pizzi, *Un amico di Erasmo. L'umanista Andrea Ammonio*, Florence, 1956.

to medical studies in England. What is more, in addition to the specific contributions he made to the encouragement and development of a higher level of medical science in England, more permanent patterns were engendered through the establishment of the College of Physicians and the founding of medical lectureships at both Oxford and Cambridge. Linacre, along with Caius and Harvey, might be named as one of the seminal influences on the development of medicine in Britain during the early modern period.

His place in the development of humanistic studies was no less significant, though in that field he had more English contemporaries of international reputation to aid him in the task. As well as Grocyn, who was a few years his senior, Linacre was supported by Colet, Lily, Tunstal, More, Pace, Latimer, Lupset, and Pole. These men established a firm basis of classical knowledge and learning which drew the praise time and again of some of the most distinguished continental humanists. Nearly all these English humanists made the journey to Italy, and came back imbued with the new learning. As a result of this we can observe a remarkable change in the way in which the continental humanists viewed the English nation.

Italian humanists at the end of the fourteenth and through the fifteenth century often took a very dim view of the cultural achievements of the English, and saw the medieval logical and scientific traditions which had penetrated Italy from Oxford as particularly barbarous[1]—witness the rather patronizing remarks of Enea Silvio Piccolomini (the future Pope Pius II) about the crudities of British life which he encountered during his diplomatic mission to the island in 1435.[2] Yet a striking reversal of this attitude took place during the early years of the sixteenth century. No longer were Britons looked on as barbarous. Both Aldus and the Italophile Erasmus praised them more than once for their polish and culture in matters literary.[3] By 1517, Erasmus could say 'if Linacre or

---

[1] See C. Dionisotti, 'Ermolao Barbaro e la fortuna di Suiseth', in *Medioevo e Rinascimento: Studi in onore di Bruno Nardi*, Florence, 1955, pp. 219–53, and E. Garin, *L'Età nuova*, Naples, 1969, pp. 139–77 ('La cultura fiorentina nella seconda metà del '300 e i "barbari britanni"', reprinted from *Rassegna della letteratura italiana*, lxvi (1960)).

[2] For an English translation, see F. A. Gragg and L. C. Gabel, *Memoirs of a Renaissance Pope*, New York, 1958, pp. 34–6.

[3] See Aldus's prefatory letter to the Proclus edition in Botfield (p. 61 n. 1), pp. 239–40, and Allen, i. 415, etc. See also Aldus's letter to Musurus prefaced to Statius, *Sylvarum libri quinque* . . . [Venice, 1502], sig. ai^v–aii^r.

Tunstal were my teacher, I should not miss Italy'.[1] Those who know the cultural situation obtaining in Europe on the very eve of the Reformation will recognize that higher praise could not be desired. Britain had come of age culturally and it was Linacre and his colleagues, all of whom had imbibed large doses of Italian humanism, who were responsible for the metamorphosis.

[1] Allen, ii. 486.

Addendum to p. 53 n. 4:

On Avanzi's humanistic interest, see esp. C. Dionisotti, 'Caldarini, Poliziano e altri', *Italia medioevale e umanistica*, xi, 1968, 151–85, at 173–9.

Linacre and Medical Humanism

RICHARD J. DURLING*

I. *Historical Perspective*

MUCH HAS BEEN WRITTEN ON THE MANY CONNOTA-
tions of the modern term 'humanism'. For the purposes of this
paper, I shall adopt the definition of humanism, or rather the older
term 'humanist', given by the late Roberto Weiss: by 'humanist' he
understands 'the scholar who studied the writings of ancient authors
. . . searched for manuscripts of lost or rare classical texts, collected
the works of classical writers, and attempted to learn Greek and
write like the ancient authors of Rome'.[1] In this narrower sense,
Linacre *was* a humanist; he studied Aristotle, Galen, and Proclus,[2]
he collected books and manuscripts (some of which appear to have
been copied for him in Florence),[3] and he possessed a complete
mastery of Greek and Latin. If, however, it be insisted with Edel-

---

* Institut für Geschichte der Medizin und Pharmazie, Christian-Albrechts-
Universität, Kiel.
[1] R. Weiss, *Humanism in England during the Fifteenth Century* (3rd edn.),
Oxford, 1967, p. 1.
[2] For his contributions to Aristotelianism which included editorial work
on the Aldine *editio princeps* and a now lost version of books 1–2 of the *Meteorologica* see Allen's note to Erasmus, *Opus Epistolarum Des. Erasmi Roterodami*, ed.
P. S. Allen, 12 vols., Oxford, 1906–58, iii. 403. Linacre's version of Ps.-Proclus'
De sphaera, his first publication, was included with a glowing testimonial to
his talents from the pen of Aldus in the *Astronomici veteres* of 1499 (Goff F–191).
I have not seen the presentation copy in Trinity College, Cambridge, MS.
936, mentioned in A. B. Emden's *A Biographical Register of the University of
Oxford to A.D. 1500*, 1958, ii. 1147–9.
[3] See his letter to the physician Giampiero Machiavelli, edited by R. Weiss
in *Miscellanea Giovanni Mercati*, vol. iv, Studi e Testi 124, Vatican City, 1946,
pp. 373–80 (facsimile, with note by T. J. Brown, in *The Book Collector*, xiii, 1964,
341). For his library, see the list of known titles in Emden, op. cit.

stein[1] that only an adherence to 'certain aesthetic, historical and philosophical views' qualifies a man for the title, then our evidence is sadly inconclusive. Linacre was not given to grandiose statements of principle or belief.

But what is *medical* humanism and who were the *medical* humanists? By common consent, medical humanism connotes a devotion to the medical classics, Hippocrates, Galen, even the Byzantine compilers, coupled with a desire to apply the infant science of philology to their interpretation. There is as yet no single adequate study of the phenomenon, and the bibliographical research necessary for it has barely begun. Nevertheless, the main contributors are well known to every student of Erasmus, who shared his friends' enthusiasm: they include Giorgio Valla, Niccolò Leoniceno, and Wilhelm Kopp (Copus). To these three we must add the name of the Florentine, Lorenzo Lorenzano (Laurentianus). Between them, as I shall show, they translated in the space of thirty years, from *c.* 1484 to 1514, roughly an eighth of Galen's output. With the publication of his Galenic versions (some of which duplicated work already done), Linacre achieved almost as much in seven years (1517–24).

Was this preoccupation with ancient Greek medicine anachronistic, as a noted student of the classical heritage seems to suggest? Dr. Bolgar has written of Linacre that 'within the limits of his own profession he was a devotee of the outdated Galenian school which the humanist doctors of his time had largely abandoned'.[2] A survey of the preliminary work carried out by Linacre's precursors and a reading of their prefaces suggest that far from being outdated, Galenism at this period was considered synonymous with progress. Far from abandoning Galen, they championed him in preference to Avicenna and his ilk. Nor, significantly, was an interest in Greek medicine restricted to the profession. To mention only Linacre's distinguished teachers, Politian and Chalcondylas, the former had virtually completed by June 1490 a translation of Hippocrates' *Aphorisms* with Galen's accompanying commentary,[3] and the latter

[1] See his paper, 'Andreas Vesalius, the Humanist', reprinted in *Ancient Medicine: Selected Papers of Ludwig Edelstein*, ed. by Owsei Temkin and C. Lilian Temkin, Baltimore, 1967, pp. 441–54.

[2] R. R. Bolgar, *The Classical Heritage and its Beneficiaries . . .*, Cambridge, 1954; repr., Harper Torchbooks, New York, 1964, p. 312.

[3] See his letter of 5 June 1490 in *Prose volgari inedite . . .*, a cura di I. Del Lungo, Florence, 1867, p. 77.

rendered (perhaps unwisely) Galen's *De anatomicis administrationibus*, though this remained unpublished until 1529.[1] Chalcondylas also assisted Lorenzano in translating the very same texts that had interested Politian.[2]

It is impossible to determine who first had the idea of translating Galen afresh. Lorenzano thought he was a lone pioneer, but if anyone deserves that title it must be Giorgio Valla. Not one of the Renaissance's greater luminaries, he nevertheless inaugurated a trend in the publication of the first of the *novae translationes*. This, appropriately, was a version of Galen's *De sectis*, published in a Milanese edition of Francesco Filelfo's *Orationes et opuscula* (1483–4) under the title: *Introductorium ad medicinam*.[3] This is the text Galen himself had recommended the beginner to read first.[4] Valla put students of Galen further in his debt by publishing in 1498, with his version of Nicephorus' *Logica* (Goff N–44), renderings of four minor treatises, namely the *De optima corporis nostri constitutione*,[5] the

---

[1] I say unwisely since this text, previously unknown to the Latin West, demands specialist knowledge which the layman Chalcondylas did not possess. For Johann Guinther's scathing comments on his predecessor's version, see my 'A Chronological Census of Renaissance Editions and Translations of Galen', *J. Warburg and Courtauld Inst.* xxiv, 1961, 230–305, 239 n. 49 (hereafter referred to as 'Census').

[2] See Lorenzano's dedicatory letter to Piero de' Medici (dated shortly before the latter's expulsion) in Hippocrates, *Sententiae cum Galeni commentis*, Florence, A. di Miscomini, 1494 (Goff H–273). His version of Galen's commentary begins (sig. b5ʳ): 'Sententiam hanc esse totius operis exordium seu simplex seu duplex sit: consensu ferme omnium interpretum creditur.' This *incipit* is not listed by Lynn Thorndike and Pearl Kibre, *A Catalogue of Incipits of Mediaeval Scientific Writings in Latin* (rev. and augm. edn.), London, Mediaeval Academy of America, 1963 (hereafter abbreviated to TK²). The whole of Lorenzano's preface repays careful reading: his artistic *credo* is decidedly humanist. For an earlier Graeco-Latin version of the commentary, see p. 83 n. 2, below.

[3] Goff P–607 (often reprinted). It was primarily intended for Niccolò, the nephew of the dedicatee Jacopo Antiquario. Niccolò had recently turned from dialectic and philosophy to the study of medicine. Valla's translation begins: 'Medicinae artis intentio quidem est sanitas: finis autem sanitatis adeptio . . .' (not in TK²). For Burgundio's medieval rendering from the Greek see p. 84 n. 3, below.　　　　[4] *Scripta Minora*, ii, 1891; repr. 1967, pp. 83–4.

[5] *Inc.* (*ed. princ.*, sig.z1ʳ): 'Quaenam optima nostri corporis confirmatio: an que temperatissima sicut multi veteres medici ac philosophi existimaverunt . . .' (not in TK²). Dedicated, as is the following, to the Venetian Agostino Barbadico (doge from 1486 to 1501). Again, Valla had been anticipated: see p. 84 n. 1, below.

De bono corporis habitu,[1] the *De inaequali intemperie*[2] (later translated by both Linacre and Leoniceno), and a fragment of a larger work, the so-called *De praesagitura* or *De praenotione*.[3] Two *spuria* were also added, one translated by himself,[4] and the other by his adopted son, Giampietro.[5] This (two trifles on uroscopy apart) is the sum total of Valla's contributions. Further translations from the pen of Lorenzano were issued posthumously (he committed suicide in 1502):[6] the *Ars medica* (already available in a version from the Greek)[7] which a Pavian professor, Pietro Antonio Rustico, published in an edition of the *Articella* of 1506;[8] the *De differentiis febrium* which

[1] *Inc.* (*ed. princ.*, sig. z2ᵛ): 'Habitus boni nomen cunctis rebus ingerere consuevimus stabilitate & solutionis difficultate . . .' (not in TK²). See p. 83 n. 6, below.

[2] *Inc.* (*ed. princ.*, sig. z3ʳ): 'Distemperantia inaequalis fit aliquando corporis animati . . .' (TK², col. 438). See p. 84 n. 2, below.

[3] This (as Kalbfleisch showed) is an excerpt from Galen's *De constitutione artis medicae*, the text printed in Kühn's edition (xix. 497–511) corresponding to i. 289–304 K. Valla's rendering begins (z6ʳ): 'De praesagitura hinc loqui constituamus: quia usus dierum ad alia . . .' (TK², col. 386). Dedicated to the physician Niccolò Masini of Cesena. See p. 84 n. 4, below.

[4] *Praesagium experientia confirmatum*; *inc.* (*ed. princ.*, sig &2ʳ): 'Cuicunque praesciscere libuerit mortis non diem modo sed etiam horam considerare expedit . . .' (not in TK², but noted by Prof. Kibre in *Speculum*, xliii, 1968, 83). Dedicated to the Venetian Senator, Constantinus Priolus.

[5] *De succedaneis*; *inc.* (*ed. princ.*, sig. &4ᵛ): 'Cum reciprocorum medicaminum notum sit librum scripsisse Dioscoridem . . .' (TK², col. 335, where Giorgio is credited with the authorship). Giampietro dedicated this slight piece to the Ferrarese notable Ludovico Bonaccioli, physician to Lucrezia Borgia, patron of Leoniceno, and author of *Enneas muliebris*, for whom see *Dizionario biografico degli italiani*, xi, 1969, 456–8 (G. Stabile).

[6] His death is discussed by his pupil Pietro Crinito in book 3, ch. 9 of his *De honesta disciplina*, Florence, 1504, recently edited by C. Angeleri, Rome, 1955. Lorenzano, Professor successively of Logic, Physics, and Medicine at Pisa, also translated Aristotle's *De interpretatione*, issued with a commentary in Venice, 8 January 1500/1 (Goff L–87). A friend of Antonio Benivieni, who originally dedicated his famous autopsies to him, and of the Florentine Platonist Francesco da Diacceto, he is perhaps best known as the subject of Botticelli's portrait now in the Pennsylvania Museum of Art. See L. Dorez, 'Le Portrait de Lorenzo Lorenzano . . .', *Bulletin de la Société française d'Histoire de la Médecine*, vi, 1907, 235–8.

[7] See my brief note in *Classical Philology*, lxiii, 1968, 56–7.

[8] Lorenzano's version begins (*Articella*, 1506, sig. I2ᵛ): 'Tres sunt omnes doctrine ordinem subsequentes. Prima ex finis cognitione per resolutionem efficitur . . .' (not in TK²). Dedicated (13 February 1500) to Francesco Pandolfini, son of Pierfilippo the elder. Francesco, we are told, had translated,

Leoniceno included in his *In libros Galeni a se . . . translatos*, Venice, 1508,[1] and finally Hippocrates' *Prognostics* with Galen's commentary published separately in Florence in 1508.[2] Leoniceno's first published contribution to the growing tide duplicated the efforts of Lorenzano: in the Venice, 1508 edition mentioned above will be found his rendering of the *Ars medica*.[3] This was soon followed up by another version which threatened the supremacy of Lorenzano, namely that of Galen's *In Hippocratis Aphorismos*.[4] Ludovico Bonaccioli, who financed the publication, duly lauds Leoniceno to the skies as the *divinus interpres*, and the obscure Tricaglia who saw it through the press speaks of him as the *dulciloquus latine medicinę concionator*. Leoniceno's friend, Ottato, in a letter of 1506 had been equally enthusiastic: 'Tu primus: verusque Galeni interpres: in te uno confidimus omnes . . .'[5] The confidence seems to have encour-

but not published, the pseudo-Galenic *Definitiones medicae*. I can find no trace of this version.

  [1] *Inc.*, Venice, 1508, fol. 25ʳ: 'Differentie febrium maxime quidem proprie ac maxime principales secundum substantiam . . .' Prefixed is a letter from Lorenzano's former colleague in Tuscany, Cesare Ottato, then in Venice, dated (*more Veneto?*) 1 January 1500. Ottato is loud in his condemnation of medieval versions (they are rather inversions)—medicine would have been better off without them. His views, he adds, are shared by their friend Francesco da Diacceto, and by Leoniceno, *vir litteratissimus & in medicina Hercules*. The latter's famous critique of Pliny, Avicenna, *et al.* is warmly praised. For an earlier Graeco-Latin version, see p. 83 n. 4, below.

  [2] The Galenic commentary begins (Florence, 1508, sig. a3ʳ): 'Medicum uti providentia (ut mihi videt) optimum est. Pro praesensione dixisse providentiam perspicuum est . . .' The posthumous editor (Augustinus Florentinus) praises Lorenzano's fidelity and style: '. . . summa interpretis fide, non indocto sermone, qui solet esse physicis rarus, in latialem linguam & eleganter & pure vertit'. Yet he was not the first: see p. 83 n. 3, below.

  [3] *Inc.*, Venice, 1508, fol. 5ᵛ: 'Tres sunt omnes doctrine que ordini inherent. Prima quidem ex notione finis que per resolutionem fit . . .' (TK², col. 1585, cites a slight variant from the 1524 edition, for which see my *A Catalogue of Sixteenth Century Printed Books in the National Library of Medicine*, Bethesda, Md., 1967, no. 1771, and the Wellcome *Catalogue of Books printed before 1641*, London, 1962, no. 2527). Leoniceno dedicated his version to Alfonso I d'Este.

  [4] The Galenic commentary begins (Ferrara, 1509, sig. H1ʳ): 'Hanc orationem sive unus sit aphorismus, sive plures, esse prooemium totius operis, pro confesso habetur apud omnes fere eius expositores . . .' Again, Leoniceno had been anticipated. See p. 83 n. 2, below.

  [5] Letter of 1 September 1506 acknowledging Leoniceno's dedication of his treatise *De virtute formativa*. Cited from the 1524 edition mentioned in n. 3, above (sig. S1ʳ).

aged Leoniceno: at any rate, further activity led to the (perhaps unauthorized) publication of four more treatises in 1514, this time beyond the Alps. From the Paris house of Henri Estienne came his versions of the *De differentiis morborum*,[1] the *De inaequali intemperie*[2] (previously rendered by Valla), *Ad Glauconem*[3] (of which a Greek text had been published in 1500 from a manuscript belonging to Leoniceno),[4] and the *De crisibus*.[5]

Thus far, the Italians had made all the running. The first contribution from the North comes from Erasmus's friend Wilhelm Kopp (Copus) for whom, be it said, Linacre had a high regard.[6] Kopp had already published a version of Book I (without the prooemium) of the Byzantine compiler, Paul of Aegina's *Epitome*, under the title *Praecepta salubria*, Paris, 1510;[7] he now fulfilled the promise expressed in that edition[8] with a translation of Galen's most important work

---

[1] *Inc.*, Paris, 1514, sig. a2ʳ: 'Primum dicere oportet quid morbum appellemus, ut libri intentio magis innotescat . . .' For an earlier translation from the Greek, see my note in *Traditio*, xxiii, 1967, 461–76, s.v. 'Census', no. 65a.

[2] *Inc.*, ibid., sig. e1ʳ [mis-signed a]: 'Intemperatura inequalis totum corpus animalis aliquando obsidet . . .' See p. 84 n. 2, below.

[3] *Inc.*, ibid., sig. f1ʳ: 'Quod quidem non communem tantum hominum naturam medicum cognoscere oportet, o Glaucon . . .' See p. 83 n. 5, below.

[4] Venice [Z. Callierges, for] N. Vlastos, 1500 (Goff G–35). My note ('Census,' p. 236 n. 32) should have read *Musurus'* letter to Z. Callierges (not Leonicenus').

[5] *Inc.*, Paris, 1514, sig. m1ʳ: 'Sive subitam in morbo mutationem, sive solum in melioramentum [*melius momentum* 1524 ed.] sive eam quae antecedit agitationem . . .' How far this is superior to Burgundio's version (see p. 82 n. 3, below) remains to be seen.

[6] See Allen, ii. 252–3 (a letter from Erasmus to Budé of *c.* 19 June 1516): 'Idem evenit apud eum [sc. Linacrum] in Copo, *cuius omnia citra exceptionem probat.*' My italics.

[7] This contains an illuminating preface, bewailing the condition of medicine, now obliterated by barbarian dregs—with the result that no man of culture and refinement would dream of touching it: Pico and Politian—*qui unus a gothorum iniuria linguam latinam vindicare potuisset*—had, alas! died prematurely, before they could do medicine justice. He, Kopp, trained in Germany by Mithridates and Celtes, then in Paris by Janus Lascaris, Erasmus, and Girolamo Aleandro, has tried to restore the ancient physicians to their former glory (Hippocrates, Galen, Rufus, Oribasius, Paul, Alexander having lain in dust). . . . He follows in the footsteps (though from afar) of Theodore Gaza and Niccolò Leoniceno.

[8] 'Dabimus operam, ut propediem Galeni quoque opera: quorum ne umbram quidem adhuc latini viderunt, non minore a Romanis quam Grecis (quantum latini sermonis inopia patitur) facilitate legantur.'

on pathology, the *De locis affectis*,[1] which he had somehow managed to complete while accompanying his master, Louis XII of France, on the latter's strenuous campaigns against the English.

This, then, is the record of Galen's 'abandonment' by the medical humanists. Between them, four men had translated afresh from the Greek a total of thirteen Galenic texts (one a fragment) and two *spuria*, by the end of 1514—three years, that is, before the publication of Linacre's *De sanitate tuenda* version, Paris, 1517. In crude terms, they had rendered just under 2,275 pages of Kühn's bilingual edition, or roughly an eighth of the Galenic corpus, excluding texts only preserved in Syriac, Arabic, or the like. One is impressed by the enthusiasm of these four men, but precisely what were they contributing? A new elegance, certainly, though not as marked as they liked to think, or others have claimed for them. Did they contribute new texts unknown to the West in the ages of barbarism? Alas, no!

For every genuine text translated by these medical humanists, there existed, had they but known, a medieval Graeco-Latin version from the pen of the barbarians they so despised. True, these were not always available in the bulky *editio princeps* of the Galenic corpus published in Venice in 1490 (Goff G–37);[2] the editor of that volume, the Brescian physician, Diomedes Bonardus, had combed the libraries of Italy for manuscripts, but all his efforts failed to reveal some of the versions from the Greek. Instead, he discovered and printed their ubiquitous rivals, the Arabic-Latin renderings of Constantine, Gerard of Cremona, Marc of Toledo, and the like. Thus, Bonardus prints Gerard's version of the *De crisibus*; that of the twelfth-century humanist Burgundio remains in manuscript, though duly appreciated by the latest editor of the Greek text, Dr. Bengt Alexanderson.[3]

---

[1] *Inc.*, Paris, 1513, fol. 4ʳ: 'Non solum recentiores medici, sed veterum quoque non pauci, corporis particulas, locos nominare consueverunt . . .' In my 'Census', s.v. 1510(?).1 I allowed myself to be influenced by the British Museum's dating of an edition *s.l.s.n.s.d.* My friend Dr. D. E. Rhodes will shortly publish a paper showing it to have been printed in Venice some ten years later. It lacks the preface referring to the circumstances of composition, found in the *editio princeps* of 1513. For a previous Graeco-Latin version of uncertain authorship, see p. 83 n. 1, below.

[2] For a partial list of contents, see M. B. Stillwell, *The Awakening Interest in Science during the First Century of Printing, 1450–1550* . . ., New York, 1970, no. 375.

[3] *Galenos.* Περὶ κρίσεων. *Überlieferung und Text* . . . Studia Graeca et Latina Gothoburgensia, xxiii, Göteborg, 1967, pp. 19–20, 32–5 and *Nachtrag*. The

Bonardus seems not to have come across the Graeco-Latin version of the *De locis affectis*,[1] and I doubt if Kopp had either.

If Bonardus overlooked some of the humanists' medieval precursors, so did earlier editors of the *Articella*. This standard university corpus, though subject to individual editorial whims, always comprised the *Ars medica* and Hippocrates' *Aphorisms* and *Prognostics*. The Latin versions were invariably Constantine's, for the text of *In Hippocratis Aphorismos* ascribed variously to Burgundio and Niccolò[2] must have been almost as inaccessible as the anonymous Graeco-Latin rendering of *In Hippocratis Prognostica* which I have just discovered in Naples.[3] Not surprisingly they printed the Arabic-Latin version of the latter, beginning 'Manifestum est quod Ypocras non utitur hac dictione scilicet previsio nisi loco pronosticationis . . .' (TK[2], col. 847).

I stress the point that the humanists may well have imagined they were pioneers, in the sense of translating from the Greek for the first time a number of texts previously only available in crabbed Latin versions from the Arabic of Hunain or his colleagues. What they cannot strictly plead is ignorance of the following, all included in the *editio princeps* of Bonardus (1490): Burgundio's rendering of the *De differentiis febrium*[4] and Niccolò's of *Ad Glauconem*,[5] *De bono habitu*,[6]

Munich MS. begins (Clm. 35, s. xiv, f. 82ra): 'Sive repentinam egritudine transmutationem sive ad melius incessionem . . .' (cf. TK[2], col. 1511).

[1] *Inc.*: 'Loca (autem) nominant . . .' (TK[2], col. 831 after Silverstein). Variously ascribed to Burgundio and Niccolò da Reggio. See my note in *Traditio*, xxiii, 1967, 461–76, s.v. 'Census', no. 60a. I can now add after an examination of Montpellier MS. 18 that its ascription of the version (printed by Bonardus) beginning 'Medicorum non solum moderni . . .' is based on a half-truth: what that manuscript contains is an Arabic-Latin version *conflated* *with* the Graeco-Latin. I plan to edit the latter, with full stylistic analysis.

[2] *Inc.* (Vat. lat. 2369, s. xiv, f. 3[r]): 'Quoniam quidem sermo hic sive unus afforismus est sive duo . . .' (cf. TK[2], col. 1296 and *Traditio*, art. cit., s.v. 'Census', no. 149a). I have since discovered another copy in Erfurt Amplon. F. 278, s. xiv, fols. 173[ra]–213[va] (not identified as Galen's commentary by Schum).

[3] Lorenzano and Leoniceno can both be forgiven for overlooking the version in Naples VIII.D.25, a.1380, ff. 85[ra]–122[rb]. *Inc.*: 'Quoniam quidem pro pronosticatione et precognitione dixit providentiam . . .' (not in TK[2]).

[4] *Inc.*: 'Differentie febrium que quidem maxime proprie sunt . . .' (TK[2], col. 429).

[5] *Inc.*: 'Quoniam quidem non solum communem universorum hominum . . .' (cf. TK[2], col. 1297).

[6] *Inc.*: 'Exeos nomen quod habitum significat . . .' (TK[2], col. 540).

De optima corporis constitutione,[1] and *De inaequali intemperie*.[2] Valla translated the *De sectis* before the appearance of Bonardus's edition, which included Burgundio's rendering:[3] he can be forgiven for not noticing that the *De praesagitura* fragment had been treated as the second part of Galen's *De praecognitione ad Epigenem*, and included in a version attributed to Niccolò in the *editio princeps* of 1490.[4]

If Linacre's precursors were not, strictly speaking, breaking new ground, what was the extent of his contribution?

11. *Linacre's Translations*

The chronology of Linacre's versions is as follows:[5]

1517 *De sanitate tuenda.* fol. Paris: G. Rubeus. Dedicated to King Henry VIII.

1519 *Methodus medendi.* fol. Paris: D. Maheu for G. Hittorp. Dedicated to King Henry VIII.

1521 *De temperamentis* and *De inaequali intemperie.* 4to. Cambridge: J. Siberch. *STC* 11536. Dedicated to Pope Leo X.

1522(?) *De pulsuum usu.* 4to. London: R. Pynson. *STC* 11534. Dedicated to Cardinal Wolsey.

1523 *De naturalibus facultatibus.* 4to. London: R. Pynson. *STC* 11533. Dedicated to William Warham, Archbishop of Canterbury.

1524 *De symptomatum differentiis. De symptomatum causis.* 4to. London: R. Pynson. *STC* 11535. [Posthumous publication.][6]

All of these texts, with the exception of the first six books of the *Methodus medendi* and the *De pulsuum usu*, had already been translated from the Greek during the Middle Ages. Niccolò da Reggio had translated the first five books of the *De sanitate tuenda* in their entirety,[7]

---

[1] *Inc.*: 'Que est optima constructio corporis nostri . . .' (TK², col. 1183).

[2] *Inc.*: 'Inequalis discrasia fit quidem . . .' (cf. TK², col. 742).

[3] *Inc.*: 'Medicinalis artis intentio quidem sanitas . . .' (TK², col. 859).

[4] *Inc.* (Bibl. nat. 6865, s. xiv, f. 184vb): 'De pronosticatione igitur consequenter dicimus . . .' (not in TK²; cf. Cesena Sin. Plut. 5, cod. 4, s. xiv, fols. 134va–135va, Paris, Académie de Médecine 51, s. xv, fols. 198^r–201^v).

[5] For details of the numerous reprints, I refer readers to my 'Census'. This shows that Linacre's versions eventually supplanted their rivals.

[6] Though mentioned on the title-page to a version by Leoniceno ('Census', 1522(?).1), Linacre's texts are not included in the two copies known to me. I therefore now assume that they first appeared posthumously in the edition of 1524, which refers to Linacre's death and benefactions.

[7] *Inc.* (Munich, Clm. 35, s. xiv, f. 2ra): 'Ea que circa corpus hominis arte una existente . . .' (TK², col. 479).

and Burgundio the sixth book,[1] as well as an epitome(?) of the first five, which is unfortunately useless for comparison purposes. The tradition of the *Methodus medendi* is equally complicated. As Linacre himself remarks in his preface, the student had previously to depend either on jejune extracts culled by some Arab—an oblique reference to Constantine's *Megategni*[2]—or on what Linacre considered barbarous and unreliable versions. One of these was Gerard of Cremona's rendering from the Arabic of all fourteen books.[3] The other was of books 7–14 only, by Burgundio from the Greek. The editor of the *editio princeps* of 1490 had printed books 1–6 in Gerard's version and the remainder in Burgundio's. Linacre's rendering of the first six books was therefore particularly valuable. The third text, the *De temperamentis*, had been translated by Burgundio, but his very literal rendering from the Greek, the beginning of which I print for the first time,[4] had been too little diffused to gain Bonardus's attention. He printed instead the ubiquitous Arabic-Latin version of Gerard.[5] The *De inaequali intemperie* had been translated by Niccolò long before Valla, Leoniceno, or Linacre: I print a specimen below. For the *De pulsuum usu*, medieval readers had had to rely on Marc of Toledo's rendering of Hunain's Arabic; the extract printed here gives one an inkling of his execrable style. Burgundio had translated the *De naturalibus facultatibus* from a better manuscript than that available to Linacre and Leoniceno. Finally, both treatises on symptoms had been rendered from the Greek, but only versions from the Arabic were included in the 1490 *editio princeps*.[6] Specimens

[1] *Inc.* (ibid., f. 32ra): 'Alterius materie sanativarum contemplationum principium in hoc libro . . .' (TK², col. 87, cites one fifteenth-century MS. only, but the text was widely diffused). For Burgundio's curious (and untypical) handling of the first five books see Koch, *CMG*, v. 4. 2, pp. xvii–xviii.

[2] Constantine's prologue begins (Boulogne-sur-Mer 197, s. xiii, f. 88ra): 'Quamvis karissime fili Johannes ingenium acutissimum . . .' (cf. TK², col. 1163). The text is included in the 1515 edition of Isaac Israeli's *Omnia opera*.

[3] *Inc.* (Vat. lat. 2375, s. xiv, f. 304ra): 'Librum de sanitatis ingenio a te et a multis . . .' (TK², col. 825).

[4] I am about to publish a critical edition of Burgundio's version with a detailed introduction on his translation technique.

[5] *Inc.* (Naples VIII.D.30, s. xiv, f. 1ra): 'Insignes antiqui medicorum et philosophorum . . .' (TK², col. 752).

[6] They are included in the six books known to medieval students as *De accidenti et morbo*. See my note in *Traditio*, art. cit., s.v. 'Census', nos. 64a, 65a, 112a, 113a.

of the former appear here for the first time, from a Wellcome manuscript.

Let us take each of Linacre's translations in turn, paying due attention to his dedicatory letters and remarks to the reader. We must also attempt to identify, where possible, the Greek manuscript(s) he may have used, for his merits must be assessed in the light of his exemplars. A detailed critique is out of the question here. A general discussion of his style and technique will be found in the following section.

In his dedicatory letter to King Henry, Linacre states that he was urged to publish his first version by the learned of Italy, Germany, and France, especially by 'the two lights of our time', Erasmus and Budé. More revealing is his letter to the reader, the most explicit statement of his stylistic aims and procedures. Particularly important is his admission that he had access to only one manuscript of the *De sanitate tuenda*, that he was fully aware of its *lacunae*, and had attempted to fill them (*suo Marte*) within square brackets. Konrad Koch, the latest editor of the Greek text (*Corpus medicorum Graecorum*, hereafter *CMG*, v. 4, 2), praises Linacre's work highly, noting that he made a number of happy conjectures which inspired Cornarius and Caius. Nevertheless, some of the defects of his exemplar are inevitably reflected in his version, though they do not seriously impair it. Koch shows that in all probability, his exemplar was a *gemellus* of Leipzig 50 (Koch's L), belonging to the inferior *b* family. The reader can obtain some idea of Linacre's performance from the following. I regret very much not being able to include a sample of Niccolò's version for comparison.

DE SANITATE TUENDA i, 1

CMG v. 4, 2 Koch

Τῆς περὶ τὸ σῶμα τἀνθρώπου τέχνης μιᾶς οὔσης, ὡς ἐν ἑτέρῳ δέδεικται γράμματι, δύο ἐστὶ τὰ πρῶτά τε καὶ μέγιστα μόρια· καλεῖται δὲ τὸ μὲν ἕτερον αὐτῶν ὑγιεινόν, τὸ δὲ ἕτερον θεραπευτικόν, ἔμπαλιν ἔχοντα πρὸς ἄλληλα ταῖς ἐνεργείαις, ἐπειδή γε τῷ μὲν φυλάξαι, τῷ δ' ἀλλοιῶσαι πρόκειται τὴν περὶ τὸ σῶμα κατάστασιν. ἐπεὶ δὲ καὶ χρόνῳ καὶ ἀξιώματι πρότερόν ἐστιν ὑγεία νόσου, χρὴ δήπου καὶ ἡμᾶς, ὅπως ἄν τις ταύτην φυλά-

LINACRE (*ed. princ.*)

Inc. Cum una sit ars, quae corpori hominis tuendo dicata sit: ut alibi a nobis ostensum est: eius primae ac maximae partes sunt due. Quarum alteram sanitatis tuendae: alteram morbi profligandi facultatem appelles. Earum contraria inter se officia sunt, siquidem illi tueri, huic immutare statum corporis est propositum. Quoniam autem & dignitate & tempore sanitas morbum praecedit: utique & nobis quem-

ξειεν, ἐσκέφθαι πρότερον, ἐφεξῆς δὲ καί, ὡς ἄν τις ἄριστα νόσους ἐξιῷτο. κοινὴ δ' ἀμφοτέροις ὁδὸς τῆς εὑρέσεως, εἰ γνοίημεν, ὁποία τίς ἐστιν ἡ διάθεσις τοῦ σώματος, ἣν ὑγείαν ὀνομάζομεν· οὐ γὰρ ἂν οὔτε φυλάττειν αὐτὴν παροῦσαν οὔτ' ἀνακτήσασθαι διαφθειρομένην οἷοί τε ἦμεν ἀγνοοῦντες τὸ παράπαν, ἥτις πότ' ἐστι. γέγραπται δὲ ἡμῖν ἑτέρωθι καὶ περὶ τοῦδε καὶ δέδεικται τῶν μὲν ὁμοιομερῶν ὀνομαζομένων ἡ ὑγεία, ψυχροῦ καὶ θερμοῦ καὶ ξηροῦ καὶ ὑγροῦ, συμμετρία τις ὑπάρχουσα, τῶν δ' ὀργανικῶν ἐκ τῆς τῶν ὁμοιομερῶν συνθέσεώς τε καὶ ποσότητος καὶ πηλικότητος καὶ διαπλάσεως ἀποτελουμένη. ὥστε καὶ ὅστις ἂν ἱκανὸς ᾖ φυλάττειν ταῦτα, φύλαξ οὗτος ἀγαθὸς ὑγείας ἔσται.

admodum haec servanda sit: prius tractare conveniet. Post autem, quo pacto commodissime morbus sit abigendus, utriusque facultatis inveniendae communis ratio est: ut quidnam ea corporis affectio sit quae sanitas dicitur, liquido constet. Quandoquidem nec praesentem servare, nec amissam restituere, si eam penitus ignores, licet. Scripsimus de hoc alibi, ostendimusque similarium quas vocant partium sanitatem, calidi, frigidi, humidi, & sicci, Symmetrian id est convenientiam inter se quandam esse. Instrumentarium vero, ex similarium ipsarum compositione, numero, magnitudine figuraque constare. Quare quisquis haec commode tueri possit: is optimus sanitatis custos fuerit.

The *Methodus medendi* (1519) is prefaced by an important letter of Guillaume Budé to Thomas Lupset. Budé tells him he had compared selected passages with the Greek exemplar (presumably the Greek *editio princeps* of 1500) and had attempted in vain to improve on Linacre's performance. He praises the translator's elegant and exquisite style, noting Linacre's preference for the *prisca scribendi vertendique severitas* in a passage to be recalled by Gesner; some later critics were to find this *severitas* excessive. Linacre's own letter to the King comments on the prolixity of the work and regrets that nobody had yet done it justice: earlier versions are unfaithful and barbaric. As for his own, he trusts his readers will pardon an occasional fault due to the sheer tedium of his task. In fact, a careful comparison of his version with Kühn's text of over 1,000 pages has revealed a number of omissions[1] but no serious mistakes. I know of no cogent evidence to suggest that he did not avail himself of the printed edition of 1500. Thus he faithfully translates its reading πολλοὺς καὶ ἑτέρους at x. 57. 18 K. ('multos etiam alios'): the true

---

[1] The more important omissions include x. 44. 7–8 K. ὥσπερ–διάλεκτον; 89. 15 ἡ διάθεσις–ἀρρωστία; 164. 12–13 κατὰ σύμβασιν–τούτῳ; 170. 5 οἶστοιχείων; 275. 16–17 χρονίζει–θεραπείαν; 278. 7–9 ὅτι–θεραπείαν; 314. 1 πῶς οὖν–τὸ αἷμα; 349. 15–18 ἐπειδὴ–πορεύεται; 396. 7 ἵνα–φθονοῦντες; 404. 13–14 ὅπερ–συνήθως; 875. 16–17 ἀεὶ–μορίοις; 1021. 8 ὁποῖον–πτέρις.

reading, given by the Aldine and subsequent editions, is πολλῷ σκαιοτέρους. Elsewhere, Linacre's version, printed with minor changes by Kühn, yields better sense than the latter's Greek. Thus at x. 228. 7 Linacre rightly reads *putant* (= οἴονται) where Kühn has οἶόν τε; at 337. 8 Linacre has *variabitur* (= ἐξαλλαχθήσεται) for Kühn's ἐξελεγχθήσεται; at 479. 1 *legerit* suggests ⟨ἀνα⟩γινώσκειν and at 552. 10 Linacre's *transpirabile* (= εὔπνουν) is clearly preferable to ἔμπνουν.

I append the openings of books I and VII.

METHODUS MEDENDI i. 1

x. 1–2. 10 Kühn

Ἐπειδὴ καὶ σύ με πολλάκις, ὦ Ἱέρων φίλτατε, καὶ ἄλλοι τινὲς νῦν ἑταῖροι παρακαλοῦσι θεραπευτικὴν μέθοδον αὐτοῖς γράψαι, ἐγὼ δὲ μάλιστα μὲν καὶ ὑμῖν χαρίζεσθαι βουλόμενος, οὐχ ἥκιστα δὲ καὶ τοὺς μεθ' ἡμᾶς ἀνθρώπους ὠφελῆσαι καθ' ὅσον οἷός τέ εἰμι προαιρούμενος, ὅμως ὤκνουν τε καὶ ἀνεβαλλόμην ἑκάστοτε διὰ πολλὰς αἰτίας, ἄμεινον εἶναί μοι δοκεῖ καὶ νῦν αὐτὰς διελθεῖν, πρὶν ἄρξασθαι τῆς πραγματείας, ἔχουσι γάρ τι χρήσιμον εἰς τὰ μέλλοντα ῥηθήσεσθαι. κεφάλαιον μὲν οὖν ἁπασῶν αὐτῶν ἐστι τὸ κινδυνεῦσαι μάτην γράψαι, μηδενὸς τῶν νῦν ἀνθρώπων ὡς ἔπος εἰπεῖν ἀλήθειαν σπουδάζοντος, ἀλλὰ χρήματά τε καὶ δυνάμεις πολιτικὰς καὶ ἀπλήστους ἡδονῶν ἀπολαύσεις ἐζηλωκότων ἐς τοσοῦτον ὡς μαίνεσθαι νομίζειν εἴ τις ἄρα καὶ γένοιτο σοφίαν ἀσκῶν ἡντιναοῦν. αὐτὴν μὲν γὰρ τὴν πρώτην καὶ ὄντως σοφίαν, ἐπιστήμην οὖσαν θείων τε καὶ ἀνθρωπίνων πραγμάτων, οὐδ' εἶναι νομίζουσι τὸ παράπαν· ἰατρικὴν δὲ καὶ γεωμετρίαν καὶ ῥητορικὴν ἀριθμητικήν τε καὶ μουσικὴν ἁπάσας τε τὰς τοιαύτας τέχνας εἶναι μὲν ὑπολαμβάνουσιν, οὐ μὴν ἐπί γε τὸ τέλος αὐτῶν ἰέναι δικαιοῦσιν.

LINACRE (*ed. princ.*)

Inc. Cum et tu saepe alias charissime Hiero: et alii quidam amici me nunc hortentur, ut sibi medendi methodum conscribam: ego sane tametsi tum vobis imprimis gratificari: tum vero posteros non nihil pro viribus iuvare studens: semper tamen fateor cunctabar ac distuli multis de causis, quas nunc quoque percommode dicturus videor priusquam id quod petitis aggrediar. Sunt enim ad ea quae post dicentur sane non inutiles. Earum igitur omnium illa praecipua fuit, quod frustra me scriptum timebam. Cum nemo prope dixerim, hac nostra aetate veritatis inquisitioni sit deditus, sed pecuniam, & civilem potentiam, et inexplebiles voluptatum delicias, omnes eousque suspiciant: ut si quis sapientiae quodvis studium sectetur, pro insano hunc habeant. Quippe qui primam ipsam & vere sapientiam, quae divinarum hum⟨an⟩arumque rerum est scientia, ne esse quidem omnino existiment. Medicinam, Geometriam, Rhetoricen, Arithmeticen, Musicen, ac reliquas id genus artes, esse quidem autument, caeterum ad finem earum studio contendendum minime censeant.

METHODUS MEDENDI vii. 1

x. 456–457. 10 Kühn

Τὴν θεραπευτικὴν μέθοδον, ὦ Εὐγενιανὲ φίλτατε, πάλαι μὲν ὑπηρξάμην γράφειν Ἱέρωνι χαριζόμενος, ἐπεὶ δὲ ἐξαίφνης ἐκεῖνος ἀποδημίαν μακρὰν ἀναγκασθεὶς στείλασθαι, μετ' οὐ πολὺν χρόνον ἠγγέλθη τεθνεώς, ἐγκατέλιπον κἀγὼ τὴν γραφήν. οἶσθα γὰρ ὡς οὔτε ταύτην οὔτε ἄλλην τινὰ πραγματείαν ἔγραψα τῆς παρὰ τοῖς πολλοῖς ἐφιέμενος δόξης, ἀλλ' ἤτοι φίλοις χαριζόμενος ἢ γυμνάζων ἐμαυτόν, εἴς τε τὰ παρόντα χρησιμώτατον γυμνάσιον εἴς τε τὸ τῆς λήθης γῆρας, ὡς ὁ Πλάτων φησίν, ὑπομνήματα θησαυρισόμενος. ὁ γάρ τοι τῶν πολλῶν ἀνθρώπων ἔπαινος εἰς μὲν χρείας τινὰς ἐπιτήδειον ὄργανον ἐνίοτε γίγνεται τοῖς ζῶσιν, ἀποθανόντας δὲ οὐδὲν ὀνίνησιν, ὥσπερ οὐδὲ τῶν ζώντων ἐνίους. ὅσοι γὰρ ἥσυχον εἵλοντο βίον, ὠφελημένοι μὲν ἐκ τῆς φιλοσοφίας, αὐτάρκη δ' ἔχοντες τὰ πρὸς τὴν τοῦ σώματος θεραπείαν, τούτοις ἐμπόδιον οὐ σμικρόν ἐστιν ἡ παρὰ τοῖς πολλοῖς δόξα, περαιτέρω τοῦ προσήκοντος ἀπάγουσα τῶν καλλίστων αὐτούς. ὥσπερ ἀμέλει καὶ ἡμᾶς οἶσθα πολλάκις ἀνιωμένους ἐπὶ τοῖς ἐνοχλοῦσιν οὕτω συνεχῶς ἐνίοτε χρόνον ἐφεξῆς πολύν, ὡς μηδ' ἄψασθαι δυνηθῆναι βιβλίου.

LINACRE (*ed. princ.*)

Inc. Medendi methodum Eugeniane charissime, quam olim in Hieronis gratiam scribendam susceperam, posteaquam illum subito longum iter ingredi coactum, non multo post diem obiisse nunciatum: ipsi quoque persequi destitimus. Tu enim mihi conscius es, neque hoc me opus: neque aliud ullum popularis aurae studio fuisse aggressum, sed quo vel amicis gratificarer: vel me ipsum simul utilissima ratione ad rem propositam exercitarem: simul ad oblivionem senii (ut Plato inquit) commentarios mihi reponerem. Quippe multitudinis laus commodum ad usus nonnullos instrumentum viventibus aliquando est, mortuis certe nihil prodest, sicut neque viventium quibusdam. Nam qui vivere in tranquillo optarunt, ac fructum ex philosophia ceperunt, & iis quae corpori curando sufficiunt sunt contenti: hiis utique impedimento non parvo est apud vulgum fama, ut quae eos a rebus pulcherrimis plus justo tranverses auferat; veluti me quoque non ignoras ab iis quae sunt molesta, sic nonnunquam taedio affectum: ut bono interdum spatio ne tangere quidem librum possim.

The *De temperamentis* followed two years later. Dedicated to Pope Leo X, with whom Linacre had long before been a fellow pupil and to whom he was recently indebted for an unspecified favour, it is a version of a book 'admittedly short, but necessary no less to philosophers than to physicians', as he remarks. Galen discusses temperaments in terms of single or paired primary qualities (hot, cold, wet, dry) and introduces a number of familiar Aristotelian distinctions (e.g. between actual and potential, innate and acquired). The work is primarily theoretical, but its discussion in book 3 of the distinction between foodstuffs and drugs has important implications for pharmacology and therapy in general. It had been widely studied in the Middle Ages in Gerard's version; few had consulted Burgundio's. Thanks to the existence of a modern critical edition by Georg Helmreich, we can identify with some ease the Greek manuscripts available to both men. Burgundio, as I shall show elsewhere, had access to the parent of our earliest and best manuscript, Laurentianus 74, 5 (Helmreich's *L*): Linacre, on the other hand, used an inferior manuscript, either Bodleian Laud. 58 (Helmreich's *O*) or its parent, Vatican gr. 282. I quote *O* since Helmreich, unaware of the true relationship of the two manuscripts, failed to collate Vat. gr. 282 in full. First, Linacre shares *O*'s *lacunae* at 77. 24 Helmreich, 83. 20–1, and 95. 1. Second, he constantly reflects *O*'s readings, e.g.

O (*Linacre*)	*Cett.* (*LMTV*)
35. 10 H. ξηρότητι (siccitate)	σκληρότητι *LT*(*V*) σμικρότητι *M*
49. 2 κινήσεως (motu)	νοήσεως
64. 6 σκληρότερον (durius)	ξηρότερον
91. 13 εἰ δ' ἐκεῖνο (At si illa)	εἰ δὲ κείνως *L*¹ (κοινῶς *L*²): εἰ δ' ἱκανῶς *MT*
98. 17 ταύτῃ (ad hunc modum)	ταυτὶ *LT* ταῦτα *M*
115. 25 καὶ διδάσκεσθαι (tum doceri)	*om.*

I print herewith book 1, chapter 1 in the two Graeco-Latin versions of Burgundio and Linacre.

DE TEMPERAMENTIS i. 1

Ed. G. Helmreich (Leipzig, Teubner, 1904; repr. 1969).

Ὅτι μὲν ἐκ θερμοῦ καὶ ψυχροῦ καὶ ξηροῦ καὶ ὑγροῦ τὰ τῶν ζῴων σώματα κέκραται καὶ ὡς οὐκ ἴση πάντων ἐστὶν ἐν τῇ κράσει μοῖρα, παλαιοῖς ἀνδράσιν ἱκανῶς ἀποδέδεικται φιλοσόφων τε καὶ ἰατρῶν τοῖς ἀρίστοις· εἴρηται δὲ καὶ πρὸς ἡμῶν ὑπὲρ αὐτῶν τὰ εἰκότα δι' ἑτέρου γράμματος, ἐν ᾧ περὶ τῶν καθ' Ἱπποκράτην στοιχείων ἐσκοπούμεθα. νυνὶ δ', ὅπερ ἐστὶν ἐφεξῆς ἐκείνῳ, ἁπάσας ἐξευρεῖν τῶν κράσεων τὰς διαφοράς, ὁπόσαι τ' εἰσὶ καὶ ὁποῖαι κατ' εἴδη τε καὶ γένη διαιρουμένοις, ἐν τῷδε τῷ γράμματι δίειμι τὴν ἀρχὴν ἀπὸ τῆς τῶν ὀνομάτων ἐξηγήσεως ποιησάμενος. ἐπειδὰν μὲν γὰρ ἐκ θερμοῦ καὶ ψυχροῦ καὶ ξηροῦ καὶ ὑγροῦ κεκρᾶσθαι λέγωσι τὰ σώματα, τῶν ἄκρως τοιούτων ἀκούειν φασὶ χρῆναι, τουτέστι τῶν στοιχείων αὐτῶν, ἀέρος καὶ πυρὸς καὶ ὕδατος καὶ γῆς· ἐπειδὰν δὲ ζῷον ἢ φυτὸν ἤτοι θερμὸν ἢ ψυχρὸν ἢ ξηρὸν ἢ ὑγρὸν εἶναι λέγωσιν, οὐκέθ' ὡσαύτως. οὐδὲ γὰρ δύνασθαι ζῷον οὐδὲν οὔτ' ἄκρως θερμὸν ὑπάρχειν ὡς πῦρ οὔτ' ἄκρως ὑγρὸν ὡς ὕδωρ. ὡσαύτως δ' οὐδὲ ψυχρὸν ἢ ξηρὸν ἐσχάτως, ἀλλ' ἀπὸ τοῦ πλεονεκτοῦντος ἐν τῇ κράσει γίγνεσθαι τὰς προσηγορίας, ὑγρὸν μὲν καλούντων ἡμῶν, ἐν ᾧ πλείων ὑγρότητός ἐστι μοῖρα, ξηρὸν δ', ἐν ᾧ ξηρότητος· οὕτω δὲ καὶ θερμὸν μέν, ἐν ᾧ τὸ θερμὸν τοῦ ψυχροῦ πλεονεκτεῖ, ψυχρὸν δ', ἐν ᾧ τὸ ψυχρὸν τοῦ θερμοῦ. αὕτη μὲν ἡ τῶν ὀνομάτων χρῆσις.

LINACRE (*ed. princ.*)

Inc. Constare animalium corpora ex calidi, frigidi, sicci, humidique mixtura, nec esse horum omnium parem in temperatura portionem demonstratum antiquis abunde est, tum philosophorum, tum medicorum praecipuis. Diximus autem & nos de iis, ea quae probabilia sunt visa alio opere, in quo de iis, quae Hyppocrates constituit elementis, egimus. Hoc opere, quod illi proxime succedit, omnium temperamentorum differentias, quot hae, qualesque sint, sive generatim quis, sive membratim dividat, invenire docebo. Sumamque ab ipsa nominum interpretatione principium. Cum nanque ex calidi, frigidi, sicci, & humidi, temperatura conflari corpora dicunt, de iis, quae summo gradu sic se habent, ipsis scilicet elementis, aere, igni, aqua, terra, intelligendum aiunt. Cum vero animal, stirpemve calidam, humidam, frigidam, vel siccam esse, non item. Neque enim ullum animal, aut calidam in summo esse posse, ut est ignis, aut in summo humidum, sicut est aqua: pari modo nec frigidum, siccumve in summo. Sed ab eo quod in mixtura pollet, appellationem sortiri, vocantibus nobis id humidum, in quo maior est humiditatis portio, siccum, in quo siccitatis. Ita vero et calidum, in quo calidum frigido plus valet, frigidum vero in quo frigidum calido praestat. Atque hic quidem nominum usus est.

BURGUNDIO OF PISA

Inc. Quoniam quidem ex calido et frigido et sicco et humido animalium confusa sunt corpora et quod non equalis omnium est in confusione particula, a veteribus viris sufficienter demonstratum est et philosophorum et medicorum nobilioribus: dicta sunt autem et a nobis super hiis que oportet in alio libro, in quo De secundum Ypocratem elementis scrutati sumus. Nunc autem, quod est deinceps illi, omnes invenire complexionum differentias, et quot sunt et quales secundum species et genera dividentibus, in hoc libro pertranseo, principium a nominum expositione faciens. Cum quidem enim ex calido et frigido et sicco et humido commixta esse dicunt animalium corpora, de summe talibus intelligere inquiunt oportere, idest elementis ipsis, aere, igne, terra et aqua. Cum autem animal vel arborem vel calidum vel frigidum vel siccum vel humidum esse dicunt, non adhuc similiter. Neque enim potest animal esse aliquod seu extreme calidum ut ignis seu summe humidum ut aqua. Similiter autem neque frigidum neque siccum ultime, sed ab habundante in commixtione fieri appellationes, humidum quidem vocantibus nobis, in quo est maior humiditatis particula, siccum autem, in quo siccitatis: similiter autem et calidum quidem, in quo calidum frigido superhabundat, frigidum autem, in quo frigidum calido. Hic quidem igitur nominum usus. (MSS. Boulogne-sur-Mer 197, s. xiii, fol. 141va; Munich Clm 35, s. xiii, fol. 114va; Vat. Barb. lat. 179, s. xiv, fol. 1ra; Wellcome 286, s. xiv, fol. 1ra.)

The *De inaequali intemperie,* included in what would appear to be the second issue of the preceding, need not detain us long. Again

Galen shows from his final remarks (vii. 752. 16–18 K.) that he considered it an essential preliminary to the reading of his works on pharmacology and therapeutics. It also looks forward to his treatises *De symptomatum causis* (746. 14 K.) and *De morborum causis* (748. 9–10 K.) where he will treat of internal and external causes of fever. It is a little difficult to understand its attraction for the three humanists Valla, Leoniceno, and Linacre: perhaps its very brevity was sufficient recommendation. There exists no modern critical edition, but a collation of Bodleian MS. Laud. gr. 58 (*O*) shows once again that this was in all probability the translator's exemplar. Thus at 733. 12 Linacre's *aliquatenus* reflects *O*'s addition of κατά τι after ἀλλοιουμένων and *medicamentis* at 734. 3 that of φαρμάκων following προσπιπτόντων, while his *multum* at 736.3 corresponds to *O*'s πολὺ (*pro* παχὺ).

DE INAEQUALI INTEMPERIE
vii. 733–734. 10 Kühn

Ἀνώμαλος δυσκρασία γίνεται μὲν καὶ καθ᾽ ὅλον τοῦ ζῴου τὸ σῶμα ἐνίοτε, καθάπερ ἔν τε τοῖς ἀνὰ σάρκα λεγομένοις ὑδέροις, καὶ τοῖς ἠπιάλοις καλουμένοις πυρετοῖς, καὶ σχεδὸν ἅπασι τοῖς ἄλλοις, πλὴν τῶν ἑκτικῶν ὀνομαζομένων· γίνεται δὲ καὶ καθ᾽ ἓν ὁτιοῦν μόριον, οἰδισκόμενον, ἢ φλεγμαῖνον, ἢ γαγγραινόμενον, ἢ ἐρυσιπελατούμενον, ἢ καρκινούμενον. τούτου δὲ τοῦ γένους καὶ ὁ καλούμενος ἐλέφας καὶ ἡ φαγέδαινα καὶ ὁ ἕρπης. ἀλλὰ ταῦτα μὲν ἅπαντα μετὰ ῥευμάτων· ἄνευ δ᾽ ὕλης ἐπιρρύτου, μόναις ταῖς ποιότησιν ἀλλοιουμένων τῶν μορίων, ἀνώμαλοι γίνονται δυσκρασίαι, ψυχθέντων, ἢ ἐκκαυθέντων, ἢ γυμνασαμένων ἐπὶ πλέον, ἢ ἀργησάντων, ἤ τι τοιοῦτον ἕτερον παθόντων. οὐ μὴν ἀλλὰ κἀκ τῶν ἔξωθεν προσπιπτόντων ἀνώμαλοι δυσκρασίαι τοῖς σώμασιν ἡμῶν πλείονες ἐγγίνονται, θερμαινομένοις, ἢ ψυχομένοις, ἢ ξηραινομένοις, ἢ ὑγραινομένοις. ἁπλαῖ μὲν γὰρ αὗται, καθότι κἀν τοῖς περὶ κράσεων ὑπομνήμασιν ἐδείκνυτο· σύνθετοι δὲ ἐξ αὐτῶν εἰσιν ἕτεραι τέσσαρες, ἢ θερμαινομένων ἅμα καὶ ξηραινομένων, ἢ ψυχομένων τε ἅμα καὶ ὑγραινομένων, ἢ ψυχομένων τε ἅμα καὶ ξηραινομένων, ἢ θερμαινομένων τε ἅμα καὶ ὑγραινομένων.

LINACRE (*ed. princ.*)	NICCOLÒ DA REGGIO
Inc. Inaequalis intemperies alias in toto animalis corpore fit, veluti in ea hydropis specie, quam graeci ἀνασάρχα[!] vocant & febribus iis, quas iidem hepialas appellant, fereque reliquis omnibus, exceptis, quas Hecticas nominant. Incidit autem & in unaqualibet parte, quum ea vel intumuit, vel Phlegmone, Gangrena, Erisipilate, Cancrove, est affecta. Huc pertinet & qui Elephas dicitur,	*Inc.* Inequalis discrasia fit quidem et secundum totum animalis corpus quandoque, quemadmodum in anasarca vocatis yderis et empielis vocatis[1] febribus et fere universis aliis preter ethicas. Fit autem et secundum unamquamque particulam ydemantem vel flegminantem vel gangrenantem vel erisipilate laborantem vel cancro. Huius autem generis [1] dictis *ed.*

& Phagedena, & Herpes. Verum haec omnia cum fluxione consistunt. Absque autem materiae affluxu, solis partium qualitatibus aliquatenus alterandis, inaequales intemperies fiunt, utique refrigeratis iis, aut deustis, aut immodice exercitatis, aut feriatis, aut aliquid id genus passis. Iam ex medicamentis iis, quae foris corpori occurrunt, inaequalis intemperies gignitur, dum id vel frigefit, vel cafefit, vel siccatur, vel humectum redditur. Quippe hae simplices intemperies sunt, veluti in iis, quae de temperamentis scripsimus, est monstratum. Compositae ex iis aliae quatuor sunt, quum corpus vel calefit simul & siccatur, vel calefit simul & humectatur, vel refrigeratur simul & siccescit, vel refrigeratur pariter & madescit.

est et ⟨qui⟩ vocatur[1] elefas et fagedena et erpes. Sed hec quidem universa cum reumatibus: absque materia vero influente, solis qualitatibus alteratis particulis, inequales fiunt discrasie [734 K.] frigefientibus vel estuantibus vel exercitantibus amplius vel ociantibus vel quid tale aliud patientibus. Attamen et ab extrorsum incidentibus inequales discrasie corporibus nostris fiunt[2] cum calefiunt vel infrigidantur vel exiccantur vel humectantur. Simplices quidem et hee sunt sicut in monumentis de crasibus monstrabatur. Composite vero ex hiis sunt alie quatuor quando ⟨vel⟩ calefiunt simul et exiccantur[3] vel calefiunt & humectantur vel infrigidantur et exiccantur vel infrigidantur & humectantur. (Wellcome MS. 286, s. xiv, fol. 132ʳ: Giunta ed. 1528, t. 1, fol. xliiʳ.)

[1] ⟨qui⟩ vocatur] vocatus *ed.*   [2] fiunt *om. MS.*   [3] quando . . . exiccantur *om. MS.*

The next version to be considered, that of the *De pulsuum usu*, was published, perhaps in 1522, by the Royal Printer, Richard Pynson. Linacre's dedicatory letter to Cardinal Wolsey contains little but the platitudes expected of a client. The treatise is brief but not unimportant: Galen here considers the role of the arteries as analogous to that of the organs of respiration, diastole being compared to inhalation, systole to exhalation. Their joint end is the conservation of the innate heat: the former cools, the latter purifies by purging the body of the sooty vapours accumulated as a result of humoral combustion (see particularly v. 161. 8–17, 163. 14–17 K.).

There exists no modern critical edition. I have compared Linacre's version with both the Aldine *editio princeps* and Kühn's text: misprints apart, the two are virtually identical. However, the Aldine text omits one or two phrases faithfully rendered by Linacre, e.g. διότι—ἠδύνατο at v. 155. 2–3 K. and ὥσπερ—πρόδηλον at 170. 16–17. At v. 152. 7, Linacre must have read or conjectured ἀλγούντων for ἀργούντων; at 167. 15 his *particula* (μόριον) is obviously right; the printed editions have μόνον. Otherwise, we find a few minor omissions, the only one worth reporting being that of εἰς τὴν καρδίαν at v. 167.1 K.

I print herewith the beginning of Linacre's version with, for comparison, Marc of Toledo's rendering of Ḥunain's Arabic:

DE PULSUUM USU

v. 149–150. 5 Kühn

Τίς ἡ χρεία τῶν σφυγμῶν; ἆρά γε ἥπερ καὶ τῆς ἀναπνοῆς, ἃς σχεδὸν ἅπασιν ἰατροῖς τε καὶ φιλοσόφοις ἔδοξεν, ἤ τις ἑτέρα παρὰ ταύτην; οὐ γὰρ δὴ ἀβασανίστως πειστέον αὐτοῖς, ἐναντιοῦσθαι δοκούντων ἄλλων τέ τινων οὐκ ὀλίγων φαινομένων, καὶ τοῦ νῦν εἰρῆσθαι μέλλοντος οὐχ ἥκιστα. στερηθέντες μὲν γὰρ τῆς ἀναπνοῆς εὐθέως ἀποθνήσκομεν, ἄσφυκτα δ᾽ ἀπεργάσῃ πολλὰ τῶν μορίων ἄνευ μεγάλης βλάβης. εἰ γοῦν ἐθελήσαις[1] ἢ τὰς διὰ τῶν βουβώνων ἐπὶ τὰ σκέλη καθηκούσας ἀρτηρίας, ἢ τὰς διὰ τῶν μασχαλῶν εἰς τὰς χεῖρας βρόχῳ διαλαβεῖν, ἀσφύκτους μὲν εὐθέως ἐργάσῃ τὰς ἐν τοῖς κώλοις ἁπάσας, οὐ μὴν παραλύσεις ταῦτα τῆς καθ᾽ ὁρμὴν κινήσεως, ὥσπερ οὐδὲ τῆς αἰσθήσεως.

[1] ἐθελήσαις *scripsi*: ἐθελήσῃς Kühn.

LINACRE (*ed. princ.*)

Inc. Quemnam esse dicat quis pulsuum usum, eundemne qui respirationis, ceu ferme tum medicis tum philosophis omnibus est visum: an praeter hunc alium? Neque enim protinus illis citraque examen est adhibenda fides, praesertim quum refragari huic sententiae, ex rebus evidentibus non paucae videantur, in primisque quod nunc subjiciam. Nam respirationem si cui adimes: illico mortem afferes. At pulsu si permultas particulas prives, non magnopere ledes. Quippe si [cf. 150 K.] vel arterias quae per inguina descendunt ad crura, vel quae per alas feruntur ad manus, laqueo complecti velis, universas quidem quae in his artubus arteriae habentur, pulsu privabis. Non tamen artubus ipsis, aut voluntarium motum adimes, aut etiam sensum.

MARC OF TOLEDO

Inc. Dixit Galienus. Oportet nos inspicere pulsus utilitatem an sit anhelitus perfectus iuxta opinionem phisicorum[1] et medicorum: tamen in maiori parte est alter: non enim decet nos credere eis absque inquisitione propter ea que dicant hoc esse: ceteri enim extimant hanc opinionem destruere. Repellitur enim & prohibetur a vero: ut nequaquam credatur esse vera non minus quam alia: quoniam quando nempe anhelitu privati fuerimus morimur incontinenti: sepe autem pulsu privantur multa membra corporis: nec tamen nocumentum incurrunt indecens. Si enim [cf. 150 K.] artarias que transeunt per inguines constringas: deinde que ad pedes aut venas que subtus asellas tendunt: demum ad eas que sunt in manibus accedas constringendas constrictione forti: venas omnes privabis pulsatiles pulsu incontinenti que sunt in manibus aut pedibus nec aliquid de motu adimetur [*in margine*: vel amittetur] voluntario: neque sensu. (Giunta ed., 1528, fol. lxxxvii[r].)

[1] philosophorum *MSS*.

Linacre's version of Galen's far more influential treatise, the *De naturalibus facultatibus*, followed in 1523. It was again published by the Royal Printer and dedicated to William Warham, Archbishop of Canterbury. To Warham, Linacre owed ecclesiastical preferment and with it the leisure necessary for his literary pursuits. In his preface, he mentions the illness which was to prove fatal, and certain business which had forced him to change his plans. Originally he had intended to dedicate to the Archbishop a version of *De elementis secundum Hippocratem*, of which the present is a logical and avowed sequel. Unfortunately this version has not survived: it would have been instructive to compare it with those of Leoniceno, Guinther, and Trincavelli.

There exists a modern critical edition of the *De naturalibus facultatibus*, again by Georg Helmreich. Linacre seems to have translated from the same Greek MS. that he had used for the *De temperamentis*. Linacre shares *O*'s lacuna at 153. 5–6 and constantly reflects its readings, e.g.

O (*Linacre*)	*Cett.* (*LMPT*)
107. 1 Η ἔχοι (habuerit)	εὕροι *L*: εὕρη *MPT*
113. 17 τῶν τελείων (perfectorum hominum)	*om.*
120. 6 τὰ δὲ κατέχει (alia teneat)	*om.*
120. 25 τῶν ἁπλῶν (simplicia)	*om.*
205. 24 πέπεισται βιαίως (creditque invitus)	π. βεβαίως
228. 20 χρόνου *O*¹: χρόνῳ *O*² (tempore)	μόνου
255. 23–4 τὸν ὁμοιότατον (quam simillimo)	τὸν ἐπιτηδειότατον

Burgundio, as I shall show elsewhere, had access to the parent of our earliest and best manuscript. I print the opening in both versions:

DE NATURALIBUS FACULTATIBUS

Scripta Minora iii. 101–102. 5 (ed. Helmreich)

Ἐπειδὴ τὸ μὲν αἰσθάνεσθαί τε καὶ κινεῖσθαι κατὰ προαίρεσιν ἴδια τῶν ζῴων ἐστί, τὸ δ' αὐξάνεσθαί τε καὶ τρέφεσθαι κοινὰ καὶ τοῖς φυτοῖς, εἴη ἂν τὰ μὲν πρότερα τῆς ψυχῆς, τὰ δὲ δεύτερα τῆς φύσεως ἔργα. εἰ δέ τις καὶ τοῖς φυτοῖς ψυχῆς μεταδίδωσι καὶ διαιρούμενος αὐτὰς ὀνομάζει φυτικὴν μὲν ταύτην, αἰσθη-τικὴν δὲ τὴν ἑτέραν, λέγει μὲν οὐδ' οὗτος ἄλλα, τῇ λέξει δ' οὐ πάνυ τῇ συνήθει κέχρηται. ἀλλ' ἡμεῖς γε μεγίστην λέξεως ἀρετὴν σαφήνειαν εἶναι πεπεισμένοι καὶ ταύτην εἰδότες ὑπ' οὐδενὸς οὕτως ὡς ὑπὸ τῶν ἀσυνήθων ὀνομάτων διαφθειρομένην, ὡς τοῖς πολλοῖς ἔθος, οὕτως ὀνομάζοντες ὑπὸ μὲν ψυχῆς θ' ἅμα καὶ φύσεως τὰ 3ῷα διοικεῖσθαί φαμεν, ὑπὸ δὲ φύσεως μόνης τὰ φυτὰ καὶ τό γ᾽ αὐξάνεσθαί τε καὶ τρέφεσθαι φύσεως ἔργα φαμέν, οὐ ψυχῆς.

Καὶ ζητήσομεν κατὰ τόνδε τὸν λόγον, ὑπὸ τίνων γίγνεται δυνάμεων αὐτὰ δὴ ταῦτα καὶ εἰ δή τι ἄλλο φύσεως ἔργον ἐστίν. ἀλλὰ πρότερόν γε διελέσθαι τε χρὴ καὶ μηνῦσαι σαφῶς ἕκαστον τῶν ὀνομάτων, οἷς χρησόμεθα κατὰ τόνδε τὸν λόγον, καὶ ἐφ᾽ ὅ τι φέρομεν πρᾶγμα. γενήσεται δὲ τοῦτ᾽ εὐθὺς ἔργων φυσικῶν διδασκαλία σὺν ταῖς τῶν ὀνομάτων ἐξηγήσεσιν.

LINACRE (*ed. princ.*)

Inc. Quum et sensus et voluntarius motus propria animalium sint, auctio et nutritio etiam iis communia, quae, propterea quod naturae ipsius sponte proveniunt, phyta gręcis, apo᾽ tu phyein idest nascendo sunt dicta: fuerint non inmerito priora duo, animę: posteriora, naturae ipsius opera. Quodsi quis etiam iis, quae naturae ipsius vi proveniunt: (Romani ea plantas stirpesve nominant) animam impertiat: atque alteram ab altera separans, hanc naturalem, illam sentientem appellet: diversa quidem quam nos minime dicit, dictione tamen utitur non perinde consueta. Nos vero claritatem maximam esse dictionis virtutem persuasi, atque eam nulla perinde re atque inusitatis nominibus viciari, prout vulgus hominum consuevit: ita nominantes, animal quidem ab anima simul et natura gubernari dicimus: stirpes a sola natura. Tum auctionem ac nutritionem naturę esse opera, animę nequaquam. Et in hoc quidem opere inquiremus, a quibus facultatibus auctio nutritioque, et si quod aliud naturae opus est, proveniant. Verum prius [102 H.] distinguamus, explicemusque oportet: de qua re singula quibus in hoc opere utemur, nomina dicantur. Fiet enim eo pacto, ut naturalium operum doctrina, una cum ipsis nominum interpretationibus, protinus tradatur.

BURGUNDIO OF PISA

Inc. Quoniam sentire quidem et moveri secundum electionem propria animalium sunt, augeri vero et nutriri communia[1] et plantis, erunt utique[2] priora anime, secunda vero nature opera. Si vero quis et plantis animam prebebit et dividens eas[3] nominabit plantativam quidem hanc, sensitivam vero[4] aliam, dicet quidem neque ipse[5] alia, dictione vero non valde assueta utetur. Set nos maximam dictionis demum bonitatem apertionem esse confitentes et hanc scientes a nullo ita ut ab insuetis nominibus corruptam, ut[6] multis consuetudo, ita nominantes[7] ab anima quidem simul et natura animalia dispensari aimus, a natura vero sola plantas et augeri demum et nutriri nature opera aimus, non anime. [Cap. II] Et[8] queremus secundum hunc sermonem a quibus fiunt virtutibus hec utique ipsa et si utique aliqua alia nature opera est. Set prius demum [102 H.] dividere[9] oportet et ostendere manifeste singulum nominum quibus utemur[10] secundum hunc sermonem et in quam ferimus rem hoc nomen.[11] Fiet autem hoc mox operum naturalium doctrina cum exposicionibus nominum. (Wellcome MS. 286, s. xiv, fol. 159: Giunta ed. 1528, t. 1, fol. ciii^v.)

[1] communia+eis *ed.* [2] itaque *MS.* [3] eam *MS.* [4] autem *ed.* [5] ipse neque *coll. MS.* [6] et *MS.*: et ut *ed.* [7] nominantes *conieci*: nominari *MS.*: nominandi *ed.* [8] Ut *MS.* [9] videre *ed.* [10] utetur *MS.* [11] τοὔνομα *add.* L(aurentianus 74, 5).

We come now to the last of Linacre's Galenic versions, published posthumously in 1524. In the present state of our knowledge of the text tradition of both *De symptomatum causis* and its sister work *De symptomatum differentiis*, we can only guess at the identity of the Greek manuscript available to the translator. In all probability it belonged to the same family as that used for the Aldine edition. Linacre's version echoes the Aldine readings at e.g. vii. 256. 16 K. (ἀτμοειδῶς for δροσοειδῶς), 266. 10–11 (τὰς κεραίας = ceraeas for the *lectio facilior* τὰ κέρατα), and 270. 2–3 (οὔτ' οὖν ἄλλην for οὔτ' ἄλλην ἀνίαν). The translator or his exemplar omitted two passages found in the *editio princeps*, namely vii. 77. 8–10 K. (αὐτὰς—ὁμογενεῖς) and 181. 2–4 (καθάπερ—περιττώματα); both involve homoeoteleuton. Other omissions may be due simply either to haste on the translator's part or to the printer's negligence. The most serious occurs on p. 118 of Kühn's edition, where six whole lines from ὥσπερ to ὁ λόγος ἦν are not translated: can Linacre have felt these references to Platonic synonyms for pain in the *Timaeus* and *Philebus* to be otiose? Surely the minor blemishes in this his last version can be explained more charitably in the light of its posthumous publication.

I append excerpts from Linacre's versions, together with the medieval Graeco-Latin renderings. The latter are here published for the first time.

DE SYMPTOMATUM CAUSIS

vii. 85–86. 7 Kühn

Τὰς αἰτίας τῶν συμπτωμάτων ἐν τοῖσδε τοῖς γράμμασι σκεψώμεθα, τὴν αὐτὴν τῷ λόγῳ τάξιν φυλάττοντες, ἣν κἂν τῷ περὶ διαφορᾶς αὐτῶν ἐποιησάμεθα. ἔστι μὲν οὖν τὰ σύμπαντα γένη τρία τῶν συμπτωμάτων. ἀλλὰ περὶ μὲν τούτου τοῦ πρώτου ὁ λόγος ἡμῖν ἐγένετο, καθὸ καὶ βεβλάφθαι τὴν ἐνέργειαν ἔφαμεν, οὕτως ἀκούειν ἀξιώσαντες, ὡς εἰ καὶ τελέως τις ἀπόλοιτο. διττῶν δ' οὐσῶν κατὰ γένος ἐνεργειῶν, τῶν μὲν φυσικῶν, τῶν δὲ ψυχικῶν, ἀπὸ τῶν ψυχικῶν ἠρξάμεθα, καὶ ταύτας τριχῆ διελόμενοι, τὰς μὲν αἰσθητικάς, τὰς δὲ κινητικάς, τὰς δὲ ἡγεμονικὰς ἐκαλέσαμεν. ἐν τοίνυν ταῖς αἰσθητικαῖς ἐνεργείαις τριττὴ τῶν συμπτωμάτων ἐστὶν ἡ διαφορά· μία μέν αὐτοῦ τοῦ πρώτου τῆς αἰσθήσεως ὀργάνου πεπονθότος· ἑτέρα δὲ τῆς αἰσθητικῆς δυνάμεως· ἡ τρίτη δὲ τῶν εἰς ὑπηρεσίαν τινὰ τοῦ πρώτου τῆς αἰσθήσεως ὀργάνου γεγονότων.

LINACRE (*ed.* 1524.)	ANONYMUS
Inc. Causas symptomatum in his libris contemplabimur, eundem sequentes disputationis ordinem, quem	*Inc.* Causas sinthomatum in hoc libro scrutemur, eundem sermoni ordinem servantes, quem et in eo qui de

de ipsorum differentiis proposuimus. Sunt igitur symptomatum genera in totum tria. Quorum de eo primum disputavimus in quo lesam esse actionem diximus. Ita nimirum intelligere lectorem censentes, etiam si prorsus periit. Cum autem duplices genere actiones sint, aliae naturales, aliae animales, ab animalibus incepimus. Easque trifariam divisimus, in sentientes, activas, et quas appellavimus rectrices. Ergo in sentiendi actionibus, triplex incidit symptomatum differentia. Una cum ipsum primum sensus instrumentum est male affectum, altera cum sentiendi facultas, et tercia cum aliquid eorum quae primo sentiendi instrumento subserviunt, male habet.

differentia eorum fecimus. Sunt quidem igitur tria omnia genera sinthomatum sed primo sermo nobis factus fuit de eo quo nocitum esse actum diximus, ita audire dignum extimantes, ut si et finaliter periret. Duplicibus autem existentibus secundum genus actibus, hiis quidem animalibus, illis vero naturalibus, ab animalibus incepimus, et hos trifariam [86 K.] dividentes, hos quidem sensitivos, illos autem operativos, illos autem ygemonicos idest principantes vocavimus. Igitur in sensitivis quidem actibus triplex sinthomatum est differentia, una quidem ipso primo sensus organo paciente, altera autem sensitiva virtute, tertia vero eis que in administracionem aliquam primi sensus organi facti sunt. (Wellcome MS. 286, s. xiv, fol. 142ᵛ.)

DE SYMPTOMATUM DIFFERENTIIS

vii. 42–43. 8 Kühn

Τίνα μέν ἐστι καὶ πόσα τὰ σύμπαντα νοσήματα κατ' εἴδη τε καὶ γένη διαιρουμένοις, ἁπλᾶ τε καὶ σύνθετα, ὁπόσαι τε καθ' ἕκαστον αὐτῶν αἰτίαι τῆς γενέσεως, ἐν ἑτέροις ὑπομνήμασι γέγραπται. λοιπὸν δ' ἂν εἴη περὶ τῶν συμπτωμάτων διελθεῖν, ἵν' ᾖ τέλειος ὁ περὶ πασῶν τῶν παρὰ φύσιν διαθέσεων λόγος. ἅπασα γὰρ οὖν διάθεσις σώματος ἐξισταμένη τοῦ κατὰ φύσιν ἤτοι νόσημά ἐστιν, ἢ αἰτία νοσήματος, ἢ σύμπτωμα νοσήματος. ὅπερ ἔνιοι τῶν ἰατρῶν ἐπιγέννημα καλοῦσιν. ἀλλὰ τοῦτο μὲν οὐ πάνυ τι σύνηθές ἐστι τοῖς Ἕλλησι τοὔνομα, σύμπτωμα δὲ καὶ πάθημα καὶ πάθος ὀνομάζουσι συνήθως ἅπαντα τὰ τοιαῦτα. σημαίνεται μὴν οὐ πάντη ταὐτὸν ἐκ τῶν ὀνομάτων, ἀλλ' ὡς ἐγὼ νῦν διαιρήσω περὶ πάντων ἑξῆς τῶν παρακειμένων ἀλλήλοις κατὰ τόνδε τὸν τρόπον ἐπεξιών. ἡ μὲν δὴ νόσος εἴρηται, κατασκευή τις οὖσα παρὰ φύσιν, ὑφ' ἧς ἐνέργεια βλάπτεται πρώτως.

LINACRE (*ed. 1524.*)

Inc. Quinam et quot numero morbi in universum sint tam simplices quam compositi generatim membratimque dividentibus, quot item cuiusque generandi sunt causas aliis commentariis prodidimus. Reliquum est de symptomatis disserere, quo de affectibus qui praeter naturam sunt,

ANONYMUS

Inc. Que quidem sunt et quot universe egritudines secundum species et genera dividentibus, simplices et composite, et quot secundum unamquamque earum cause generationis, in aliis submemoracionibus scriptum est. Reliquum autem utique de sinthomatibus erit pertransire, ut sit omnis nobis absolvatur disceptatio. Omnis igitur corporis affectus qui a naturali statu recessit, vel morbus est, vel morbi causa, vel morbi symptoma. [. . .] Quod etiam pathos et pathema graecis nominare in usu est. Sane non idem omnino significatur per iam dicta nomina, sed sicuti ipse nunc distinguam, de omnibus deinceps quae propinqua inter se sunt, ad hunc modum disserens. Ergo dictum est morbum esse corporis statum quendam pręter naturam, a quo functio lęditur primum.

perfectus sermo qui de omnibus que preter naturam dispositionibus. Omnis denique dispositio corporis desistens ab eo quod secundum naturam egritudo est, vel causa egritudinis, vel sinthoma egritudinis. Quod quidam [43 K.] medicorum supergermen vocant. Sed hoc quidem [nomen] non valde aliquod consuetum est grecis, sinthoma vero et paxionem nominant consuete omnia talia. Significatur quidem demum non omnino idem ex nominibus, sed ut ego nunc dividam de omnibus deinceps que adiacent sibi invicem secundum hunc modum tractans. Egritudo quidem utique dicta est constructio quedam existens preter naturam, a qua energia nocetur prime. (Wellcome MS. 286, s. xiv, fol. 139ᵛ.)

III. *Technique*

The translator of a difficult technical text can make any number of standard responses. He can coin a new term, give an old one a new meaning and new life, use two or more synonyms, transcribe and gloss, or take refuge in circumlocution. We shall examine Linacre's neologisms, doublets, glosses, and periphrases in turn.

Linacre coined new terms only as a last resort. In his preface to the *De sanitate tuenda*, he writes: '. . . [voces] quasdam rursus aliquando novem, sed cum praefatione, & ubi latinas non invenio quibusdam graecis utar, sed quae usitatam latinis inclinationem maxime recipiant'. If he introduces *symptoma, phlegmone, apotherapia*, and *symmetria* in that work, it is in good company and with Horace's dictum in mind.[1] Neologisms, in fact, are rarely needed, for Linacre's *copia verborum* is truly Erasmian in scope.[2] With all his friend's calculated abandon, he exploits to the full the resources of a language now enriched by more than 1,500 years of pagan, patristic, and scholastic activity. Side by side with genuine *Ciceroniana*, we find Plautian vulgarisms, Apuleian conceits, and the indispensable coinages of Saints Augustine, Gregory of Tours, Irenaeus, and Jerome. It goes

[1] *Ars poetica* 52–3.
[2] See D. F. S. Thomson, 'The Latinity of Erasmus', in *Erasmus, Studies in Latin Literature and its Influence*, ed. T. A. Dorey, London, 1970, pp. 115–37.

without saying that he owes a special debt to didactic writers such as Celsus, Columella, Pliny, Varro, Vitruvius, and the Seneca of the *Naturales Quaestiones*.

To late authors, he is indebted for the following substantives: *absumptio, adhaerentia, apparentia, densitudo* (Gloss.), *deustio, elusiones, fermentatio, gulositas, imparitas* (Boethius), *indocilitas, invaletudo, novatio* (Tertullian), *perpensio* (Augustine), *ruditas*. Late Latin adjectives include: *appetitorius, constrictorius, expulsorius, inputrescibilis, indicibilis, instrumentarius, interpretabilis, medicatorius, morbificus, nutritorius, scientificus, tractatorius*. Late verbs include: *collimo* ('examine'), *garrulor* (the deponent is attested for Saint Gregory of Tours), *gracilesco, inaugeo* (doubtfully attested for Ulpian), *nigrefio, obtenebro* (Eccl.). There are a few late adverbs, such as *contentiosius* (Ps.-Quintilian), *inoffense, inevitabiliter, sensibiliter, speciatim*. But the medieval legacy is no less apparent: we find among substantives, *accessorium* ('symptom'), *elixatio, fluxibilitas, notabilitas, perspiratio, pugnantia* (n.f.), *resultus* (4th decl.), *sanguificatio, transpiratus* (4th decl.). Amongst adjectives he adopted *acquisiticius, adsciticius, aegritudinalis* (Albertus Magnus), *alteratrix, attractatorius, auferibilis* (Albertus Magnus), *dilatabilis, dolorificus, excrementicius, excretorius, exhalabilis, experimentalis, flatulentus* and *flatuosus, imaginatrix, indicatrix, insectilis, nerveus, pulsatilis, ratiocinatrix, retentrix*.

There remain, however, a number of forms which cannot be traced in the standard published lexica or in the files of the *Mittellateinisches Wörterbuch*.[1] It would be rash to claim all of these for Linacre, for there are two largely uncharted centuries between the terminal date of the *Wörterbuch* and Linacre's literary activity—two centuries in which translators as industrious as Niccolò da Reggio had wrestled with identical problems. I would put in a separate category neologisms which are deliberately modelled on, as they are provoked by, *Greek* neologisms, such as: *erysipelatosus, oedematosus, phlegmonosus* (ἐρυσιπελατώδης, οἰδηματώδης, φλεγμονώδης), *membranificus, nervificus*, and *ossificus* (χονδρο-, νευρο-, ὀστοποιητικός), and *aeratio* (ἀέρωσις, a hapax). Much less startling are the new coinages in *-trix*, Cicero's beloved suffix: *affectrix, attractrix, concoctrix, decretrix, excretrix, finitrix, gustatrix, impultrix, odoratrix, propultrix, recordatrix, refectrix, segregatrix, tractrix*. Other favoured suffixes are *-ivus* and *-orius*, witness *convulsivus, deiectorius, detersivus* and *detersorius*,

[1] I am grateful to Dr. Theresia Payr, Redaktor, *Mittellateinisches Wörterbuch*, for kindly searching its unpublished files.

gustatorius, humectatorius, propulsorius, recuratorius, renutritorius, tactorius, tenuatorius. Also noteworthy are *auctilis, crustificus, excrementosus, halituosus, nidorulentus, sciticius, transpirabilis.* As for substantives, *contrectatus* (4th decl.), *deligatura, demotiones, friabilitas, hirtitas* (! for δασύτης), *intercidentia* (n.f.), *itatio* (! for βάδισις), and *transpiratio* deserve mention. Few of the innovations involve verbs or adverbs, a finding which reflects that of Plezia[1] for medieval neologisms as a whole: I noted only *alterasco* (also used by Leoniceno), *obnigresco* and *diminute* (translating both ἀμυδρῶς and ἐλλιπῶς).

Linacre often attempts to render a nuance or even an ambivalence in his original by employing two or three exact or near-synonyms. This is a feature known after Rönsch[2] as *Doppelübersetzung* and has recently been studied extensively in two late Latin translators of Greek medical texts, Caelius Aurelianus and Cassius Felix.[3] Though Linacre can only have known of their work, if at all, at second hand (Caelius was not published until 1529), the similarity of his response is striking. Of medieval translators of scientific texts, the only one to my knowledge for whom this device is characteristic is Robert Grosseteste. The synonyms or near-synonyms are linked by conjunctives or disjunctives. Thus we find in Linacre: ἀκρίβεια = morosa perpensio discussioque; δυσπάθεια = indolentia & tolerantia; ἔνδειξις = indicium ac documentum; κατὰ τὸ πρός τι = in respectu collationeque; παραδέχεσθαι = transmittere ac recipere; προσφῦσαι = adiungere agglutinareque; σκέμμα = perpensio aestimatioque; φθορά = corruptela interitusque. Alternative renderings include: ἀνάδοσις = digestio sive distributio; διαπνοή = transpiratio vel perspiratio vel perflatus; ἕλικες = orbes spiraeve; κακοήθη = maligna, contumacia rebelliave; πρόσθεσις = appositio vel adiunctio; πρόσφυσις = agglutinatio sive adherentia; ὑγιεινόν = salubre aut sanitati accommodum. To be distinguished from the above are instances of rhetorical *abundantia* or pleonasm. Thus, amongst adverbs, we find: ἀδιδάκτως = sua sponte citraque doctorem; ἀθρόως = propere et multum, *non sensim et paulatim*; ἁπλῶς = absolute citraque exceptionem; ὄντως = vere prorsusque;

---

[1] Plezia, M., 'Remarques sur la formation du vocabulaire médiolatin en Pologne', *Bulletin Du Cange*, xxxix, 1970, 193–8. Adverbs and verbs accounted for only 7 per cent and 10 per cent respectively of the medieval neologisms sampled.

[2] Rönsch, H., 'Die Doppelübersetzungen im lateinischen Texte des cod. Boernerianus der Paulinischen Briefe', *Zeitschr. f. wiss. Theol.* xxv, 1882, 488 ff.

[3] Bendz, G., *Studien zu Caelius Aurelianus u. Cassius Felix*, Lund, 1964.

τελέως = perfecte atque ad consummationem. Compare ἀπαθές = inpatibile omnisque affectionis expers; ἀρετή = perfectio bonitasque; μοχθηραί = culpabiles ac vitiose.

Linacre does admit Greek loan words, but sparingly and only with a helpful gloss or definition. He is also, as we shall see, careful to alert the reader to the precise sense of a word in a given context, distinguishing the different meanings of, e.g., ῥῖγος. Thus we find: ἀθέρωμα (x. 82. 14 K.) = atheroma *idest tuber cui pulticule simile quid inest quam graeci Atheram dicunt*; ἀνατομικόν τι θεώρημα (*De Temp.* 76. 24 H.) = speculatio quaedam anatomica *idest quae ad corporum dissectionem pertinet*; ἀτροφίαν (x. 68. 12 K.) = atrophiam *idest affectum in quo corpus non nutritur* (the verb ἀτροφεῖν is similarly glossed in the *De sanitate tuenda* at 102. 6 and 141. 28 Koch); τὸ κέρχνειν (vii. 173. 11 K.) = cerchnos grece dicitur. *Est autem non tussis sed exiguus quidem ad tussiendum impetus*; κλύδων (vii. 69. 4 K.) = clydon aliquis *sive fluctuatio cum sonitu*; ὁ λάρυγξ (*Scr. Min.* iii. 224. 2) = larinx, *ea est arteriae que aspera dicitur pars summa*; τοῖς μαρασμώδεσιν (x. 469. 1 K.) = qui marasmo *idest senili ariditate* macescunt; μεθόδου (53. 20 Koch) = methodi, *idest sicut veteres interpretantur*, viae et rationis; πληθώρας (96. 4 Koch) = plethoras idest succorum aequabiliter se habentium redundantiam (the adjective πληθωρικός is similarly glossed at x. 512. 7 K.); σκίρρον (33. 5 Koch) = scirros (hi sunt duricies quaedam non sensiles); τεινεσμός (x. 82. 5 K.) idest desidendi assidua cupiditas. With these compare: ἀπονευρώσεις (x. 411. 9 K.) = nervea tenuitas musculorum quam aponeurosin graeci vocant; ἀποφλεγματισμοί (x. 903. 16 K.) = quae pituitam *per os* evocant; ἐμπλαστικωτέρας οὐσίας ἐστίν (x. 981. 13 K.) = eius substantia in cutis meatibus herere est apta. Emplasticoteron graeci vocant; καρπῷ (x. 334. 6 K.) = articulo brachii summaeque manus medio (less happily rendered by *vola* at vii. 735. 5 K.; classical Latin has no single term for wrist, *carpus* being a late import); τὸν πυλωρόν (*Scr. Min.* iii. 214. 7) = exitum ventriculi quo loco cum intestino committitur, pylorum gręci vocant; ῥίγους (85. 13 Koch) = concussio commotioque totius corporis inaequalis, quod gręci ῥῖγος vocant (cf. *infra* 105. 29 Koch, where Linacre adds: Appello nunc rigorem, nec illum vehementis frigoris sensum, nec duritiem, sed inequalem totius corporis concussum & turbationem. There is a similar gloss at x. 679. 12 K.); οἱ δὲ ὑπόσφαγμα πεπονθότες (vii. 99. 11 K.) = quibus autem ex plaga ruptę recenter sunt in prima tunica venae.

Finally, certain Greek terms could only be rendered in round-about fashion. Typical circumlocutions include: ἀναρριχᾶσθαι (62. 21 Koch) = per funem manibus apprehensum scandere; στιμμίζεσθαι (192. 32 Koch) = cum stibio oculis gratiam conciliare; χνοωδέστατος (125. 11 Koch) = minutissimum instar pollinis; χύλωσις (*Scr. Min.* iii. 213. 18) = conversio ciborum in cremorem. 'Analytic' translations are also common, e.g. ἀσύνθετος = compositionis expers; ἀτμοειδῶς = halitus vice (likewise δροσοειδῶς = roris vice); δυσιατότερον = ad sanandum rebellius; δύστηκτος = aegre liquabilis; εὔθραυστος = fractioni obnoxius; εὐμνημόνευτος = facile recordabilis (Eccl.); σκιατροφία = umbratilis consuetudo.

IV. *Reputation*

Linacre's contemporaries and immediate successors had the highest regard for his talents and achievement. Erasmus awaited with impatience the publication of Linacre's version of the *De sanitate tuenda*, assured, as he wrote to his friend Budé, of nothing but perfection: 'Nihil ab eo viro expecto non absolutissimum omnibus numeris.'[1] Nor was he to be disappointed. In his letter to Ambrogio Leone, another medical humanist, Erasmus praised its fidelity, clarity, and style: 'Est apud Britannos vir undiquaque doctissimus Thomas Linacrus, tibi iam olim ex Aldi nostraque praedicatione cognitus, tuae professionis ac, ni fallor, aetatis. Is idem agit quod tu [Leone was to publish in 1519 a translation of the Byzantine physician Joannes Actuarius' *De urinis*]: multis annis elimatas lucubrationes suas vicissim aedit in lumen. Prodiit Galenus περὶ τῶν ὑγιεινῶν *tanta fide, tanta luce, tanto Romani sermonis nitore redditus*, ut nihil usquam desyderet lector Latinus; imo nihil non melius reperiat quam apud Graecos habeatur.'[2] He writes to Gilles Busleiden in much the same vein: 'Mitto dono libros Galeni [the *De sanitate tuenda* again] opera Thomae Linacri melius Romane loquentes quam antea Graece loquebantur . . .'[3] More perceptive and considered is his thumbnail sketch of Linacre's style included in the *Dialogus Ciceronianus*, first published in Basle in 1528:

Sed Thomam Linacrum non verebor proponere? NOSOP. Novi virum undiquaque doctissimum, sed sic affectum erga Ciceronem, ut

---

[1] Allen, ii. 479 (21 February 1516/17). He had already alerted readers of his edition of Jerome (1516) to the forthcoming publication (ibid. ii. 139).
[2] Ibid. iii. 403 (15 October [1518]).
[3] Ibid. iii. 597 (*c.* 21 May 1519).

etiam si potuisset utrumlibet, prius habuisset esse Quintiliano similis quam Ciceroni, non ita multo in hunc aequior, quam est Graecorum vulgus. Urbanitatem nusquam affectat, ab affectibus abstinet religiosius quam ullus Atticus, breviloquentiam et elegantiam amat, ad docendum intentus, Aristotelem et Quintilianum studuit exprimere. Huic igitur viro per me quantum voles laudum tribuas licebit, Tullianus dici non potest, qui studuerit esse dissimilis.[1]

In fact, as we have already seen, Linacre's vocabulary is distinctly eclectic. If, in Erasmus's eyes, Linacre has a fault, it is his perfectionism, which delayed publication of his important labours: '. . . sine fine premis tuas omnium eruditissimas lucubrationes, ut periculum sit, ne pro cauto modestoque crudelis habearis, qui studia huius seculi tam lenta torqueas expectatione tuorum laborum . . .'[2]

For all Erasmus's genius, I am inclined to attach greater weight to the judgement of his professional colleagues. Leonhart Fuchs, professor of Tübingen, published a number of medical commentaries in addition to his famous herbal. One of these deals with Galen's *De sanitate tuenda*.[3] In a revealing preface addressed to Nicholaus Biechner, Abbot of Zweifalten, he explains at some length why he has ventured to criticize and emend Linacre's version of the text: he did this, he says, not from envy or ambition, indeed he prefers Linacre to all other translators of Galen for his remarkable mastery of both tongues, Greek and Latin: 'Diligentem praeterea de interpretis latini conversione censuram adiecimus, idque nullis sane ambitionis aut invidiae stimulis agitati . . . Linacri autem viri doctissimi gloriae tantum abest ut invideamus, ut potius eum, absit invidia verbis, omnibus interpretibus Galeni, propter insignem tum in Graecis, tum in latinis literis cognitionem, anteferamus' (fols. *3^{v}–4^{r}). He points to the *De emendata latini sermonis structura* as proof of Linacre's erudition, and continues: 'Hoc itaque in praesentia dixisse sat est, Linacrum diligentia & orationis puritate omnes post se reliquisse interpretes . . .' but he cannot help adding a rider:

[1] *Opera omnia Desiderii Erasmi Roterodami* . . ., vol. ii, Amsterdam, 1971, 676. 14–679. 12. Very similar is Erasmus's appreciation of Jean Ruelle, physician to Francis I, whose version of Dioscorides had been published in Paris in 1516: 'De Ruello quid sentis? NOSOP. Quod peritissimo rei medicae dignum est, in vertendis Graecis religiosae fidei. *Hoc laudis maluit quam haberi Tullianus*' (ibid. 675; italics mine). Leoniceno, of course, had no stylistic pretensions: 'Leonicenus medicus erat, non rhetor' (ibid. 668. 3–4).

[2] Allen, iv. 570 (letter to Linacre, 24 August 1521).

[3] Tübingen, U. Morhard, 1541 (Wellcome 2615).

Linacre's version is often so obscure as to be unintelligible, without recourse to the original. Hence Linacre has been blamed for excessive *severitas* and *gravitas*.[1]

Agostino Ricci's judgement is similar: writing in the same year, he acknowledges Linacre's pre-eminence but claims it is impossible to do Galen complete justice in Latin; despite Linacre's diligent attention to style, it still helps to consult the Greek. If this is true for Linacre's versions, it could be said far more of all others.[2] Ricci, in common with other Renaissance editors, prints Linacre's renderings in preference to those of his rivals, with valuable marginalia pointing out his occasional omissions. But the most significant verdict was pronounced by Conrad Gesner. In his invaluable, though occasionally inaccurate, catalogue of Galenic translators and translations prefixed to the 1562 Froben edition of Galen's collected works, he wrote:

Thomas Linacer natione Anglus, philosophus & medicus utraque lingua doctissimus, & politissimi stili, magnam scriptis suis laudem & gratiam apud omnes eruditos meruit, ita ut grammaticus optimus, & prestantissimus Galeni interpretum merito habeatur ... Transtulit aliquot Galeni libros *eleganti & exquisito* sermone, ut Guilhelmus Budeus gravissimus censor de eo praedicat, ita ut *multo plus priscae scribendi vertendique severitati, quam nostri temporis indulsisse licentiae lascivienti* animadvertatur ... [There follows a list of titles] Quod si quid in eius translationibus emendari potest aut potuit, exemplarium forte

[1] Ibid. (fol. *4^v): 'Constat saepe in eius interpretatione tantam subesse obscuritatem, ut nisi graeca adhibeas, fieri non posse ut recte intelligas. Hinc est quod plerisque etiam aliis bonis & doctis viris severitas illa nimia Linacri & gravitas improbetur ...' Fuchs and his readers, of course, would recall that it was precisely this *severitas* that had appealed to Budé.

[2] 'Galeni autem tantus est in graeco idiomate dicendi candor, atque venustas, ut nunquam fieri posse credam, ut quisquam integre eam omnem latinis verbis referat. Quamobrem etsi Linacrus inter recentiores doctos in hoc vertendi munere clarissimus omni studio contendit ut quam candidissimo stilo hos libros in latinum transferret; semper tamen qui graeca ante oculos habebunt, ex illis non nihil luminis & claritatis ad hasce res comparabit quod & multo magis (absit calumniandi suspitio) de omnibus aliorum versionibus liceat pronuntiare' (*Galeni Operum omnium sectio quinta* ..., Venice, 1541, sigs. A3^v–4^r). Ricci's edition has not had the attention it deserves; it is based partly on a collation of Greek MSS. not available to the Aldine editors (e.g. Ermolao Barbaro's MS. of the *Methodus medendi*). I plan to devote a separate monograph to Ricci shortly.

quibus usus est culpa fuerit; nam diligentiam, iudicium, & Graecae linguae peritiam, vix usquam in eis desiderari arbitror.[1]

Linacre's competence, then, has never been in serious doubt. His successors could only make minor improvements, often in the light of Greek manuscripts unavailable to him. They respected his work too much to repeat it.

[1] *Cl. Galeni Pergameni Omnia, quae extant, in Latinum sermonem conversa . . . His accedunt nunc primum Con. Gesneri Praefatio & Prolegomena tripartita, De vita Galeni, eiusque libris & interpretibus . . .*, Basle, 1562, fols. C† 3ᵛ–4ʳ.Gesner lists without comment the versions of Giorgio Valla, Lorenzano and Kopp, criticizes Giampietro Valla's version of the pseudo-Galenic *De succedaneis* with a curt 'parum feliciter', but praises Leoniceno: 'Nicolaus Leonicenus Vicentinus . . . inter primos & praecipuos purioris elegantiorisque medicinae assertores, & Galeni interpretes . . .' (fol. C† 3ʳ).

Addendum to p. 82 n. 1:

Dr. Rhodes' paper has now been published: Dennis E. Rhodes, 'An Unidentified Edition of Galen', *Festschrift für Claus Nissen. Zum siebzigsten Geburtstag 2. September 1971* (ed. by Elizabeth Geck and Guido Pressler), Wiesbaden, 1973, pp. 575–83. Dr. Rhodes concludes (p. 581) that the undated edition of *De locis affectis* 'was printed at the press of Philippus Pincius at Venice . . . probably after 1515 and certainly before 1524'.

Linacre's Lands and Lectureships

JOHN M. FLETCHER*

I. *The Academic Background*

DURING THE CENTURY AND A HALF PRECEDING
Thomas Linacre's election as a Fellow of All Souls College, Oxford,
the opportunities available to European students to complete a
medical course at some recognized university had greatly increased.
Throughout Europe, and especially in the Holy Roman Empire,
new foundations had brought the possibility of a university education to many students who might previously have been deterred by
distance and the expense of travel from attending one of the famous
early academic centres. Almost all these new universities possessed
from the start the coveted privilege of awarding degrees in all four

* Reader in the History of European Universities, Department of Modern
Languages, University of Aston, Birmingham.

Acknowledgements. The preparation of this paper has been encouraged by the
interest of the Principal and Fellows of Linacre College, Oxford, in the life of
the great scholar from whom their College takes its name. Its production has
been made possible by the assistance given by several librarians and archivists.
I am especially grateful for the co-operation of the archivists of the Mercers'
Company, London, of St. John's College, Cambridge, of Brasenose College,
Oxford, and of All Souls College, Oxford. Mr. N. C. Buck and Mr. W. T.
Thurbon of St. John's College, Cambridge, kindly answered repeated questions and investigated material available at the College. Miss Margaret
Pelling gave much practical and valuable advice in the final presentation of
the text. I must express my appreciation above all of the help given to me by
Dr. J. R. L. Highfield and Mr. John Burgass, librarian and assistant librarian
of Merton College, Oxford; they provided shelter, food, and co-operation during my many visits to the College archives. The documents and extracts
printed in this present paper are reproduced by kind permission of the Warden
and Fellows of Merton College, the Master and Fellows of St. John's College,
and the Mercers' Company.

faculties, arts, theology, law, and medicine. A few earlier foundations, where the faculty of medicine was not recognized or had simply a nominal existence, acquired during this period the right to award degrees in medicine; Perugia, for example, at first essentially a university devoted to the study of civil and canon law, received permission to grant academic qualifications in arts and medicine in 1321.[1]

Despite this rapid expansion of provision for the teaching of medicine in old and new foundations, the situation at the close of the medieval period remained little different from what it had been at the end of the thirteenth century. Almost without exception the new faculties made little impact on the learned world of the fourteenth and fifteenth centuries. The statutes of the College of Spain in Bologna, revised in 1375–7, lament that 'ab experto vidimus male haberi posse Hispanos volentes audire scienciam medicine'.[2] Haller, for all his admiration of the early history of the University of Tübingen, can find little to say of the medical faculty there. He states that had he not been able to discuss the life of Johann Widmann, the humanist and medical scholar who passed some time at the University, he would have found 'für das erste Menschenalter ... überhaupt gar nichts'.[3] Historians of the other German universities have been hardly more fortunate; small numbers and infrequent promotions were, it seems, common. Krabbe writes of Rostock: 'Die Zahl der Lehrer der Arzneiwissenschaft war auch verhältnissmässig eine weit geringere, als die Zahl der Theologen und der Rechtslehrer.'[4] Although the University of Toulouse claimed to have possessed all four faculties from its foundation, a roll with the names of approximately 1,400 masters and students submitted to Clement VII in 1378 contained the name of only one medical student, described as a master in grammar and scholar in medicine.[5] French universities, with the exception of Paris and

---

[1] H. Rashdall, *The Universities of Europe in the Middle Ages*, ed. F. M. Powicke and A. B. Emden, 3 vols., Oxford, 1936, ii. 41.

[2] B. M. Marti, *The Spanish College at Bologna in the Fourteenth Century*, Philadelphia, 1966, p. 142.

[3] J. Haller, *Die Anfänge der Universität Tübingen 1477–1537*, 2 vols., Stuttgart, 1927–9, i. 134.

[4] O. Krabbe, *Die Universität Rostock im funfzehnten* [sic] *und sechzehnten Jahrhundert*, Rostock, 1854, pp. 247–8.

[5] The roll is no. 697 in M. Fournier, *Les Statuts et privilèges des universités françaises*, 4 vols., Paris, 1890–4, vol. i.

Montpellier, were dominated by the doctors and students of civil and canon law. The three 'new' faculties of arts, medicine, and theology at Angers had to struggle even to obtain equality with the older law faculties in the appointment of University officials.[1] In 1500 as in 1300 the medical schools of the Italian universities and of Montpellier provided the best and most consistent medical education in Europe.

If the impact of these new medical schools had been so small, one might wonder why older foundations were so eager to expand themselves by the erection of such faculties and why new foundations tried to secure the right to award degrees in all faculties. The answer may, of course, lie partly in the customary medieval concern with prestige; new and 'incomplete' universities were envious of the right of promotion in arts, law, theology, and medicine possessed by such older centres as Paris or Oxford.[2] Probably of more importance were the advantages that even a small and weak medical faculty could bring to a local community. Most of the universities of the later medieval period were 'territorial' foundations. They were usually erected in response to a demand from some local prince, city, or region, and although having traditional cosmopolitan pretensions, catered essentially for local needs. Such a university, even if it produced only a handful of graduates in medicine, could provide medical care for the local nobility and burgesses who were willing to pay for this, and although it might be able to employ only one lecturer of repute, this qualified physician was at least available to treat the family of the local prince who had often been responsible for the original foundation. This is probably why the faculties of medicine maintained their existence even where it is hardly possible for us to trace any significant contribution made by them to the study of the subject or to the numbers of qualified graduates. It is notable that the Faculty of Medicine at Paris, although it never enjoyed a reputation such as that possessed by the Faculties of Arts and Theology, produced doctors who have been described as 'a wealthy and influential body of men'.[3] Clearly, in a city so closely associated with one of the most splendid royal courts of Europe, attracting rich noblemen

[1] Ibid., nos. 493 ff.
[2] See, for example, the complaint of the University of Toulouse against the position of Oxford and Cambridge while itself claiming the right to a faculty of theology: ibid., no. 640.
[3] Rashdall, op. cit. i. 435.

and prelates from France itself and from abroad, the services of trained physicians would always be required and could be afforded. At the University of Vienna, also closely associated with the Imperial court, the medical faculty contained 'nur eine geringe Anzahl activer, wirklich lesender Mitglieder'; in the period 1400–65 about forty doctors gave lectures. Few of these had anything more than a local reputation.[1] Yet this small faculty was able to secure a notable victory over the University lawyers in 1417 when a ducal decision placed the medical doctors before the licentiates in law in official academic processions, contrary to previous custom.[2] Clearly the influence at court of certain of the medical regents was a thing not to be underestimated. Sometimes their absence from the University meant that a course of lectures was not completed. One may find, for instance, in the records of the Senate at the University of Freiburg frequent references to the University's rebuking of its salaried medical lecturers for their overzealous concern with the local noble houses at the expense of their university teaching duties. In Germany in particular, where the local princes still retained considerable political importance and prestige, the income that could be obtained from catering for their needs was sufficient to attract at least native medical doctors to the local universities and to maintain the existence, even though at a much reduced level, of a traditional medical faculty.

The universities of Germany had another advantage which encouraged the continuance there of medical faculties. The majority of their students were enrolled in the Faculty of Arts. Even at a university such as Cologne, with its traditional connection with Duns Scotus and the Dominican theological school, the arts faculty accounted for from seventy to ninety per cent of the student body.[3] The connection between the medical faculty and the Faculty of Arts was very close during the medieval period. Montpellier, where the artists never became a body of any significance, is perhaps an exception to this, although even in this case the early statutes of the medical faculty allow graduates in arts to shorten the course for medical degrees.[4] In the Italian universities, too, graduates in arts

[1] J. Aschbach, *Geschichte der Wiener Universität*, Vienna, 1865, pp. 326–7.
[2] Ibid., p. 316.
[3] See the estimate in H. Keussen, *Die alte Universität Köln*, Cologne, 1934, p. 295.
[4] See Fournier, op. cit. ii, nos. 885, 910.

were permitted to proceed more quickly to their degrees in medicine.[1] It was perhaps the overwhelming predominance of the lawyers
rather than of the arts students at the foundation of most of the
universities of Spain and provincial France that prevented the
growth there of really important medical faculties. Already by 1263
the *Siete Partidas* of Alfonso X, el Sabio, King of Castile, were allowing the payment at Salamanca of salaries of 500 and 300 maravedis
each to four lawyers; the masters of logic, grammar, and physic were
each allocated 100 maravedis only.[2] Where, as in Germany, students
in the Faculty of Arts formed the majority from the very foundation
of the University, there was a greater chance that a few scholars
each year would proceed to study medicine after obtaining an arts
degree. This was encouraged, as at Montpellier and the Italian
universities, by the statutes of the medical faculties. At Ingolstadt
in 1472, for example, the course for the lower degree was fixed at
three years, but bachelors of arts had this time reduced by six
months and masters of arts by one year.[3] We shall find the assumption that a medical student would first have completed the M.A.
course, when we examine the regulations made by Linacre for his
own medical lectureships.

The close association of the Faculty of Arts and the Faculty of
Medicine did have great dangers, especially where the repute of the
university as a whole rested essentially on its work in speculative
logic and philosophy. Medicine 'was taught as a philosophy with
maximal reliance on established authority and minimal concern with
observation and experimentation'.[4] Kaufmann quotes two interesting examples from Ingolstadt of medical doctors who achieved some
local fame, the first by a commentary on Aristotelian logic and the
second by his work later in the faculty of arts.[5] Even more striking
evidence of the approach of these medical scholars towards their
subject is given by the chance survival at Heidelberg of a statement
by doctor Heinrich von Munsingen. In 1430 he submitted to the
University a long defence of his treatment of a wounded scholar who

[1] For Bologna see Rashdall, op. cit. i. 247.
[2] Ibid. ii. 81.
[3] K. Prantl, *Geschichte der Ludwig-Maximilians-Universität*, 2 vols., Munich,
1872, ii. 41–2.
[4] C. H. Talbot and E. A. Hammond, *The Medical Practitioners in Medieval
England: A Biographical Register*, London, 1965, p. ix.
[5] G. Kaufmann, *Geschichte der deutschen Universitäten*, 2 vols., Stuttgart,
1888–96, ii. 477.

later died. It is a scholastic proof, with references to prescribed authors and with syllogistic arguments, demonstrating the author's familiarity with the methods of the Faculty of Arts.[1] The absence of such a powerful tradition of logical and philosophical speculation in the Italian universities may explain why they were better able to encourage the practical study of medicine,[2] but, as I have mentioned, even here the connections between arts and medicine were strong, and the influence of astrology upon medical practice was of considerable importance.[3] The 'new learning' of the fifteenth century was especially hostile to the study of scholastic philosophy and the logic of the schools. It is not surprising that its proponents also attacked the use of such philosophical and logical methods in the faculties of theology and medicine. The clash was especially acute in those northern universities (such as Paris and Oxford) where these methods were deeply entrenched. Linacre showed his awareness of the problem in the detailed arrangements he made for the establishment of his lectureships.

From the previous discussion, it seems that the establishment and continuance of a successful medical faculty depended, other things being equal, on three factors. First, in universities where the Faculty of Medicine had by the close of the medieval period a tradition of regular promotions and teaching, the very existence there of a recognized *studium* in medicine would tend to attract students and masters often from considerable distances. Such a factor could not, of course, ensure the permanent fame of the faculty, but it could prevent its sudden decline, or carry it through lean times. The remarkable history of the medical faculty of the University of Montpellier, which from at least the thirteenth until the eighteenth century continued to attract students from France and from abroad, must owe something to this factor. Secondly, skilled physicians could command a high salary; a thirteenth-century doctor demanded a fee of 100 golden ducats a day to treat the Pope.[4] They would, as already suggested, be attracted to universities adjacent to social centres where rich noblemen, ecclesiastics, or merchants regularly gathered

---

[1] E. Winkelmann, *Urkundenbuch der Universität Heidelberg*, 2 vols., Heidelberg, 1886, i. 124 ff.

[2] For the study of anatomy at Bologna, see Rashdall, op. cit. i. 244–6.

[3] Ibid., pp. 242–3.

[4] Ibid., p. 236 n. 3. According to Rashdall, 'marvellous stories' were told of this practitioner's wealth and professional exactions.

in some numbers. Finally, and most important from the academic point of view, was the question of the ability of the university itself to compete for the services of the better physicians. Clearly if these could obtain high salaries by the treatment of wealthy patients there would be little incentive for them to devote themselves to academic lecturing in return for little reward. Any university, therefore, that wished to attract highly qualified lecturers, especially if they were to travel from some distance, had to provide adequate remuneration first to bring them to the university and secondly to keep them there. In considering the state of the European medical faculties at the close of the medieval period, these three factors must be borne in mind.

The newer foundations of the fourteenth and fifteenth centuries could not, of course, depend on any tradition of long continuance or success to attract students and masters to their medical faculties. They could usually offer some employment for students and graduates since they were founded for the most part in regional capitals. The newer faculties followed the precedent set by their predecessors, and attempted to obtain control over the practice of medicine in their local communities.[1] But no new faculty could hope to attract students unless regent doctors in medicine provided regular lectures. In universities adopting a constitution derived from that of Paris, this was done by compelling every graduate in medicine to spend some time at the university as a lecturer after he had obtained his degree. This method was unpopular with medical doctors because it required them to spend time at a university, with no further chance of academic promotion, when they might have been pursuing a lucrative career in the world outside. Furthermore the regency system did not guarantee the appointment of any exceptional lecturer, as all graduates, regardless of their abilities, were expected to teach. For the new foundations of the fourteenth and fifteenth centuries, however, it had a greater disadvantage. These new universities wished to attract lecturers with an already established reputation; they could not wait for the gradual emergence of their own teachers, even where this was possible. In addition, the increase in the number of universities, most of them with medical faculties, meant that each was competing for talent that was scarce.

[1] For example, by a bishop's decree of 1404 all doctors practising in the diocese of Worms had to be approved by the Heidelberg medical faculty. See Winkelmann, op. cit. ii. 18.

Accordingly most new universities abandoned the traditional regency system, and offered salaries to qualified lecturers willing to take appointments as university teachers in medicine.

This movement is most easily seen within the universities of the Empire. The new universities here were quick to claim that they had been founded 'ad instar Parisiensis', but rapidly became dominated by small groups of salaried lecturers.[1] Medical doctors were usually prominent members of these groups. Their salaries were generally less than those of the lawyers and theologians but greater than those of the artists. At Ingolstadt, for example, the lecturers on the *Decretum* usually received 120 florins yearly, those lecturing on the *Liber sextus* or the *Clementinae* or on civil law 130 florins, and the lecturers in arts, 40 florins. The medical lecturers normally received about 80 florins.[2] As we have already noted, the use of this system throughout the Empire did not succeed in building up strong medical faculties that could rival those of Italy or Montpellier. It did, however, encourage individual medical doctors to seek employment in these new universities. A chair at Ingolstadt was held in 1526 by Leonhard Fuchs, 'der hervorragendste unter den Medicinern jener Periode';[3] Peter Luder, trained in Italy, taught at Basle and assisted in the preparation of the medical faculty's statutes;[4] Johann Widmann, a graduate of Pavia, was attracted to Tübingen.[5] These few examples from many show how the universities of the Empire could attract qualified graduates in medicine, especially those who had been trained in Italy. Naturally Germans formed the majority of those so employed. However, it was also possible to attract by salaried chairs distinguished teachers from other countries. Galeazzo de Santa Sophia from Padua and Michael Falconis from Montpellier both taught medicine at the University of Vienna.[6] The influence of such scholars on the universities at which they were employed was considerable. Not only did they bring with them the medical skills they had acquired abroad, but those who had studied in Italy usually had as well some familiarity with the 'new learning' and helped to disseminate this in the univer-

---

[1] See my essay, 'Wealth and Poverty in the Medieval German Universities with Particular Reference to the University of Freiburg' in *Europe in the Late Middle Ages*, ed. J. R. Hale, J. R. L. Highfield, and B. Smalley, London, 1965, pp. 410–36.

[2] Prantl, op. cit. i. 29. [3] Ibid., p. 197.

[4] E. Bonjour, *Die Universität Basel*, Basle, 1960, p. 95.

[5] Haller, op. cit. i. 134. [6] Aschbach, op. cit., p. 327.

sities of the Empire. The establishment of salaried chairs in medicine throughout the Empire in the later medieval period did, therefore, achieve some modest success.

It is noticeable that almost all the distinguished medical doctors of the later medieval period had spent at least part of their period of study in Italy or at Montpellier; Thomas Linacre was in this respect no exception. Some credit for the remarkably long predominance of Italy and Montpellier must, as already suggested, be attributed to the fact that there the tradition of medical study was deeply implanted. The early contribution of Salerno to the history of medicine can hardly be overestimated.[1] Italy was conveniently placed to receive the medical texts of the Islamic world, and the names of important physicians appear in the records of its university towns well before established faculties of medicine develop. In 1214 a 'Medicus Vulnerum' was offered 600 *librae* to come to Bologna as a public surgeon.[2] At an early date this general interest in medicine was concentrated in the universities by the foundation of specific faculties of medicine. By the last quarter of the thirteenth century there is definite evidence of graduations in medicine at Bologna.[3] Other Italian universities of this century, some having only a fleeting existence, also show that lectures in medicine were given by graduate doctors. There are references to such courses being organized in Vicenza, Arezzo, Padua, Naples, Siena, and Piacenza.[4] In these universities, and in those that were founded at a later date in Italy, the arts course was regarded as a preparation for the study of medicine rather than for the study of theology. Until a comparatively late date, the higher faculties of an Italian university consisted only of those of civil and canon law, and medicine. These early efforts to set up medical faculties show that there was a demand for medical treatment from the merchants of Italian towns, and for certain scholars and doctors prepared to study and lecture in the faculties.

Italian cities vied with each other in their efforts to attract highly qualified lecturers. Their motives were, of course, not simply academic; a well-known lecturer could bring with him his own students

---

[1] See the note in Rashdall, op. cit. i. 85-6, and P. O. Kristeller, 'The School of Salerno: Its Development and its Contribution to the History of Learning', *Bulletin of the History of Medicine*, xvii, 1945, 138-94.

[2] Rashdall, op. cit. i. 235.

[3] Ibid., p. 237.

[4] Ibid. ii. 7, 8, 12, 24, 31, 37.

and draw to the city when he began to lecture an even greater
number of scholars. To an Italian city, especially one damaged by
competition or a decline in trade, such an influx of young men could
act as a considerable economic stimulus. The effect of this policy of
seeking to attract eminent doctors was to increase the salaries which
the latter could acquire, and so to enable them to pick such a position as best suited themselves. It is not surprising that few, comparatively, responded to the attempts of northern universities to
attract them to what was, both literally and metaphorically, a colder
climate. The willingness of Italian cities to pay high salaries to
regent doctors in medicine ensured the continuance there of medical
education by well-qualified lecturers. A famous physician such as
Dino del Garbo could obtain a comfortable livelihood as a university
lecturer. He taught at Bologna, Padua, Florence, and Siena; the last
city paid him 100 florins per annum for his services to its university.[1]
This factor alone would be sufficient to explain the predominance
in the medical field of the Italian schools.

The fame of the University of Montpellier as a centre of medical
education is more unusual and interesting. No doubt its position
gave it particularly early and ready contact with the Islamic learning of Spain and the Mediterranean. Islamic tradition has been
given as the reason for the development at Montpellier of a separate
university of medicine.[2] The lecturing staff at the University was
obtained in a manner that has more in common with the Paris than
the Bologna model. By the statutes of 1340, each candidate for the
doctoral degree was compelled to swear that he would remain at
Montpellier as a medical lecturer for a period of two years after
obtaining his qualification.[3] The system at Montpellier, therefore,
possessed in the fourteenth century all the disadvantages connected with the necessary regency system already discussed. It is
interesting to see that, by the close of the medieval period, modifications were being introduced. Louis XII in 1498, speaking of the
University as being 'par aucun temps destituée et dépourvue', provided an annual grant for the payment of four doctors lecturing in
medicine and for the repair of the schools.[4] It would seem that the
inadequacies of the regency system had begun to be felt at Montpellier by the late fifteenth century, with consequent damage to the

---

[1] Ibid. ii. 33 n. 3.   [2] Ibid. ii. 121 n. 3.
[3] Fournier, op. cit. ii, no. 947 *quater*, sect. LVIII.
[4] Ibid., no. 1209.

University's reputation. The introduction of salaried chairs seems, however, to have revitalized the faculty. During the sixteenth and seventeenth centuries Montpellier continued to attract medical students from several European countries, and it can claim to have produced many of the most prominent physicians of that period.

Thomas Linacre could not have had first-hand knowledge of all the problems connected with the teaching of medicine in European universities. His own career, however, must have given him an insight into the different methods adopted by various institutions, and especially into the difficulties that English students of medicine had to face. Linacre was elected a Fellow of All Souls College, Oxford, in 1484.[1] Since he was later to take the degree of Master of Arts, he must by this date have been well advanced in the study of arts; the college statutes required its Fellows to be between seventeen and twenty-six years old and to have spent at least three years at Oxford before admission.[2] Linacre was still a Fellow of the college in 1495, but had in the meantime travelled in Italy. Since he was admitted to the doctorate in medicine at Padua in August 1496, he must have obtained his M.A. degree and spent some years in the study of medicine before this date.

It is interesting to notice here some of the problems faced by Fellows of All Souls College wishing to study medicine. The statutes of the college provided places for those intending to study arts, theology, and law; no provision was made for medical students. Those members of the college ambitious to obtain the doctorate in medicine could, however, study informally while working for degrees in other subjects or while necessary regents in arts. A further obstacle may have been the founder's regulation that all masters of arts must take orders within two years after the completion of their necessary regency. Medical doctors at this date often preferred to retain the right to marry later if they so wished. Nevertheless, we are advised by E. F. Jacob that 'the early interest of the college in medicine needs more emphasis than it has yet received'.[3]

---

[1] The biographical details used in this study are taken from A. B. Emden, *A Biographical Register of the University of Oxford to A.D. 1500*, 3 vols., Oxford, 1957–9, or from J. K. McConica, *English Humanists and Reformation Politics under Henry VIII and Edward VI*, Oxford, 1965, unless otherwise stated.

[2] *Statutes of the Colleges of Oxford*, 3 vols., Oxford/London, 1853, i, *All Souls College*, p. 20.

[3] *The Victoria History of the Counties of England: Oxfordshire*, 10 vols., London, 1907–72, iii. 176.

The assumption that Linacre acquired an interest in medicine only after visiting Italy and coming into contact with humanist scholars there does not seem justified by the evidence. Amongst the Fellows of All Souls College who were predecessors of Linacre, there were three medical doctors: Stephen Barworth, who was admitted in 1450, Nicholas Halswell, admitted 1468, and John Racour, admitted 1467. William Goldwin, admitted in 1455, obtained at least the lower degree in medicine. Nicholas Halswell may have been a contemporary of Linacre's at the college. Nor was Linacre the only medical scholar produced by All Souls College at the close of the fifteenth century. John Game, admitted 1488, and Richard Bartlatt, admitted 1495, both obtained the doctorate in medicine in the early years of the sixteenth century.

This evidence suggests that before, during, and after Linacre's tenure of his college fellowship there was a lively tradition of medical study at All Souls. Of greater significance is the fact that all the scholars mentioned, with the exception of Stephen Barworth, are known to have bequeathed medical texts to the college library as if expecting the continuance of, and encouraging, the study of medicine there. However, despite this informal support, it is very suggestive that not one of these medical scholars is known to have obtained his doctorate while a Fellow of the College. Apparently all had to leave before they had completed the course. This may be one of the explanations for Linacre's eagerness to travel to Italy and for his successful attempt to obtain there the doctorate in medicine. The restrictions imposed by the statutes of his college may have been one of the first obstacles encountered by Linacre in his efforts to obtain a medical qualification.

He could also hardly have been unaware of the state of the Faculty of Medicine at Oxford, which we shall consider below. In Italy he visited the university towns of Florence, Rome, Padua, and possibly Bologna. He must have been impressed by the strength of the medical faculties of these universities and, especially at Padua,[1] by the reputation of contemporary teachers in this subject. In his arrangements for his own medical lectureships, Linacre was clearly drawing on his experiences in both Oxford and Italy.

The English universities were both dominated, constitutionally and numerically, by the masters and students in arts. It seems,

[1] See J. H. Randall, Jr., *The School of Padua and the Emergence of Modern Science*, Padua, 1961.

therefore, that many graduates were produced who, in the opinion of academics of the fifteenth century, were properly fitted to continue with the study of medicine. Yet at neither university did they do so in any considerable numbers. At Oxford, for instance, during the whole of the fifteenth century fewer than forty students are known to have obtained the M.D. degree. During the same period, the university is known to have awarded some 500 doctorates in theology, of which about half went to secular students.[1] Such a number of promotions in theology is certainly very unusual and distinguishes Oxford from continental universities apart from Paris. The reason for the predominance of secular theological doctorates at Oxford is no doubt associated with the prestige of the University in this particular field, but it must also owe something to the character of the provision made by earlier benefactors for the study of theology. Most of the Oxford colleges were endowed to encourage scholars to work for the doctorate in theology or law. Where provision was made for the study of medicine it was usually of a permissive rather than a compulsory nature; that is, certain fellowships were available to medical students, rather than being exclusively reserved for them.

Both the English universities suffered from being provincial rather than national centres. Neither had close associations with a local court or ecclesiastical see of great importance. This may have helped Oxford and Cambridge to retain an independence from secular or episcopal control, but it brought major disadvantages to medical students. The right to practise exclusively in Oxford or Cambridge could not be compared with the opportunities presented by a medical career in London. Linacre himself had little close association with Oxford after his return from Italy, preferring to pursue his medical work at the Court and amongst the wealthy nobility and citizens of the capital.

The effects of this situation on the teaching of medicine were very considerable. Not only were few students positively encouraged to study for medical degrees, but those who did succeed in obtaining the doctorate were reluctant to spend any more time in Oxford than was absolutely necessary. The statutes of the University expressly allowed masters of arts to depose, that is to give their opinion as to the suitability of the candidate, when students applied for the

---

[1] This analysis is based on my study of the names recorded in A. B. Emden's *Biographical Register*.

doctorate in medicine.[1] Clearly the University was obliged to legislate for occasions when there were not sufficient members of the medical faculty available to express an adequate opinion. The university registers also show that there were occasions when no regent doctor was present to preside at the ceremonies associated with the award of a degree in medicine. Several entries allow masters of arts to perform the functions here that should have been undertaken by a medical doctor.[2] The small size of the faculty and the haphazard and inconsistent nature of the instruction offered must have been grave deterrents to all but the most enthusiastic students of medicine. The situation certainly reflected little credit on either Oxford or Cambridge, both of which had possessed the privilege of awarding medical degrees from the earliest years of their foundation.

It did not require much foresight to see what had to be done to remedy the position. Already at Oxford, the University itself, even in the Faculty of Arts, had begun to make modifications to its traditional lecture system. Appeals had been made in the fifteenth century to various wealthy noblemen and prelates for endowments to set up salaried chairs in the arts subjects.[3] At Magdalen College, founded in 1448, William of Waynflete had provided money to pay lecturers in philosophical subjects who could lecture without charge to members of the University as a whole as well as to scholars of their own particular college. Linacre must have been familiar with the arrangements made for the Oxford Lectureship in Theology established by the Lady Margaret in 1502. It is not surprising that, with his experience of Italian conditions, Linacre saw that salaried lectureships in medicine were the only way in which Oxford and Cambridge could ensure the continued availability of instruction. What is unusual is the tenacity with which he pursued his plans, the detailed instructions he left to his lecturers, and the length of time it took to transform his intentions into practice.

11. *The Acquisition of Property*

Linacre had finally returned to England by 1499, when he gave

[1] S. Gibson (ed.), *Statuta antiqua Universitatis Oxoniensis*, Oxford, 1931, p. 31.

[2] See for example entries in *The Register of Congregation 1448–1463*, ed. W. A. Pantin and W. T. Mitchell, Oxford Historical Society, Oxford, 1972, pp. 174, 371.

[3] The question is discussed at length in my forthcoming book on the Faculty of Arts at Oxford, 1400–1520.

lectures, probably in London, which Thomas More attended. His relations with the universities do not seem at this time to have been very close. Anthony Wood suggests that he did teach medicine at Oxford, for he states that he 'was incorporated into his own University and read a shagling lecture in that faculty', but gives no evidence for this statement. Linacre's close association with the Court, first as tutor to Prince Arthur, then as physician to Henry VIII, and finally as tutor to Princess Mary, drew him towards the London circle of humanist scholars. His close friends were William Grocyn, William Latimer, Thomas More, William Lily, John Colet, and Cuthbert Tunstal, all well known for their connections with London and the Court rather than for their prowess in academic fields alone.

Linacre, however, retained some connection with the academic world because much of his work in both the medical and grammatical fields was of fundamental importance to the university curriculum. As he established himself amongst the leaders of those scholars aiming at the reform of the teaching of grammar, and as a reputable translator from the Greek of the works of Proclus and of Galen, the University of Oxford could not ignore his accomplishments. In a letter that can be dated to the close of the year 1521, the University speaks of him as 'novum Latinae linguae parentem',[1] and reports with enthusiasm of Lupset's lectures on his translation of Proclus. Linacre, unlike other humanist scholars concerned only with the study of Greek and Latin literature, and able to pursue their interests without direct reference to the university curriculum, was dependent upon the reaction of academics to his proposals.

For the last four or five years of his life, Linacre was a well-established figure. As a physician in London he treated many of the most prominent personages of the day, including William Warham and Cardinal Wolsey. During these years he accumulated ecclesiastical preferments of some value. It must then have seemed possible for him to think of giving the necessary financial support to plans that may have been many years old.

At the time of Linacre's return to England and the establishment of his reputation in London, the institution of public lectureships was, as already indicated, being strongly advocated in academic

---

[1] Oxford, Bodleian Library, Bodley MS. 282 (S.C. 2949), fol. 44ᵛ. A translation is printed by J. N. Johnson, *The Life of Thomas Linacre*, ed. R. Graves, London, 1835, pp. 180–2.

circles.[1] The growing influence in northern Europe of scholars
trained in Italy or deriving their attitudes from the 'new learning'
of that country gave a considerable impetus to this movement.
Public lectureships were at this later time seen not merely as a
supplement to assist in the better provision of education in the
traditional medieval academic subjects, but as a means by which the
educational content of these subjects could be modified or new subjects introduced into universities still dominated by the medieval
faculties. In this way humanists outside Italy, where many universities still held firmly to the medieval curriculum especially in arts,
medicine, and theology, hoped to infiltrate their ideas into the
academic world without the risk of a full-scale confrontation with
the strongly entrenched masters and doctors. In the interesting
attempts to establish humanistic studies in the University of
Vienna, particularly famous in the medieval period for the strength
and vigour of its Faculty of Arts, one can see very clearly the pursuit
of this policy by German humanists. They first appealed to the
Emperor for finance to establish a chair 'in arte humanitatis', and
then attempted to incorporate lectures given by the holder of this
position into the normal curriculum of the Faculty of Arts. These
moves were resisted by the Faculty. Conrad Celtis, 'der deutsche
Erzhumanist', next made strenuous efforts to create a college for the
study of 'poetry', separate from and outside the jurisdiction of the
Faculty of Arts. Lectureships were to be set up in poetry, eloquence,
and mathematics. This project also failed.[2] More successful were the
plans to establish trilingual colleges in certain major European universities, with the particular aim of encouraging a greater interest
in Greek and Hebrew.[3]

At Oxford the movement to establish such lectureships had
received a new impetus with the foundation of Corpus Christi
College in 1517. By his statutes Bishop Fox, the founder, provided
three lecturers in Latin, Greek, and theology who were required to
deliver lectures that would be open to the entire University.[4] For
the first time at Oxford there was to be permanent instruction in

---

[1] See above, p. 120.

[2] The details of these attempts are set out in G. Bauch, *Die Reception des
Humanismus in Wien*, Breslau, 1903.

[3] See P. S. Allen, 'The Trilingual Colleges of the Early Sixteenth Century'
in *Erasmus: Lectures and Wayfaring Sketches*, Oxford, 1934.

[5] The statutes are summarized in *The Victoria History of the County of Oxford*,
iii. 219–20.

a large number of subjects closely associated with humanistic studies. At about the same time the powerful Cardinal Wolsey began to take an interest in these plans. Great excitement was caused in the University when the Cardinal while visiting Oxford in 1518 announced his intention of providing a number of public lectureships at his own expense. How far these ambitious plans were put into practice remains doubtful, but certain scholars were sent to Oxford by the Cardinal in an effort to extend the influence of the 'new learning' there.[1] The whole scheme was quickly submerged in the more grandiose plans to erect Cardinal College and was finally taken under royal patronage with the fall of Wolsey. These efforts to introduce humanistic scholarship into the University of Oxford were closely followed by the London supporters of the 'new learning', who threw their political weight behind such proposals and who by letters kept in touch with their colleagues with similar interests in the University. At Cambridge, the foundation of St. John's College, with its emphasis on the study of Greek and Hebrew, was an attempt by another of the London humanists, John Fisher, to establish humanistic learning in that university. Fisher's close association with the Lady Margaret was to bring considerable benefits to Cambridge and to the supporters of the 'new learning' there.[2] The second decade of the sixteenth century saw, therefore, a determined effort by the humanists to establish their influence within both English universities. As one of the most prominent figures in London and at the Court, Linacre must have been in close touch with these plans and sympathetic to those seeking to implement them.

It is not possible to say exactly when Linacre began to draw up concrete proposals for the establishment of public lectureships in medicine. The letter already mentioned,[3] which he received from the University in 1521, may possibly indicate that by the close of that year some rumour of his intentions had reached Oxford. Certainly in 1523 the University was again writing to him urging that he should implement the plans he had made for the setting up of these lectureships. This letter speaks of 'lectiones magnificas, quas

[1] Wood's attempt to enumerate the lectureships and their incumbents is given in his *Historia et antiquitates universitatis Oxoniensis*, 2 vols., Oxford, 1674, ii. 34–6.

[2] These developments are discussed in more detail in McConica, op. cit., pp. 78–80.

[3] See above, p. 121.

tuis impendiis hic legendas destinasti' and hopes that Linacre will not be distracted by 'ulle cogitationes tue tam multe aut tam varie'.[1] The documents in Merton College seem to show that the period during which Linacre was most active in the acquisition of property that was to provide the financial basis for his lectureships fell between 1520 and his death in 1524. It would appear that he had waited until his own position in London was well established before expending money on the acquisition of lands, and it may be that he was then encouraged to take these steps by the apparently cordial reception given at both Oxford and Cambridge to the new college and university lectureships in humanistic subjects.

Linacre's efforts to acquire lands with which to endow his lectureships involved him in complicated legal disputes and financial arrangements which are not of immediate concern to us. Most of the documents illustrating his involvement in these affairs are preserved in Merton College and with others are calendared as an appendix to this study. Here I shall consider in detail only the transactions by which Linacre acquired the actual properties that were to pass later to St. John's College, Cambridge, and Merton College, Oxford. I shall also be concerned to show how speedily the purchase of the various lands was accomplished, and how closely the London humanists were associated with Linacre at this stage of his plans.

Before discussing these documents, it is perhaps relevant to note that on 14 January 1515 Linacre passed on to Thomas More, John Davy, John Babham the son of John Babham, and Richard Hardyng certain lands 'in parochiis de Ffeversham et Boughton subtus Le Blee in comitatu Kancie'.[2] The purpose of the gift is noted as 'ad inde perimplendum ultimam voluntatem mei prefati Thome Lynacre'. Could it perhaps be that at this date Linacre was already considering the possibility of a large-scale endowment, and ensuring that important Londoners would be involved in the execution of his policies? Certainly both More and Hardyng figure prominently in the legal activities which were later to accompany the acquisition of his lands.

The bulk of the property obtained by Linacre came eventually to Merton College, and the documents associated with the purchases are now preserved there. His first and most substantial acquisition

---

[1] Oxford, Bodleian Library, Bodley MS. 282 (S.C. 2949), fol. 60. A translation is printed by Johnson, op. cit., pp. 269–72.
[2] Calendar no. 1.

was the manor of Traces in Kent. This land was the subject of an indenture made on 8 November 1520 between Lewis Clyfford and Linacre, although Clyfford had entered into an obligation concerning the lands as early as 21 September 1519.[1] By this indenture, the manor of Traces together with lands and other rights in 'Newenton, Hartlepp, Stokbury, Upchurche, Reynham, Tong, and Morston' and elsewhere in Kent were purchased by Linacre for the sum of £216. Clyfford agreed to transfer the estates for Linacre's use to Richard Pace, Cuthbert Tunstal, Thomas More, William Shelley, John Drewe, and John Clement.[2] Here we have an important collection of laymen and ecclesiastics, influential in London and at the Court, and sympathetic to humanistic studies. Tunstal, More, and Shelley reappear later as executors of Linacre's last will. Tunstal, Master of the Rolls, already had behind him a distinguished diplomatic career, was well known as a humanist, and was soon to become Bishop of London. Thomas More, a King's Councillor since 1517, had already produced his *Utopia*. William Shelley was a well-known London lawyer. Of the others, John Clement was a close associate of Colet and More and was later to follow Linacre in the study of medicine; Richard Pace, Secretary to Henry VIII, was another of More's influential friends. John Drewe has not been identified.

Linacre next acquired what is perhaps the best known of his possessions, his house in Knight Rider Street, London. On 30 September 1522 Richard Hyll and Linacre made an indenture noting that the Stone House in Knight Rider Street had been sold to Linacre for £46. 13s. 4d.[3] This was followed by a deed transferring the house and its garden to Linacre, Tunstal, Pace, Roger Drewe, John Chambre, Roger Denton, John Stokesley, More, Shelley, Francis Poyntz, and Clement on 8 January 1523.[4] The new names that appear in this list offer further evidence of the breadth of Linacre's connections with London humanist society. Roger Drewe is possibly the scholar of the same name who was admitted Fellow of All Souls College, Oxford, in 1512.[5] Roger Denton has not been identified. John Stokesley was a royal chaplain and was later to follow Tunstal as Bishop of London. Francis Poyntz, an experienced royal servant, was later associated with the translation into English of some of Erasmus's works. For a year or so, until his death, the Stone House was Linacre's home in London; after which, as we shall see, the

---

[1] Calendar no. 2.   [2] See Appendix A1.   [3] See Appendix A2.
[4] Calendar no. 3.   [5] Information from Dr. A. B. Emden.

'chappell and the chamber over the chappell' passed to the College of Physicians of which he had been the first President. The remainder of the property eventually came to Merton College. By this division, Linacre probably thought that his lecturers at Oxford would retain some connection with the College of Physicians. He may also have hoped that the house would occasionally provide accommodation for his lecturers when in London. At a much later date, the Stone House was used as a lodging in London by the Warden of Merton College.[1]

On 14 November 1522 Linacre acquired from Thomas Elmeston property known as 'Sevans lande' and 'Bulles',[2] and on 4 February 1523 these lands passed to Linacre and the same associates who had earlier been involved in the transfer of the Stone House.[3] Payment for the estates was received from Linacre on 5 February 1523.[4] These same associates also received from John Potett (or Pott) on 7 February 1523, land in the parish of 'Bobbyng'.[5] Property at Frognall was acquired on 18 June 1523 from William Bloor at a cost of £130. This indenture also brought to Linacre small pieces of land at 'Newenton beside Sydyngborne' and in 'Hertlep'.[6] Shortly afterwards, on 20 August 1523, Bloor passed over the lands to Linacre, Tunstal, Pace, More, Shelley, and Richard Hardyng 'yoman',[7] and on 5 November of that year released to the same group his rights in these estates.[8] Finally, two small pieces of land at 'Warndale in the parissh of Newenton besides Sydyngburn' and in the 'parissh of Stokbury' were purchased from Thomas Crips on 3 October and 23 November 1523.[9] An obligation by Crips dated 23 November and a receipt dated 20 September for a payment by Linacre to him also survive in the Merton records.[10] These are the most important purchases made by Linacre, but he must also have made a few lesser acquisitions in Tong, for a short document in the Merton archives lists 'parcells of lond' bought there for a total sum of 3s. 5¼d.[11]

Linacre's attempt to acquire lands did not pass entirely without challenge. In Michaelmas term 1520, there was a legal suit by which Linacre, Pace, Tunstal, More, Shelley, John Drewe, and Clement sought to recover the manor of Traces from John

[1] J. M. Fletcher, *Registrum Annalium Collegii Mertonensis, 1521–67*, Oxford Historical Society, Oxford, 1974, p. 225.

[2] See Appendix A3.   [3] Calendar nos. 4 and 5.   [4] Calendar no. 6.
[5] See Appendix A4.   [6] See Appendix A5.   [7] Calendar no. 7.
[8] Calendar no. 8.   [9] See Appendices A6 and A7.
[10] Calendar nos. 9 and 10.   [11] See Appendix A8.

Halys,[1] seisin being granted on the failure of a witness to appear. On 2 December they appointed their attorney to receive the property from the sheriff of Kent.[2] This, however, is almost certainly a fictitious action, an example of the legal procedure known as common recovery. Some genuine legal difficulties, however, were experienced concerning the Stone House in Knight Rider Street, and Frognall. The challenge to Linacre's purchase of the Stone House was easily resolved. Apparently the right of Richard Hyll to sell the property was challenged by William Gysnam. Documents at Merton College set out the claims of both parties.[3] The problem seems to have been resolved by the formal sale of the property[4] by Gysnam to Hyll and then Gysnam's renunciation of his rights in the Stone House and adjacent property.[5] With Frognall the trouble seems to have arisen from the need to obtain legal recognition of the sale of the land. 'Lerned councell' advised Linacre to take various steps to protect his rights;[6] William Bloor expressed his willingness to assist Linacre and apologized for any delay in enrolling the documents at London.[7] These legal difficulties do not seem to have seriously impeded Linacre's gradual acquisition of lands intended for his endowment, although their repercussions may later have involved the estate in expensive legal battles.[8]

The estates and money which passed to St. John's College, Cambridge, are more easily described. By the time of Linacre's last Will, it had been determined that property in London known as the Bell and the Lantern in Adling Street,[9] and other lands held by Thomas Cony, fletcher, of London, were to come to St. John's College. In the archives of the College is preserved the indenture between Cony and Linacre dated 12 December 1523, which sets out the terms of the agreement regulating this property.[10] Linacre also gave to the College a considerable amount of money. It is probable that this large sum was partly raised by the sale of certain of his own lands just before he died. The Merton archives contain documents that suggest this. These record that on 12 September 1523, Linacre sold land in the parish of 'Ffeversham and Boughton under the Blee' to Rauff Symonds, citizen and fishmonger of London, for £85,[11] and that shortly afterwards on 1 May 1524 he sold property in Knight

---

[1] Calendar no. 11 and probably no. 13.   [2] Calendar no. 12.
[3] Calendar nos. 14 and 15.   [4] Calendar no. 16.   [5] Calendar no. 17.
[6] Calendar no. 18.   [7] Calendar no. 19.   [8] See below, p. 138.
[9] Now Addle Hill.   [10] See Appendix A9.   [11] Calendar no. 20.

Rider Street to William Mortymer 'citezein and brawderer' of London for £30.[1] Again we see Linacre completing arrangements for his Cambridge lectureships at a very late date; as with the setting up of the Oxford lectureships, his concern for this endowment can be dated only to the last years of his life.

Nevertheless, the surviving documents at Oxford and Cambridge indicate that Linacre's plan to establish lectureships in both universities was no sudden, haphazard scheme but a well-thought-out policy. His lectureships at both Oxford and Cambridge should be seen as part of the important efforts of London humanist scholars to introduce their educational ideas into the universities, efforts which have perhaps been obscured by the sudden onset of the Reformation, but which are of considerable importance to the history of education in Tudor England.

III. *The Establishment of the Lectureships*

Linacre died on 20 October 1524. His last Will, dated 19 June 1524, as printed by Johnson[2] poses important problems to the historian in that it contains no mention of the property acquired during the previous years and little reference to his proposals concerning the medical lectureships he wished to found. This lacuna in our knowledge has prevented any adequate discussion of Linacre's intentions and has made it difficult to understand the later behaviour of his executors.

The problem is resolved by a document now in the archives of Merton College, Oxford.[3] Endorsed 'ultima voluntas Thome Lynacre in medicinis doctoris', this long roll declares itself to be 'my last wyll as to the disposicion of all my maners, landes, and tenementes wyche I or any other parson or parsones have or hath to my use in the countie of Kent, in the citie of London, or elswhere wyth in the realme of England'. Since these lands formed the endowments to finance the Linacre lectureships at both Oxford and Cambridge, it would appear that Linacre made two Wills. The first, printed by Johnson, provided for minor gifts to the physician's relations and friends, set out the procedure to be followed at his funeral, and made various donations to churches in compensation for unpaid tithes.

[1] Calendar no. 21.
[2] Johnson, op. cit., pp. 343–5. See also Appendix B1.
[3] See Appendix B2.

The much longer and more important Merton document, here printed for the first time, was intended to set out the complex details for the endowment and continuance of his medical lectureships in both universities. It enables us now properly to evaluate Linacre's part in the history of medical education in England, and to reconsider the subsequent policies of those given responsibility for the actual establishment of the lectureships.

When the much needed new complete life of Thomas Linacre is written, its author must consider why this important Will has been so long overlooked and overshadowed by that printed by Johnson. We cannot here be concerned with these problems except to suggest that the very existence of a printed version may have precluded proper search for another document. The recently discovered Will is important to the present discussion in that it provides a full account of the proposed lectureships, and the basis on which later documents, discussed below, were founded. The Will is dated 18 October 1524, that is only two days before Linacre's death, and must represent his final thoughts concerning the shape of his lectureships. First are listed in full the estates noted above, which were acquired by Linacre to provide the financial support for his proposals. Then the reason for Linacre's concern with the problem of medical education is bluntly stated. Although the study of medicine 'is right mete and expedient for thenhabitanntes in every cominaltie to the comfort of the people and remedy of many maladies', and a supply of trained physicians should be assured, the Universities of Oxford and Cambridge had been unable to produce this. The reason given is that there was a 'lak of lectures and instruccions'. Nor had there been any 'substanciall' or 'perpetuall' lectures in medicine founded.

The Will then instituted for Oxford two permanent lectureships, the 'more lecture' and the 'lesse lecture', terms which were later to be translated as 'lectio superior' and 'lectio inferior'. These were to be established as soon after Linacre's death as was thought convenient by the executors of the Will, Cuthbert Tunstal, Bishop of London, Thomas More, John Stokesley, canon and prebendary of St. Stephen's Chapel, Westminster, and William Shelley, Serjeant at Law and Recorder of London. It is interesting to see that Linacre chose neither an essentially academic nor an essentially ecclesiastical body to be responsible for the completion of his proposals. He further placed future responsibility for the control of his Oxford

lectureships not with any university body, but with a lay organization, the Mercers' Company. With the king's permission, the lands
and estates already mentioned in Kent, together with part of the
Stone House, Linacre's own home, were to be passed on to the
Company, which would then administer the endowments, appoint
the lecturers, and decide where and when the lectures were to be
given. If the Company were unwilling to accept this responsibility,
then the lands were to be offered to any corporate body approved
by the executors. Although Linacre's plans here were not carried
out, his approach to the Mercers' Company is of the greatest interest.
Dr. McConica has well emphasized the 'close tie between reforming
clergy in London and this influential group of merchants'. John
Colet, a close associate of Linacre, had strong family connections
with the Company and already had placed the management of his
foundation of St. Paul's School in the Mercers' hands.[1] Here is
another important example of London humanists following a common policy in the realization of their 'programme' to reform and
improve educational opportunities in England. Linacre himself may
have been somewhat uncertain about the choice of the Company,
however, since references to it in his Will appear to have been
inserted in gaps left in the original draft.

The Oxford lectures were to be read by graduates, 'masters of
arte at the leest'. Linacre was clearly not optimistic that even
generous provision could at first induce highly qualified medical
doctors to remain as lecturers at the university. As was usual in the
sixteenth century, his provisions recognized the close association between the Faculty of Arts and the Faculty of Medicine. The senior
lecturer was to receive an annual payment of twenty marks. His
teaching programme was to cover, by reading every day 'a dowble
lecture of Galyen and noon other', six books of the *De sanitate tuenda*
'for his ordynary', and three books of the *De alimentis* 'for his afture'
lecture, and also, as 'ordynary' lectures, fourteen books of the *De
methodo medendi*, and as 'after' lectures the first five books of the
De simplicibus medicamentis. The junior lecturer was to be paid
£6. 13s. 4d. annually and was to read for his 'ordynary' lectures
three books of the *De temperamentis*, three books of the *De naturalibus
potentiis*, six books of the *De morbis et simtomatis*, and two books of the
De differentiis febrium, and for his 'aftur' lecture six books of the *De*

---

[1] McConica, op. cit., pp. 48, 102.

locis affectis and then Hippocrates' *Prognostica* with the commentary by Galen. This lecturer was to be given preference when appointments to the senior position were made provided that he was found 'most able, mete, and convenyent'. To provide an income for his two sisters, Linacre restricted the senior lecturer's stipend to the sum of £11 and postponed the establishment of the junior lectureship during their lifetimes. Should one sister die, any surplus income was to be used at the discretion of his executors.

The lecturers were to receive their salaries in two equal amounts, at the Feasts of St. Michael (29 September) and of the Annunciation (25 March). They were strictly instructed to consider when lecturing only 'litterall' questions and not those which 'Galien calleth logicall'. One may see here the influence on Linacre of humanistic views and his hostility to the practice in most medieval universities of mingling the logical studies of the Faculty of Arts with the studies of the medical faculty. It is also noticeable that no reference to well-known medieval authorities such as Isaac or Bartholomew the Englishman is made. The books mentioned were to be covered during a period of two and a half years or three years at the most. In this way, a medical student could quickly obtain from the two lecturers alone a good grounding in what were then considered to be some of the essential elements of medical knowledge.[1] Should either lecturer fail to deliver his lectures as instructed, he was to forfeit a certain part of his salary.

The arrangements made for the establishment of a single lectureship in the University of Cambridge are not so complex. Linacre notes that he has already made an agreement with the Master and Fellows of St. John's College and has paid to them a certain sum of money. His Will provided for the completion of these arrangements so that the lecturer could commence his duties at the next Feast of the Annunciation. St. John's College was to appoint a graduate of the University of Cambridge, who was to be at least a master of arts, to deliver the lectures. The College was also to determine the time and place for the lectures. As salary the lecturer was to receive £12 annually paid in two equal instalments at the Feasts of St. Michael and the Annunciation. His lectures were to follow the pattern stipulated for those given by the senior lecturer at Oxford, and he too

---

[1] The books prescribed for study at Oxford are noted briefly in Rashdall, op. cit. iii. 156, and the longer list for Montpellier in the fourteenth century in ibid. ii. 127.

was to avoid the treatment of logical questions; his course was to be completed in two and a half or, at the most, three years, after which time the lectureship was to remain unfilled for six months while the income was taken by St. John's College as compensation for its work in administering the benefaction.

The Will concludes with permission to the executors to interpret any difficulty arising from its contents. Linacre also leaves the chapel and the chamber over the chapel in his house in Knight Rider Street to the College of Physicians to be used for their discussions and examinations of practitioners. A short final paragraph bequeaths £6 yearly to Linacre's sister Alice and £5 to his sister Joan. The Will is witnessed by Thomas Bentley, Willyam Partryche, Willyam Latymere (Latimer), John Castell, and John Wylforte.[1]

The copy of Linacre's last Will that has come down to us shows every sign of speedy drafting as a rough version; alterations and corrections are very frequent. Nevertheless it does throw considerable light on the attitudes of the humanists of the London circle in which he moved. It also enables us to judge how far his executors were able to remain faithful to the very complete arrangements made by Linacre for the establishment of his medical lectureships as they later made efforts to carry out their obligations.

The way was already clear for the executors to carry out their work. On 12 October, a few days before Linacre's death, the necessary royal permission to allow the estates to pass into mortmain had been obtained.[2] It is rather puzzling that the Merton version of the last Will, dated 18 October, still speaks as if the obtaining of this licence were necessary. The royal consent concerned all three lectureships, that at Cambridge as well as those at Oxford. The grant is specifically directed to the Mercers' Company although there is no evidence that Linacre intended the Company also to control the lectureship at Cambridge. The dating of this concession would suggest that Linacre's intentions were known in detail before his Will of 18 October was drawn up, and I shall return to this point below.

[1] Thomas Bentley and William Latimer both appear in Dr. Emden's *Biographical Register*, the first as a Fellow of New College, medical doctor, and President of the Royal College of Physicians, the second as a close friend of Linacre with whom he shared a strong interest in humanistic studies.

[2] Johnson, op. cit., pp. 330–3.

The establishment of the single lectureship at Cambridge was not to cause much difficulty for Linacre's executors. An agreement[1] made on 14 June 1524, between Linacre himself and the Master and Fellows of St. John's College, 'concernyng a free lecture of phesike contynually here after to be kypt, redde, and mayntened', had paved the way for the implementation of Linacre's proposals. This agreement provided for the reading of a public lecture in the 'comen scoles' by some suitable lecturer chosen by the Master of St. John's with the advice of the senior masters of certain colleges not named in the document. The appointment of the lecturer is to follow the pattern adopted at the University of Oxford. Linacre here states that, as endowment, he has on the day of the conclusion of this agreement passed to Cuthbert Tunstal £200 to be retained by him until the Master of St. John's takes steps to set up the lectureship. The Master agrees that, when the money is handed over, he will make between Linacre, himself, and an unnamed abbot and convent a further agreement to the following effect: first, that the money donated by Linacre is to be used to purchase lands in Lincolnshire or elsewhere to provide an annual income to finance the lectureship. The Master of St. John's and the heads of one or two other colleges are then to choose a lecturer before the Feast of St. Michael to give the lecture 'yerly and daily at all conveynt days' at such time as shall be most suitable for medical students. The lecturer is to hold at least the B.A. or M.A. degree. Secondly, the Master of St. John's is to pay the lecturer a salary of £10 a year in three instalments. Thirdly, regulations are made for the replacement of the lecturer if necessary and for payment of *pro rata* amounts to a substitute for any time spent in lecturing. Fourthly, the unnamed abbot and convent are given the responsibility of ensuring that the College carries out its obligations under the agreement. Finally, as compensation for its work in carrying out the provisions of the agreement, the College is to receive fifty shillings annually from the income to be derived from the lands purchased by Linacre's donation. Oversight of these arrangements is given to Cuthbert Tunstal and after his death to the Chancellor of the University of Cambridge.

This agreement was followed on 19 August by an indenture between Linacre, Tunstal, More, Stokesley, and Shelley on the one

[1] See Appendix B3.

part and Nicolas Metcalf, Master of St. John's College, on the other.[1]
Here it is noted that Linacre, by his last Will dated 17 June 1524,
has left two pieces of property in London, the Bell and the Lantern,
to the College, and, further, that Linacre has given, on the day of
the present indenture, £209 to the College over and above the
amount of nineteen marks which he has agreed to donate at the
following Feast of All Saints (1 November). This money is to be
used to purchase property and the income so coming to the College
is to provide for the payment of an annual salary of £12 to the
lecturer, who is to be appointed by the Master and seven senior
Fellows of the College. In every fourth year following the establishment of the lectureship, there is to be a period of six months during
which no lectures are given. During this time, between the Feast
of the Annunciation and that of St. Michael, the salary normally
paid to the lecturer shall come to the College itself as compensation
for its efforts. If the College carries out its obligations under this
indenture, it will not incur the loss of the £400 by which it has
bound itself. A further document at St. John's College of the same
date records this obligation of £400 and the reason for it.[2]

It is clear that in its arrangements for appointing and paying the
lecturer, and in its method of ensuring some separate income for the
College, this indenture is considerably different from that made
by Linacre in June. There are also minor variations from the
proposals set out in October in Linacre's last Will, discussed above.
These probably represent simply those modifications to his original
intentions which had to be made speedily as his death approached.
Of more interest is the reference in the indenture to a last Will dated
17 June 1524. As has been pointed out, the Will printed by Johnson
is dated 19 June 1524. Is one to assume that there was another Will,
dated 17 June, by which Linacre first made arrangements for the
disposal of his estates and the endowment of his lectureships at
Oxford and Cambridge? This seems probable for two reasons: first,
it would seem appropriate for Linacre to make such a Will as a close
accompaniment to that he was to make two days later containing
more personal details. Secondly, as noted above, the royal licence
needed for a grant into mortmain had in fact been given before the
date of his last Will of 18 October. It would appear, therefore, that
the main outlines of Linacre's plans were known before this last Will

---

[1] See Appendix B4.   [2] See Appendix B5.

was made. Any arrangements made by the Will of 17 June one must assume were superseded by those set out in the Will of 18 October. Discussions with St. John's College seem, in fact, to have been completed just before Linacre's death. The College archives have a record, dated 18 October, of the receipt of the sum of £221. 13*s*. 4*d*. from Linacre.[1] This is stated to be 'pro fundacione lecture in medicinis' as agreed in the indenture of 19 August. Later evidence indicates that the benefaction from Linacre had duly been received. There is no mention of the lectureship in the College statutes of 1530, but by the time of the version of 1545, the payment and duties of the Linacre lecturer are incorporated in the college regulations.[2] The detailed arrangements for the lectures, closely following those set out in the indenture and in Linacre's last Will, are also contained in the statutes presented to the Royal Commissioners in the nineteenth century.[3]

Linacre's choice of St. John's College as a recipient of his generosity is interesting. The College had made no provision for the study of medicine at its foundation in 1511. The statutes, codified in 1530, mention only the possibility of inviting doctors of medicine to reside in the College as pensioners.[4] However, Fisher was another member of the London 'humanist circle' I have often had occasion to mention. As Bishop of Rochester he had frequent and easy access to the capital and as chaplain to the Lady Margaret he had the ear of the Royal Court. His influence on the Lady Margaret's efforts to establish at Cambridge foundations that would enlist the support of the 'new learning' for the improvement of the Church was most profound. In his statutes for St. John's College, Fisher made for the first time at Cambridge serious efforts to provide proper instruction in the classics for students preparing for degrees in arts and theology. Linacre must have been familiar with Fisher's plans. It would be most apt if lectureships intended to replace the previous scholastic interpretation of medical texts with a close textual study in line with the humanists' aims were located in this new foundation. These were probably the motives that influenced Linacre. At

[1] See Appendix B6.
[2] J. E. B. Mayor, *Early Statutes of the College of St. John the Evangelist in the University of Cambridge*, Cambridge, 1859, pp. 171, 253–5.
[3] *Documents Relating to the University and Colleges of Cambridge*, 3 vols., London, 1852, iii. 276–7.
[4] Mayor, op. cit., p. 84.

Cambridge at least the timely completion of his plans before his death left few problems for his executors.

Unfortunately the early history of the lectureships at the College is very vague, but two important if tantalizing pieces of evidence suggest that appointments to the position were made shortly after Linacre's death. First, the brass in the College chapel that records the death in 1528 of Christopher Jackson, elected a Fellow in April 1525,[1] notes that he had held the lectureship. Its wording is interesting: 'Christophorus Iacsonus, socius huius collegii et artium ac medicae lectionis a doctore Linacro institutae professor, e sudore Britannico adhuc iuvenis moritur atque hic sepelitur anno 1528° die 2° Iulii' (see Plate III). The style and form of this inscription seem contemporary; we should also perhaps expect a specific mention of Jackson's appointment as Linacre lecturer if the endowment was still fresh in the minds of his colleagues. As Linacre's instructions required, Jackson was also qualified as a lecturer in arts and therefore a proper person to hold the lectureship. Secondly, Baker in his history definitely states of George Daye, fourth Master of the college: 'In his younger years he had studied physic and was the first that held the Linacre lecture.' As a footnote to this comment, Baker adds: 'Anno 16, 17 etc. Hen. 8[vi]', which is to say that the lectureship was first held in the regnal year beginning April 1524.[2] It does not seem possible to check the accuracy of either of these statements from contemporary evidence, but it does appear correct to assert that a tradition of the college assumed that appointments to the Linacre lectureship in medicine were made in the mid 1520s. Linacre's executors do not seem to have had to involve themselves deeply in the establishment of the Cambridge lectureship.

The establishment of the Oxford lectureships, a far more complicated and more important part of Linacre's programme, was much more difficult. Linacre's last Will imposed upon his executors the full weight of the duty of seeing that his intentions here were implemented. Apart from the general statements that he had made to the University, there is no indication that serious negotiations, as at Cambridge, had begun before his death. Linacre's executors were closely connected with both London and the Court; they were also very busy men. Tunstal, More, and Stokesley were at the centre of

[1] T. Baker, *History of the College of St. John the Evangelist, Cambridge*, ed. J. E. B. Mayor, 2 vols., Cambridge, 1869, i. 282.

[2] Ibid. i. 112.

political events in the crucial years following Linacre's death; frequently they were sent abroad as royal ambassadors. Tunstal, the most important figure, was especially involved in affairs of state during these years; his translation to the see of Durham in 1530 was followed by his appointment as President of the Council of the North. Tunstal's Register as Bishop of Durham[1] makes no mention of his concern with Linacre's Will, nor has his biographer[2] paid much attention to the problem of why action to implement Linacre's plans was so delayed. There may have been divisions amongst the executors as the progress of the royal divorce issue began to split the intellectual community. Whatever the reason for inaction, no attempt seems to have been made to implement the terms of Linacre's Will until 1532. On 25 September of that year, the Acts of Court of the Mercers' Company record that it was 'ordeyned and agreed that a chist of evidence of certen londs late doctor Lynacres pretended to be geven to this Compeny shalbe receved and kepte in this hous'.[3]

Apparently the executors now came upon an unexpected snag. The Mercers' Company refused to accept the responsibility of endowing the lectures according to the terms of Linacre's Will. We know that a definite refusal was made because this is explicitly stated later in the document by which Linacre's estates passed to Merton College.[4] Unfortunately nothing appears to have survived to indicate why this refusal was made. It is not difficult, however, to suggest practical problems that might have stood in the way of implementing Linacre's proposals. Given the climate of the early 1530s it is not surprising that an important trading company, with close links with Europe and with the Royal Court, was reluctant to become involved in academic affairs. Efforts by Henry VIII to win support from prominent academics for the royal policy towards the papacy were turning problems that ten years earlier could have been considered as purely educational into political issues. An obligation to become entangled at this date in close negotiations with the University of Oxford could clearly have been a source of

---

[1] *The Registers of Cuthbert Tunstall, Bishop of Durham 1530–59, and James Pilkington, Bishop of Durham 1561–76*, ed. G. Hinde, Surtees Soc., vol. clxi, Durham, 1952.

[2] C. Sturge, *Cuthbert Tunstal*, London, 1938.

[3] London, Mercers' Company, Acts of Court 1527–1560, fol. 49.

[4] See Appendix B9.

some embarrassment to the Mercers' Company. In the 1530s the attack on monastic property and in 1535 the visitation of the universities must in any case have cast doubt on whether endowments at Oxford and Cambridge would be allowed to stand. This was not the most propitious time to take on the responsibility for the administration of an academic benefaction.

Despite the transfer of the deeds of Linacre's lands to the Mercers' Company, Tunstal may have continued to administer the property, perhaps because of the Company's reluctance to carry out Linacre's instructions. Certainly, after his recovery of the deeds in 1542 noted below, the Bishop's agent received the income from the estates. By chance there survive at Merton College accounts[1] for 1543–4. Here Tunstal's servant, William Hebelthewayte, records the income and expenditure for the manors of Traces and Frognall. It is interesting to note that two payments, each of fifty shillings, were made at Easter and Michaelmas to Linacre's sister. This must have been Joan, as a payment of five pounds annually to her was required by Linacre's last Will. Of more importance is the surprisingly small amount, 4s. 6½d., held by Hebelthewayte after making all the payments required of him. It is impossible to say whether the expenditure of this year was exceptionally high; legal payments certainly absorbed some of the income. It appears possible, however, that the income available annually to Linacre's executors may not have been as high as he himself had anticipated. Although the accounts refer only to the manors of Traces and Frognall, these were the most substantial of Linacre's acquisitions and it is unlikely that the other estates would produce any considerable increase in income. Perhaps the need to provide annuities for first two and then one of Linacre's sisters proved too heavy a charge on his estate and as long as even one sister had to be supported in this way there was insufficient money available to carry out his wishes. This cannot yet be claimed as more than a suggestion to explain the executors' apparent reluctance to establish the lectureships. It is also interesting to see that when the lands eventually came to Merton College, reduced payments were allocated to the lecturers and it seemed usual there, despite the terms of both Linacre's Will and Tunstal's agreement with the College, to appoint one lecturer only. Was the income then available insufficient to provide stipends for two lecturers? Unfortunately the answer to this question cannot be readily re-

[1] See Appendix B7.

covered from the documentary evidence available at the college. Considerable research would have to be done in the Merton archives before it would be possible to plot accurately the income received in the late sixteenth and seventeenth centuries from the lands previously held by Linacre.[1] However, if this work could be done, and it could be shown that the lands then produced less than Linacre anticipated, there would be strong grounds for asserting that one of the reasons compelling his executors to delay the establishment of the Oxford lectureships was that during the lifetime of even one surviving sister, the lands did not produce an income adequate to support a lecturer. Also, if it were possible to determine the date on which Linacre's sister Alice died, this might be shown to have influenced Tunstal in the next stage of his attempts to establish the lectureships. Joan but not Alice was alive in 1543–4. It was in 1540 that a further move had been made, an approach to Brasenose College. Had Alice died before 1540, some six pounds should have been available each year to add to any surplus income from Linacre's estates. This could have been the event which stimulated the negotiations that were concluded by May 1540.

The refusal of the Mercers' Company to carry out Linacre's plan left with his surviving executors the responsibility of finding another institution willing to undertake this task. The matter was now becoming urgent. Thomas More had been executed in 1535; John Stokesley died in 1539. Tunstal, the most important surviving executor, was born in 1474 and now in his fifties must have viewed his own future with anxiety; the difficulties of steering a careful course through the political disturbances of the period were becoming more apparent as attitudes towards questions of religious faith began to harden. Linacre's original plan was abandoned. Instead, Tunstal took up the arrangements made for the Cambridge lectureship and adapted them to the needs of Oxford. He attempted to induce an Oxford college to accept the lands left by Linacre and with the income establish the medical lectureships as required by his last Will.

By 6 May 1540 negotiations were so well advanced as to enable Tunstal to conclude an indenture[2] with the Principal of Brasenose College and the Warden of All Souls College, to set up the lectureships. Following the outline of Linacre's last Will, this indenture

[1] From information kindly supplied by Dr. J. R. L. Highfield.
[2] See Appendix B8.

describes the lands left by Linacre and his intention of improving the teaching of medicine at Oxford and Cambridge. Tunstal then states that following the death of the other executors, he is left with responsibility for 'the hole trust for the performannce of the last will of the seid Thomas Lynacre'. Accordingly, he grants to the Principal and Scholars of Brasenose College for the establishment of the two lectureships the property entrusted to him, which he states is now valued at £24. 10s. The junior lecturer is to read from nine until ten every morning during term time those books allocated to him by Linacre's Will, which are here named without division into 'ordinary' and 'after' lectures as in the Will itself. The treatment of the material is to be as Linacre wished, and payment of £5 is to be made to the lecturer each year in three instalments. The lecturer is to complete his course in two and a half years or three at the most. No time of day is specified to the senior lecturer for the delivery of his course. The books allocated to this lecturer and the method of treatment are again the same as those mentioned in Linacre's Will, but again without the division found there. A salary of £10 is to be paid to this lecturer. It is perhaps significant that the two payments were considerably less than those originally allocated by Linacre. Both lecturers are to read for three-quarters of a year from the Feast of St. Michael (29 September) to the Feast of the Nativity of St. John the Baptist (24 June) and are then to spend the remaining time in recreation and in the preparation of their future lecture course. With the exception of minor details, it is apparent that Tunstal is carrying out here the terms of Linacre's Will itself.

Arrangements for the election of the lecturers are, however, considerably modified to provide for the changed situation. Responsibility is now given to the Principal of Brasenose, the Warden of All Souls, and the holder of the senior lectureship to nominate two candidates 'well lerned in phisik, maisters of arte at the lest' whenever the position of junior lecturer becomes vacant. These two are to be nominated, one from Brasenose, one from All Souls, or, if no Fellow from either college is found suitable, from other halls and colleges of the University, and presented to Tunstal, if he is readily available, to appoint one of them to the position. If he is not available, or after his death, the choice is to be made by the University Commissary or his deputy in consultation with such doctors of medicine and theology as are available. The chosen lecturer is then to be received by Brasenose College. Promotion to the position of senior lecturer is to be granted to the junior lecturer on any vacancy, with the approval of the two college heads in consultation with doctors of medicine. If the position of senior lecturer cannot be filled in this way, then the programme of nomination as provided for the junior lectureship is to be followed here also. Arrangements are made for the college heads each to ensure that the other carries out his obligations as defined by this indenture, and Brasenose is allocated an annual sum to compensate the College for its efforts in supervising the endowment.

The indenture itself presents few problems. Tunstal is clearly attempting to adapt Linacre's proposals to a new situation while remaining loyal to the essential details of the lecturing programme Linacre had set out in his Will. However, the abandonment of Linacre's policy of entrusting the endowment and its control to a lay body was an important step away from the earlier humanist schemes for educational reform. The offer of the estates and the lectureships to a college rather than to the University also seems a departure from Linacre's intentions as suggested by his earlier letters and by the general tone of the Will itself. Perhaps Tunstal thought that by this date the relative strength of the colleges within the University was so pronounced as to make it more suitable to rely on a college foundation to carry out the appointment and supervision of the lecturers. Whatever the motives behind this movement away from Linacre's original intentions, the indenture with Brasenose and All Souls is an important indication of how the Linacre lectureships were finally to be established.

The circumstances surrounding the drawing up of this indenture do present more serious difficulties. The choice of Brasenose and All Souls as colleges to administer the endowment is, to say the least, very surprising. Neither college was well known for the production of qualified medical doctors, although, as mentioned above, there is evidence for some study of medicine at All Souls College in the fifteenth century. By the terms of their statutes, neither college was encouraged to provide fellowships specifically for medical students. There was little possibility, therefore, that holders of the lectureships under the terms of this indenture could ever be more than masters of arts with an interest in medicine. It certainly was not Linacre's intention that his lectureships should never be held by fully qualified doctors in medicine, yet here Tunstal seems to be accepting such a situation. It may be that realization of this fact was

one of the reasons for the eventual failure to implement the arrangements made in this indenture. The association of All Souls College
with the scheme is perhaps not too difficult to understand since
Linacre himself had, of course, close connections with that foundation. Brasenose College had, however, made little mark on academic
history by this date and could not be compared in size with other
colleges. But there is one significant development that may have
influenced Tunstal's choice. In 1538 the President of Corpus Christi
College, John Claymond, himself a well-known humanist, had
founded six scholarships in Brasenose. These scholars were instructed
to attend the Greek lectures delivered in Corpus Christi College.[1]
As already observed, it was in such a way, by the establishment of
colleges and individual endowments associated with the 'new learning' or with separate branches of it, that the English humanists of
the early sixteenth century attempted to infiltrate the universities
and introduce their own educational concepts. Claymond's scholarships were the first considerable accession of strength to Brasenose
since its foundation and must certainly have increased interest in
humanist studies within the College. Can Tunstal's association
with Brasenose be seen as a further effort to strengthen the College
and especially the element there favourable to humanist policies?
Since there appears to survive, beyond the indenture itself, no
evidence of these negotiations, one can only make these tentative
suggestions as to why Tunstal made such a choice and why he in
this way abandoned some of Linacre's original proposals for the
administration of his Oxford lectureships.

Even more disappointing is the absence of evidence to indicate
why and when these new plans were in turn abandoned. Certainly,
for Tunstal, the following years were a period of intense diplomatic
activity. The royal progress through the North in 1541 was followed by negotiations and then war with Scotland from 1542 until
1545. Perhaps the two colleges themselves were reluctant to administer an endowment in an academic field with which they were not
over-familiar. Perhaps, with one sister still living, Linacre's estates
were not producing an adequate amount. Whatever the reasons, the
later history of the lectureships shows that the scheme of 1540 was
never in permanent operation, and from the absence of reference to
it in the archives of both Brasenose and All Souls Colleges, it is
probable that it was never instituted.

[1] *Victoria History of the County of Oxford*, iii. 209.

Tunstal, however, must have been confident that he would soon be able to establish the lectureships in some form, for on 25 September 1542 he took a decisive step to gain control of the documents concerning Linacre's lands. On this date his servant, William Hebelthewayte, appeared before the court of the Mercers' Company to deliver a letter from the Bishop requesting the Company to return to him the 'cheste of evydence of doctor Lynackors' which had been retained by the Company for the past eleven years. The Company agreed to the request provided that acknowledgement of the receipt of the chest from them was properly made.[1] This decision marks the end of the association of the Company with the Linacre endowment and suggests that Tunstal now thought that the end of his long career as executor of Linacre's Will was in sight.

This may have been because negotiations had begun with Merton College. Again there is no evidence to indicate why Tunstal made this choice, but it certainly appears more understandable than his earlier efforts to involve Brasenose and All Souls. Merton was one of the very few Oxford colleges to have produced medical doctors of some importance in any number. During the medieval period, its medical graduates were often to be found in the employment of the royal family and in noble households. More recently, John Chambre, Warden of the College from 1525 until 1544, had served as physician to Henry VIII and had co-operated with Linacre in setting up the College of Physicians in London. Tunstal must have been familiar with Chambre, since the latter spent much of his time at Court. It may be that the credit for first interesting Tunstal in passing on to Merton the Linacre endowment should go to Chambre in the years before and after his retirement from the Wardenship of the college. The reputation enjoyed by the College as a centre for medical study must certainly have been known to Tunstal. Anthony Wood also gives credit to the Warden who succeeded Chambre, Thomas Raynold, for influencing Tunstal in Merton's favour.[2] There was every reason for Tunstal to be aware of the position of Merton within the University of Oxford; apart from his own personal knowledge, he would as Bishop of Durham have come into contact with the College estates in his diocese. College officials paid regular visits to Embleton, Ponteland, and Stillington, and the Bishop was occasionally involved in Merton affairs when incumbents of College livings were changed.

---

[1] London, Mercers' Company, Acts of Court 1527–1560, fol. 157^v.
[2] A. Wood, op. cit. ii. 41.

By December 1549 Tunstal was ready to conclude an agreement with Merton College to establish the lectureships. It is important to record that by this date, according to a note in the indenture made later with the College, Linacre's sister, Joan, was dead, and so her annuity was no longer a charge on his estates. On 1 December he formally donated Linacre's lands to Merton College and appointed his proctor to carry out the transfer.[1] On the 5th, the College named its own representative to receive the property.[2] On the 10th, an indenture was made between the Bishop and the Warden and Fellows of Merton which was to form the basis for the future regulation of the Linacre lectureships within the College.[3] It was agreed that two lectureships were to be established as required by Linacre's last Will; the senior lectureship was to be endowed with a stipend of £12 per annum and the junior with one of £6. Both payments, it is stated, had been reduced from the original £13. 6s. 8d. and £6. 13s. 4d. since the revenues from the estates could not produce these amounts. The lectures were to be delivered as required by Linacre. However, in the 1562 entry of an indenture also of 10 December 1549 in the Registrum Annalium, noted below, these important changes are made. Elections from among suitable candidates, holding at least the M.A. degree, were to be made by the Warden of Merton and the seven or eight senior Fellows of the College. Linacre's wish that courses should be of three years' duration was respected, but his requirement that a 'double' lecture should be read daily was specifically abandoned. Instead Tunstal declared that both lecturers were to read every day for an hour and a quarter or at least for one 'greate houre'. Linacre's texts and method of treatment were also preserved, but the distinction between 'ordinary' and 'after' lectures was not maintained. The indenture contained provisions for the use of deputies and for the punishment of negligent lecturers; holders of the lectureships were to be allowed to practise medicine if this did not interfere with their delivery of the programme of lectures. Finally, the College agreed to make a statute within six months embodying the provisions of the indenture.

This indenture was followed on 2 January by a letter of attorney from Tunstal giving to Merton College the power to collect arrears of rent and similar monies owing to the property.[4] The legal details were concluded on 25 July 1550 by the issue of letters patent from

---

[1] Calendar no. 22. [2] Calendar no. 23.
[3] See Appendix B9. [4] Calendar no. 24.

the Warden and Fellows entered in the Liber Statutorum, recognizing their obligations.[1] Linacre's intentions are stated as obliging his executors to give the manor of Traces and other lands 'alicui collegio seu corpori corporato' for the establishment of two lectureships in medicine. Also in this document we have mention of the association of another executor with Tunstal; the Bishop and John Shelley are described as those 'qui supervixerint ac soli superfuere vivi tempore huius concessionis' and both are described as participating in the indenture of the previous December. In return for the grant of the manor of Traces and other lands, the Warden and Fellows bind themselves to keep the conditions of the indenture, now described as between Tunstal and the College, and to any interpretation of Linacre's Will the Bishop has made or may make in the future. The College agrees to have these terms placed in its statute book and read out together with its other statutes three times each year. An indenture was also copied into the Registrum Annalium in July 1562, by order of the Warden and Fellows 'ut inde semper liqueat quibus legibus ac conditionibus ipsi lectores sint astricti'.[2] Although it is dated also 10 December 1549, this indenture between Tunstal and the College differs considerably from that of the same date, previously noted, and records important changes, discussed above, in the arrangements for the lectures. This second indenture probably represents an attempt to adapt Linacre's ideas to the changed conditions of the Edwardian University.

With the production of the legal documents of transfer, the indenture, and the letters patent, it might have seemed that the last act in the long drama of the Linacre lectureships had closed. Indeed, it would appear that Merton College quickly began to manage its newly acquired property; on 28 December 1549, shortly after Tunstal's donation, the Stone House was leased to Edmund Crispin for a period of twenty-one years.[3] There was, however, to be one final scene before the actual appointment of any lecturer. The years from 1550 until his death in 1559 were tragic ones for the aged Bishop of Durham. Again he was brought into the centre of political activity and faced with a number of agonizing choices as the gulf between Catholic and Protestant widened. In October 1552 he was

[1] Calendar no. 25.
[2] Fletcher, *Registrum Annalium Collegii Mertonensis*, p. 220.
[3] Calendar no. 26.

deprived of his see, but was reinstated on the accession of Queen Mary. The reign of Elizabeth began with Tunstal absent from the coronation and at odds with the Archbishop of Canterbury. His refusal to take the Oath of Supremacy was followed in September 1559 by a second deprivation and his consignment to the Archbishop of Canterbury who lodged him in Lambeth Palace.

During these years there does not appear to have been any action taken to appoint at Merton College a Linacre lecturer. However, on 24 November 1559, the college register records: 'Admissus erat Georgius Iamis ad lectionem inferioris lectionis Linacri per litteras venerabilis viri domini Cuthberti Tonstawle, nuper Dunelmensis episcopi, a domino custode presentibus omnibus sociis in domo custodis.'[1] The Bishop had died on 18 November, so that the issue of these letters must have been among the last of his actions. Perhaps at the end, reflecting on his long and involved career, Tunstal had come again to think of his early friendship with Linacre and his obligations to him. Certainly at the close of his life, Linacre seems to have been in his mind; the Bishop's (undated) last Will requests his burial by the side 'of my old friend, doctor Linacre' should he happen to die in London.[2] It was perhaps fitting that, since he had been concerned with proposals to establish the Linacre lectureships at Oxford for the last thirty-five years, one of Tunstal's final actions was to ensure the actual appointment of a lecturer. George James was the first of a series of appointments at Merton, but unhappily Tunstal did not live to see this fulfilment of his obligation to Linacre.

Conclusion

I have traced here from the surviving documentary evidence the growth of Linacre's conception of establishing medical lectureships at Oxford and Cambridge and the steps taken by him and by his executors to ensure that his proposals could be carried out. The involvement in these plans of several of the most prominent scholars and politicians of the period, at a time when educational, religious, and political issues were placing powerful pressures on all, brought the question of the establishment of the lectureships into the arena of national affairs. I have not attempted to follow the careers of those

[1] Fletcher, *Registrum Annalium Collegii Mertonensis*, p. 192.
[2] C. Sturge, op. cit., p. 377: 'iuxta sepulchrum Thomae Linacri medici veteris amici mei'.

involved except inasmuch as they were associated with the actual fate of the lectureships. Any future general study of this period must, however, consider the wider issues here only touched upon. Are there more significant reasons than those suggested for the delay in the actual establishment of the Oxford lectureships? How deeply was the Mercers' Company involved in the political life of the country, and in the negotiations that forced the movement away from Linacre's original policy? Did Tunstal offer the lands to any other corporate bodies apart from those mentioned above? Could the estates bequeathed by Linacre produce, in the second half of the sixteenth century, sufficient revenues to provide adequate remuneration for really qualified medical lecturers at Oxford and Cambridge? These are some of the issues that the emergence of more documentary evidence and the work of other historians may further elucidate. It has not been my intention here to discuss these issues in depth.

It may be claimed, however, that the general outlines of the history of the establishment of the Linacre lectureships at Oxford and Cambridge are now clear. With the consideration of this new evidence, Tunstal's role becomes a little more understandable and he can no longer be accused of a total lack of urgency in his concern with his obligations as Linacre's executor. Linacre's plans themselves and their relation to the general educational problems of the times now become less shadowy, and he himself perhaps emerges as an important innovator so far as the state of medical education in this country is concerned. Certainly the association of Linacre with the London humanist circle and their plans for the introduction of the 'new learning' into the English universities is clearly shown. In short, the evidence here discussed for the first time modifies our previous view of all those involved with Linacre's plans and their execution: their actions appear more intelligible and our attitude to their personal difficulties must now be more sympathetic.

APPENDIX AI. Indenture between Thomas Linacre and Lewis Clyfford respecting property in Kent, and further provisions concerning this property.

Merton College, Oxford. Record no. 1437. The remains of a seal. 8 November 1520.

This endenture made the VIIIth daye of November the XIIth yere of the reign of our sovereign lord, kyng Henry the VIIIth, bytwene Thomas Lynacre, clarke, doctor of phisike too the kyngs highnes on the oon partie and Lewes Clyfford esquyer on the other partie witnessith that the seid Lewes Clyfford hath bargayned and sold and by thes presents clerly bargaynyth and sellith unto the seid Thomas Lynacre his heires and assignes the maner of Traces with the appurtenants in Newenton in the county of Kent and all his londes, tenements, rents, revercions, servyces, and hereditaments in Hartlepp, Stokbury, Upchurche, Reynham, Tong, and Morston or ellswher within the seid county which be or have ben known, letten, reputed, or taken as parcell of the seid maner, to have and to hold all the seid maner of Traces and all other the premysses with thappurtenants to the seid Thomas, his heires and assignes for ever. And the seid Lewes covenantith, waranteth, promyseth and assurith to the seid Thomas and his heires that the seid maner of Traces and other premysses bargayned and sold by the seid Lewes to the seid Thomas by thes presents ben of the clere yerly valore of XII li. over and above all yerly charges and reprices. And ffarther the seid Lewes covenantith and granntith unto the seid Thomas by thes presents that he the seid Lewes his heires or assignes byfore the fest of Ester next comyng after the date herof shall make or cause to be made to the seid Thomas Lynacre, Richard Pace, secretory to our seid sovereign lord[1] the kyng, Cuthbert Tunstall, master of the rolls, Thomas More, esquyer counceller to our seid sovereign lord the kyng, William Shelley, gentylman, John Drewe, clarke, and John Clement, ther heires and assignes, to the use of the seid Thomas and his heires a sure good, sufficient, lawfull, and indefesible estate of and in the seid maner of Traces and all other the londes, tenements and other premysses as shall be devised by the seid Thomas, his heires or assignes or his or ther lerned councell at the egall costs and charges in the lawe of bothe the seid parties the same estate to be dyscharged of all fformer bargeyns, former sales, joynters, dowres, statutes, marchannts statutes of the staple, juggements, execucions, lyvereys out of the kyngs handes, intrucions, alienacions without the kyngs license, ffees, annuyties, rents, charges, the arrerages of all rents and servyces, and all other charges and incombrannces except oonly the rents and servyces of old tyme to the chyff lordes of the ffee due and acustomed, and rents of old tyme goyeng out of the premysses or eny parte of them which after the date herof shall growe and be due. And ffarthermore the seid Lewes covenantyth and granntith unto the seid Thomas by thes presents thatt he the same Lewes and Benett his wyff his heires or assignes and Nicholas

---

[1] 'lord' inserted above the line.

Clyfford, now beyng son and heire apparannt of the seid Lewes, and all and
every other person or persons eny thyng havyng or cleynyng of and in the
premysses or eny parte of the same too the use of the seid Lewes, Benett his
wyffe, the seid Nicholas or eny of them or of the heires of eny of them shall
at all tymes herafter when and as often as he or they or eny of them shalbe
reasonable requyred doo suffer or cause to be doon all and every thyng that
shall be devysed by the lerned councell of the seid Thomas, his heires or
assignes, at the egall costs and charges in the lawe of bothe seid Thomas and
Lewes or of ther heires for the ferther suerty of the seid Thomas, master
Richard Pace, Cuthbert Tunstalle, Thomas More, William Shelley, John
Drewe and John Clement, ther heires and assignes to be had of and in the
premysses and every parte therof be hit by recoverye, yf eny wrytt for the
same maye be soffered to passe the kyngs courte of Channcerye, ffyne, feffment,
relese with warannte of the seid Lewes, Benett, and Nicholas or eny of them
ayenst all men or otherwyse waranntice of the seid other persons oonly
except. And ffarther the seid Lewes hathe bargayned and sold and by thes
presents clerly bargaynyth and sellith to the seid Thomas and his heires all
and synguler charters, dedes, evidences, ffynes, court rolls, terrers, mynyments, and escrippts the seid maner of Traces and other premysses and every
parcell therof oonly concernyng or belongyng and covenantith and granntith
by thes presents to delyver all the same evidence whiche the seid Lewes or
eny other person or persons to his use or by his delyvere hathe or have or
may reasonable combye to the seid Thomas or his assignes byfore the seid
ffest of Ester next comyng. And ffarthermore the seid Lewes covenantyth and
granntith by thes presents to the seid Thomas and his heires that he the seid
Lewes byfore the seid ffest of Ester next comyng after the date herof shall
bryng in to the kyngs court of Channcerye all dedes, charters, evidence,
ffynes, wrytyngs, and mynyments whiche he or eny other person or persons
to his use or by his delyvere and to his knolege hathe or have or whiche
byfore the seid ffest of Ester shall com to the handes or possession of the seid
Lewes, Benett, Nicholas or eny of them concernyng as well the seid maner
of Traces londes, tenements, hereditaments, and other premysses byfore
bargayned and sold or eny parcell therof as other maners, londes, and tenements the same dedes, charters, evidences, ffynes, wrytyngs, and mynyments
at the sute and costs of the seid Lewes and his heires to be copied and
exemplified in the seid court of Channcerye after the fforme of a vidimus and
after the seid dedes, charters,[1] evidences, ffynes, wrytyngs, and mynyments
soo exemplified all the seid dedes, charters, evidences, ffynes, and other wrytyngs to be redelyvered to the seid[2] Lewes and his heires or assignes without
eny cleame to be made to the same by the seid Thomas Lynacre, his heires
or assignes, and the exemplificacion of the seid evidence shall be delyvered to
the seid Thomas or his heires or assignes byfore the seid ffest of Ester. And
the seid Lewes covenantith and granntith by thes presents to the seid Thomas
Lynacre that the same Thomas his heires and assignes shall clerly, peseably,
and quyetly have, hold, possess,[3] occupye, and inyoye the seid maner of Traces
and other the premysses byfore bargayned and sold and every parcell therof

---

[1] MS. 'channters'. [2] 'seid' inserted above the line. [3] MS. 'possed'.

without[1] lett, interupcion, expolcion, vexacion, or eny inquyetyng by the seid Lewes or his heires or by the seid Benett or Nicholas or eny person or persons cleymyng to the use of the seid Lewes or his heires or the seid Benett or Nicholas or eny of them or eny title from them[2] or eny of them. And ffarther the seid Lewes covenantith and granntith by thes presents to the seid Thomas Lynacre and his heires that he the seid Lewes shall byfore the seid ffest of Ester next comyng at the egall costs and charges in the lawe of the seid Thomas and Lewes or of ther executours make or cause to be made to the seid master Richard Pace, Cuthbert Tunstall, Thomas More, William Shelley, John Drewe and John Clement and ther heires[3] suche a sure, sufficient, and lawfull estate of and in the moite of the maner of Bobbyng with thappurtenants in the county of Kent as shall be devised by the lerned councell of the seid Thomas or his heires to the uses and intents herafter folowyng, that is to saye that yf the more parte of the seid maner of Traces and other the premysses byfore bargeyned and sold after the rate of the very valure therof by the yere be[4] recovered uppon a good and just title or evicted out or ffrom the possession of the seid Thomas his heires or assignes without ffraude or coven of the seid Thomas his heires or assignes, that then immedyatly after suche recovere or eviccion the seid master Richard Pace, Cuthbert Tunstall, Thomas More, William Shelley, John Drewe and John Clement ther heyres or assignes shall stand and be seased of and in the same moite of the seid maner of Bobbyng with the appurtenants to the use and behoffe of the seid Thomas Lynacre his heires and assignes for ever, provided alwaye and it is agreed bytwene the seid parties that the seid Thomas Lynacre, master Richard Pace, Cuthbert Tunstall, Thomas More, William Shelley, John Drewe, and John Clement or eny of them, ther heires or assignes or the heires or assignes of eny of them survivyng shall assign and chose whiche moite in severalte they will take, and after suche assigment and choyse had the seid Thomas, master Richard Pace, Cuthbert Tunstall, Thomas More, William Shelley, John Drewe, and John Clement shall have and reteyne the same moite so assigned and chosen in severalte to the use of the seid Thomas Lynacre and his heyres and too and for the perfourmance of the last will of the same Thomas Lynacre in the same moite. And yf it happen eny parte or parcell of the seid maner of Traces and other the premysses byfore bargayned and sold not amountyng to the more parte of the yerly valure of the seid maner of Traces and other the premysses be recovered appon a good and just title or lawfully evicted out or from the possession of the seid Thomas Lynacre his heires or assignes without ffraud or coven of the seid Thomas his heires or assignes, that then immediatly after suche recoverye or eviccion the seid master Richard Pace, Cuthbert Tunstall, Thomas More, William Shelley, John Drewe, and John Clement ther heires and assignes shall stand and be seased of as moche of the seid moite of the seid maner of Bobbyng suche as the seid Thomas his heires or assignes will chose, accept, and take other then the dwellyng place of the seid maner of Bobbyng or the syte therof as the seid londs and tenements beyng parcell of the seid maner of Traces and other the premysses byfore bargayned and sold soo beyng recovered or devicted out or

---

[1] Altered from 'with'.   [2] 'them' inserted above the line.
[3] 'heires' inserted above the line.   [4] 'be' inserted above the line.

ffrom the possession[1] of the seid Thomas, his[2] heires or assignes shall amount
unto after the rate of the yerly valure therof to the use and behoff of the seid
Thomas Lynacre his heires and assignes and of the residue of the seid moite
of the maner of Bobbyng to the use of the seid Lewes Clyfford his heires and
assignes for ever. And ffarther it is agreed bytwene the seid parties that the
seid Thomas Lynacre shall have the oon halff of all the rent that was due of
the seid maner and other premysses at the ffest of Seynt Mychell tharchanngell
last paste to his owne use and behoff, ffor the whiche bargayne and sale and
for all the covenants of the seid Lewes well and truly to be observed, fulfylled,
and kept the seid Thomas hathe content and payed to the seid Lewes at the
insealyng of thes indentures CCXVI li., wherof the seid Lewes Clyfford
knolegith hymselff well and truly contentyd and satisfied and therof dys-
chargith and acquyetyth the seid Thomas Lynacre and his executors by thes
presents. And where the seid Lewes by his dede obligatory baryng date the
daye of thes presents standyth bounden to the seid Thomas Lynacre in the
som of CCCC li. sterlyng payable to the same Thomas Lynacre his heires,
executors or assignes in the ffest of Crystmas next comyng as in the same dede
obligatory more playnly maye appere, neverthelesse the seid Thomas Lynacre
covenantith and granntith by thes presents to the seid Lewes that yf the same
Lewes his heires executours or assignes truly fulfyll, observe, performe, and
kype all and every of the covenants, grannts, and promyses above specified on
the parte of the seid Lewes truly to be fulfilled, observed, performed, and
kept, and also yf all the promyses, warannties, and assurannces of the seid
Lewes in thes indentures conteyned be trewe, that then the seid dede obligatory shalbe voyd and of none effect or ells it shall stand in his full strenght
and vertue. In witnesse wherof the parties aboveseid to thes indentures enter-
channgeable have sette ther seales the daye and yere aboveseid.

Per me Lewys Clyfford.

Reverse:
(1) Indentura Trasis et al' inter Lynacre et Clyfford.
(2) Indentura Tracys et al' inter Thomam Lynacre et Clyfford pro vendi-
tione terrarum Traces.
(3) A modern note summarizing the contents of the document.

APPENDIX A2. **Indenture between Thomas Linacre and
Richard Hyll respecting the Stone House and adjacent
property in London.**

Merton College, Oxford. Record no. 1447. The remains of a seal.
30 September 1522.

This endenture made betwene Thomas Lynacre, clerk, on that oon partie and
Richard Hyll of London, gentilman, on that other partie, witnesseth that the

---

[1] MS. 'possion'.   [2] 'his' inserted above the line.

same Richard Hyll for the somme of XLVI li. XIII s. IIII d. sterlings to hym by the seid Thomas Lynacre before hande payde, wherof the same Richard Hyll holdesth hym wele and truly contented and payde and therof acquyteth and dischargeth the seid Thomas Lynacre by these presents, hath bargayned and sold and by these presents clerely bargayneth and selleth to the seid Thomas Lynacre oon messuage called the Stonehouse and oon gardein to the same messuage adioynyng and apperteynyng, sett and beyng in the parissh of Seint Benet of London in a strete called Knyghtryder Strete, betwene the tenements perteynyng to the cathedrall church of Seint Paule of London of the parties of est and south and the tenement of William Gysnam, otherwyse called William Guysnam of London, gentilman, in the which oon Thomas Waren sumtyme dwelt and in the which oon William Lewes afterwards dwelled in part and the tenements late of the pryour and covent of the hous, pryory or hospitall of our blissed lady of Elsyng in part on the west partie and the heigh strete called Knyghtryder Strete on the north partie, in the which messuage and gardeyn adioynyng one William Lytton, squyer, late dwelled, and also hath bargayned and sold to the seid Thomas Lynacre all and every the dedes, charters, evydences, and mynuments concernyng the seid messuage and gardyn that the seid Richard Hyll or any other persone or persones to his knowlech have or hath. And the seid Richard Hyll covenanteth, grannt- eth, promytteth, and byndeth hym by these presents that he and all and every other persone and persones havyng any astate, title, or interesse to of or in the seid messuage and gardein or to of or in any part or parcell of the same by with or from the same Richard Hyll or to his use shall onthisside the fyrst day of Marche nowe next comyng make or do to be made to the seid Thomas Lynacre and to Cuthbert Tunstall, Richard Pace, Roger Drewe, John Chambre, Roger Denton, John Stokysley, clerks, Thomas More, knyght, William Shelley, sergeaunt atte lawe, Ffranncys Poynts and John Clement, gentilmen, and to their heires and assignes to the use of the same Thomas Lynacre and of his heires to the performannce of the last wyll of the same Thomas Lynacre as sufficiannt and a lawfull astate in the lawe of and in the seid messuage and gardeyn by ffeoffament, ffyne, recovere, releesse, or other- wyse as shalbe advysed by the lerned counceill of the seid Thomas Lynacre of his heires, executors, or assignes with warrantes of the seid Richard Hyll and his heires ayenst the abbott of Westminster and his successors, and also that the same Richard Hyll shall onthisside the seid fyrst day of Marche nowe next comyng delyvere or do to be delyvered to the seid Thomas Lynacre to his heires or assignes all and every such dedes charters evidences and mynu- ments as the same Richard Hyll or any other persone or persones of his delyverannce or to his knowlege have or hath concernyng the seid messuage and gardeyn or any part or parcell of the same. In witnesse wherof the seid parties to these endentures channgeably have sett their sealls. Yoven the last day of Septembre the XIIIIth yere of the reign of kyng Henry the VIIIth.

Per me Ricardum Hyll.

APPENDIX A3. **Indenture between Thomas Linacre and Thomas Elmeston respecting property in Kent.**

Merton College, Oxford. Record no. 1518. The remains of a seal. 14 November 1522.

This endenture made betwene Thomas Lynacre, clerk, on that oon partie and Thomas Elmeston of Reynham in the countie of Kent, yoman, on that other partie witnesseth that the seid Thomas Elmeston hath bargayned and sold and by these presents clerely bargayneth and selleth to the seid Thomas Lynacre all and every the landes and tenements, medes, leeses, woods, pastures, rents, reversions, and services with their appurtenans called Sevans lande, the which he late purchased of oon Vyncent Ffynche, gentilman, and also all his lands and tenements, medes, leeses, woods and pastures, rents, reversions and services with thappurtenans called Bulles, the which the seid Thomas Elmeston late purchased of oon   ¹ Bulle   , sett, lying, and being in the parisshes, townes and ffelds of Newenton, Hertlep and Halstone in the countee of Kent. And also the seid Thomas Elmeston hath bargayned and sold and by these presents clerely bargayneth and selleth to the seid Thomas Lynacre all and every the dedes, charters, evydences, and mynuments concernyng the forseid lands and tenements, medes, leeses, woods, pastures, rents, reversions, and services with their appurtenans or any part or parcell of the same. And the same Thomas Elmeston covenanteth, grannteth, promytteth, and byndeth hym by these presents that he and alle and every such persone and persones havyng any astate, title, or interesse of or in the seid lands and tenements and other the premisses or of or in any part or parcell therof by or fro the seid Thomas Elmeston or to his use shall onthisside the ffest of Seint Andrewe thappostle nowe next comyng make or do to be made to the seid Thomas Lynacre and to other persones such as the same Thomas Lynacre woll name and assigne and to his and their heires to the use of the same Thomas Lynacre and his heires a sufficiant and lawfull astate in the lawe of and in all and every the seid lands and tenements and other the premisses with their appurtenans with lyke warrantice and after lyke forme as the seid Thomas Elmeston hath of and in the same of the forseid Vyncent Ffynche. And furdermore the same Thomas Elmeston covenanteth and grannteth by these presents that he shall onthisside the seid ffest of Seint Andrewe delyvere or do to be delyvered to the seid Thomas Lynacre to his heires or assignes all and every such dedes, charters, evidences, and mynuments as he the same Thomas Elmeston or any other persone or persones of his delyverannce or to his knowleche have or hath concernyng the seid lands and tenements and other the premisses or any part or parcell of the same. And the seid Thomas Lynacre covenanteth and grannteth and also byndeth hym by these presents that he for the forseid lands and tenements called Sevans with their appurtenans shall atte makyng of the seid astate of and in the same to the seid Thomas Lynacre and other persones and to their

¹ Blanks in the MS. before and after 'Bulle'.

heires after the forme aboveseid pay or do to be payd to the seid Thomas
Elmeston to his executors or assignes XXIIII[1] li. sterlings, and overe that shall
atte same tyme pay or do to be payd to the seid Thomas Elmeston to his
executors or assignes for such costs and charges as he hath spent and payd
in and upon certein bildyngs and reparacions of parcell of the same londs and
tenements called Sevans VI li. XIII s. IIII d. and overe that shall atte same
tyme pay or do to be payd to the seid Thomas Elmeston to his executors or
assignes asmoch money for the forseid lands and tenements called Bulles with
their appurtenants as the same lands and tenements overe all charges be in
value after the rate of twenty yeres purchase. And the seid Thomas Lynacre
covenanteth and guaranteth by these presents that the seid Thomas Elmeston
his executors and assignes shall have free libertie and licence att all tymes
convenyent onthisside the ffest of the Nativite of Seint John Baptist nowe
next comyng to have free entre and issue with horses and cartes into and fro
all and every the forseid lands, tenements, and woods called Sevans there to
take and from thens to carye to their owne use all and every such wode as
the same Thomas Elmeston hath doon to be felled within the same. And the
same Thomas Elmeston covenanteth and grannteth by these presents that
he at his owne costs shall onthisside the seid ffest of the Nativite of Seint John
Baptist sufficianntly hedge and enclose all and every the hedges and dyches
of the wodes and groves wherin the seid wode nowe lyeth felled for savyng
of the spryng fro beests. In witnesse wherof the seid parties to these endentures channgeably have sett their sealls. Yoven the XIIIIth day of Novembre
the XIIIIth yere of the reigne of kyng Henry the VIIIth.

                                                                    Carkeke

Reverse:
(1) Sevans et Bulles land. Elmstone vendidit Thome Lynacre.
(2) A modern note summarizing the contents of the document.

**APPENDIX A4. Indenture between Thomas Linacre and
others, and John Potett alias John Akent, respecting property in Kent.**

Merton College, Oxford. Record no. 1438. The remains of a seal.
7 February 1523.

Sciant presentes et futuri quod ego Iohannes Potett, alias dictus Iohannes
Akent, civis et ffruterer London', dedi, concessi et hac presenti carta mea
confirmavi Thome Lynacre, clerico, Cuthberto permissione divina London'
episcopo, Ricardo Pace, Rogero Drewe, Iohanni Chambre, Rogero Denton,
Iohanni Stokesley, clericis, Thome More, militi, Willelmo Shelley, servienti
ad legem, Ffrancisco Poyntz, Iohanni Clement, gentilmen, et Ricardo Hardyng, yoman, totum illud messuagium et gardinum annexum continentes per

                    [1] Written with XX above IIII.

estimacionem dimidiam acram terre cum suis pertinentiis, situata, iacentes et existentes in parochia de Bobbyng in comitatu Kanc' ad regiam viam ibidem versus austrum et orientem ad terram heredum Lodowici Clyfford, armigeri, versus occidentem, et ad terram heredum Iohannis Goddyn versus aquilonem, habend' et tenend' predictum messuagium et gardinum cum suis pertinentiis prefatis Thome Lynacre, Cuthberto episcopo, Ricardo Pace, Rogero Drewe, Iohanni Chambre, Rogero Denton, Iohanni Stokesley, Thome More, Willelmo Shelley, Ffrancisco Poyntz, Iohanni Clement et Ricardo Hardyng, heredibus et assignatis suis ad usum eiusdem Thome Lynacre heredum et assignatorum suorum ad inde perimplendum ultimam voluntatem eiusdem Thome Lynacre de capitalibus dominis feod' illis per servicia inde debita et de iure consueta. Et ego vero predictus Iohannes Potett et heredes mei predictum messuagium et gardinum cum suis pertinentiis prefatis Thome Lynacre, Cuthberto episcopo, Ricardo Pace, Rogero Drewe, Iohanni Chambre, Rogero Denton, Iohanni Stokesley, Thome More, Willelmo Shelley, Ffrancisco Poyntz, Iohanni Clement et Ricardo Hardyng, heredibus et assignatis suis ad usum predictum contra omnes gentes warrantizabimus et imperpetuum defende- mus per presentes. In cuius rei testimonium huic presenti scripto meo sigillum meum apposui. Datum septimo die Ffebruarii anno regni regis Henrici octavi quartodecimo.

Carkeke

Reverse:

(1) Memorandum quod possessio et seisina de et in messuagio et gardino infrascriptis deliberata fuit per infrascriptum Iohannem Potett infra- nominato Ricardo Hardyng decimo die Ffebruarii anno regni regis Henrici octavi quartodecimo in presencia Iohannis Smyth, Iohannis Day, Roberti Wynge, Ricardi Materesse, Roberti Boyes, Willelmi Skylton, Iohannis Treules et multorum aliorum.

(2) Bobbyng Kaysstrete.

(3) A modern note summarizing the contents of the document.

APPENDIX A5. Indenture between Thomas Linacre and William Bloor respecting property in Kent.

Merton College, Oxford. Document no. 1523. The remains of a seal. Signed by William Bloor. 18 June 1523.

This indenture made betwene Thomas Lynacre, clerk, on the one part and William Bloor of Reynham in the countie of Kent, gentilman, on the other part, witnesseth that the seid William for an hundred and thirty pounds sterlings by the seid Thomas to the seid William before hand payde, wherof the same William holdeth hym wele and truly payde and the seid Thomas therof to be quyte and discharged by these presents hath bargayned and sold and by these presents clerely bargayneth and selleth to the seid Thomas and

to his heires all that his messuage called Ffrognall and all his lands and
tenements, medowes, leeses, woods, underwoods and pastures, rents, reversions and services sett, lying, and being in the parissh of Newenton beside
Sydyngborne in the countie of Kent, which the seid William Bloor purchased
and bought of Thomas Draper of Erithe in the countie of Kent, gentilman,
and also one parcell of lande conteynyng by estimacion two acres of lande
lying in the parissh of Hertlep in the seid countie at a place called Goldhord
which the same William also purchased and bought of the seid Thomas
Draper, and also clerely bargayneth and selleth to the seid Thomas Lynacre
and to his heires and assignes all and every the dedes, charters, evidences, and
mynuments concernyng oonly the forseid messuage, lands, and tenements
and other the premisses or any part or parcell of the same. And the seid
William Bloor covenanteth, grannteth, promytteth, and byndeth hym by
these presents that he and all and every other person and persons havyng any
astate, title, possession or interest to of or in the seid messuage, lands, and
tenements and other the premisses with their appurtenants or to of or in any
part or parcell therof by or from the seid William Bloor or to his use shall
onthisside the last day of the moneth of August next comyng make or do to
be made to the seid Thomas Lynacre and to other persons such as the same
Thomas will name and assigne and to his and their heires to the use of the
same Thomas Lynacre and of his heires and assignes at the costs and charges
of the seid Thomas Lynacre or of his executors as sure sufficient and lawfull
astate in the lawe of and in all and every the forseid messuage, londs, and
tenements and other the premisses by recovere, ffyne, ffeoffament, release
with warrantie of the seid William Bloor and of his heires or otherwyse as
shalbe advysed by the lerned counceill of the seid Thomas Lynacre or of his
heires or assignes discharged of all and every statutes of the staple, statutes
merchannts, recognisannces, annuitees, ffees, joyntors, dowers, ffynes, issues,
amerciaments, condempnacions, jugements, execucions, encombrannces,
intrusions, arrerages of rents, former bargaynes and former sales, and of all
and every other charge and charges made, begon, grannted, or conveyed by
the seid William Bloor or his ffeoffes, except the rents and services to the
cheiff lords of the ffee from hensforthward to them hereafter to be due, so that
the seid advyse of the seid lerned councellors in that behalf be had and
declared to the seid William Bloor before the last day of Apryll nowe next
comyng.[1] And ferthermore the seid William Bloor covenanteth, grannteth,
promytteth, and byndeth hym by these presents that he shall onthisside the
last day of Septembre next comyng delyvere or do to be delyvered to the seid
Thomas Lynacre his heires or assignes all and every such dedes, charters,
evidences, and mynuments the which the seid William or any other person
or persons of his delyverannce or to his use or knowlege have or hath which
he before the same last day of Septembre shall or may come by or unto
concernyng onely the seid messuage lands and tenements and other the
premisses with their appurtenans or any part or parcell of the same, and also
that the seid William shall onthisside the same last day of Septembre delyvere
or do to be delyvered to the seid Thomas Lynacre to his heires or assignes
true and hooll copies to be made and writen at the costs and expences of the

---

[1] 'before the last . . . comyng' inserted above the line.

seid Thomas Lynacre or his executors of all and every such dedes, charters, evidences, and mynuments concernyng aswell the forseid messuage, londs, and tenements and other the premisses or any part or parcell of them and other londs and tenements of the seid William Bloor ioyntly. And ferthermore the same William Bloor covenanteth and also will and grannteth by these presents that the seid Thomas Lynacre his heires and assignes may receyve and take to his and their owne propre use all and every the rents and fermes that have growen of the forseid messuage, lands, and tenements with thappurtenants in the seid parisshe of Newenton and Hertlep sithens the ffest of Seint Mighell tharchanngell last past[1] and shall growe and be due at the ffest of Seint Mighell tharchanngell next comyng, to be perceyved and taken by the hands of the ffermors of the same messuage, lands, and tenements and other the premisses without any lett, contradiccion, or trouble of the seid William or his heires or assignes or of any other person or persons. And also that the seid messuage, lands, and tenements with their appurtenants or any part or parcell of them be not nor is holden in cheiftie of our soveraigne lord the kyng otherwise then in socage as of his maner of[2] Myddelton in the seid countie of Kent or of his maner of Chestens in the hundred of Myddelton. And also that the seid messuage, lands, and tenements with thappurtenants or any part or parcell of them be not nor is charged nor chargeable with any yerely rent or service to any person or persons but oonly with the cheiff rents and services therof due to the kyng and other lords by reason of their maners or seignouries and rents comenly called romescote, except onely an yerely rent of eight busshells of barley which is due and payable to Nicholas Clyfford, squyer, sone and heire of Lewes Clyfford, deceessed. And ferthermore the seid William Bloor covenanteth and grannteth by this indenture that yf in any tyme duryng his naturall lyf the seid messuage, lands, and tenements and other the premisses or any part or parcell therof fortune to be lawfully evycted, devested, or taken out of or from the possession of the seid Thomas Lynacre his heires or assignes by reason of any condicion, ryght, or title of any persone or persones havyng cause or begynnyng before the makyng of this present indenture and no defaute, covyn, or collucion by the seid Thomas Lynacre his heires or assignes in that behalf had or used, then the seid William Bloor his heires or executors within the tyme of forty dayes next after notyce gyven to the seid William Blower of the seid eviccion shall pay or cause to be payde to the seid Thomas Lynacre his heires or assignes, that is to say to hym or them from whos enheritannce and possession the[3] lands and tenements or part or parcell therof shalbe evycted such somme of lawfull money of Englond as then shall amount or extend to the full value of the issues and profetts of the same lands and tenements in XX[ti] yeres for and in recompense and satysfaccion of the same lands and tenements so evicted. And the seid Thomas Lynacre grannteth and agreeth by this indenture that it shalbe leefull to the seid William Bloor his executors and assignes at any tyme or tymes convenient before the ffest of Pentecost next comyng to cary and take from the seid lands and tenements all such trees and tymbre nowe being felled and lying upon the same, and also all other goods of the same William

---

[1] 'past' inserted above the line.   [2] 'of' inserted above the line.
[3] 'the' inserted above the line.

Bloor nowe lying or being upon the same, and that in the meane season the same trees, tymbre, and goods shall and may lye and be upon the same lands and tenements this indenture or the seid astate to be made in forme above written notwithstondyng. And for all and singuler covenants, promyses, and grannts above written on the behalf of the same William Blower to be wele, truly, and fully performed, observed, and kept on the behalf of the same William he byndeth hym his heires and executors by this present indenture to the seid Thomas Lynacre and his executors in the somme of two hundred marks sterlings. In witnesse wherof the seid parties to these indentures channgeably have sett their sealls. Yoven the XVIIIth day of June the XVth yere of the reigne of kyng Henry the VIIIth.

Reverse:

(1) Bloer. Indentura pro Frognall. 15 H. VIII.

(2) A modern note summarizing the contents of the document.

APPENDIX A6. Indenture between Thomas Linacre and Thomas Crips respecting property in Kent.

Merton College, Oxford. Record no. 1442. The remains of a seal. 3 October 1523.

This endenture made betwene Thomas Lynacre, clerk, on that oon partie and Thomas Crips of Newenton besides Sydyngburn in the countie of Kent, carpenter, on that other partie witnesseth that the seid Thomas Crips for the somme of XLVI s. VIII d. sterlings by the seid Thomas Lynacre to the seid Thomas Crips before the[1] hande payde, wherof the same Thomas Crips holdeth hym wele and truly contented and payde and therof and of every part therof acquyteth and dischargeth the seid Thomas Lynacre by these presents, hath bargayned and sold and by these presents clerely bargayneth and selleth to the seid Thomas Lynacre and to his heyres and assignes two acres of errable lande with thappurtenants lying and beyng at Warndale in the parissh of Newenton besides Sydyngburn in the countie of Kent betwene the lands of John Copynger, gentilman, on the parties of est and south and the lands of the seid Thomas Lynacre on the west partie and the lands of the seid Thomas Lynacre in part and the lands of Thomas Dyggs, gentilman, in part of the north partie. And also the same Thomas Crips hath sold and by these presents selleth to the seid Thomas Lynacre and to his heyres and assignes all and every dedes, charters, evidences, and mynuments concernyng the seid two acres of lande with thappurtenants, and also the seid Thomas Crips covenanteth, grannteth, promytteth, and byndeth hym by these presents that he and all and every other person and persons havyng any astate, title, or interesse to of or in the seid two acres of lande or to of or in any part or parcell of the same shall onthisside the ffest of Alle Seynts nowe next comyng make or do to be made to the seid Thomas Lynacre and to

---

[1] 'the' inserted above the line

other persons such as the same Thomas Lynacre woll name and assigne and to their heyres and assignes to the use of the same Thomas Lynacre and of his heyres and assignes a ssure sufficient and lawfull astate in the lawe of and in all the same two acres of lande with thappurtenants by recovere, ffyne, ffeoffament, release, or otherwyse with warrantee of the seid Thomas Crips and of his heyres dyscharged of almanere charges, arrerages of rents, former bargaynes and sales, and other encombrannces except the cheiff rents and services of the cheiff lords therof hereafter to be due as shalbe advysed by the lerned counceill of the seid Thomas Lynacre of his heyres and assignes. And also that he the same Thomas Crips shall onthisside the seid ffest of Alle Seynts nowe next comyng delyvere or do to be delyvered to the seid Thomas Lynacre to his heyres or assignes alle and every the dedes, charters, evidences, and mynuments the which the seid Thomas Crips or any other persone or persones of his delyverannce or to his knowlege have or hath or that he may come by or unto concernyng the seid two acres of lande or any part or parcell of the same. And also that the same Thomas Lynacre his heyres and assignes shall peasibly have, holde, and enioye the seid two acres of lande with thappurtenants without any laufull expulsion or interupcion of any person or persons. And the seid Thomas Lynacre for hym and his executors woll and grannteth by these presents that yf the seid Thomas Crips wele and truly performe, observe, fulfille, and kepe all and every covenants, grannts, and promyses aboveseid, the which on his partie owen to be performed, observed, fulfilled, and kept in manere and forme above rehersed, that than an obligacion of the date of these presents wherin the seid Thomas Crips is hold and bound to the seid Thomas Lynacre in fyve marks sterlings shalbe voyde and had for nought, and els hit shall stond in full strenght and vertue. In witnesse wherof the seid parties to these endentures channgeably have sett their sealls. Yoven the III^de day of Octobre the XVth yere of the reigne of kyng Henry the VIIIth.

Reverse:
(1) Duabus acris terre in parochia de Newington.
(2) Cryps.
(3) A modern note summarizing the contents of the document.

APPENDIX A7. Indenture between Thomas Linacre and Thomas Crips respecting property in Kent.

Merton College, Oxford. Record no. 1365. The remains of a seal. Signed by Thomas Crypse. 23 November 1523.

This endenture made betwene Thomas Lynacre, clerk, on that oon partie and Thomas Crips of Newenton besides Sydyngborne in the countie of Kent, carpenter, on that other partie, witnesseth that the seid Thomas Crips for the some of XLVI s. VIII d. sterlings by the seid Thomas Lynacre to the seid Thomas Crips before the hande payde, wherof the same Thomas Crips holdeth

hym wele and truly contented and payde and therof and of every part
therof acquiteth and dischargeth the seid Thomas Lynacre by these presents,
hath bargayned and sold and by these presents clerely bargayneth and selleth
to the seid Thomas Lynacre and to his heires and assignes one acre and half
an acre of lande with thappurtenants lying and beyng in the parissh of Stokbury in the countie of Kent, betwene the lands of Richard Tate, gentilman,
on the est partie and the kyngs heighwey on the south partie and the lands of
Thomas Alayn on the west partie and the londs of the seid Thomas Lynacre
on the north partie. And also the seid Thomas Crips hath sold and by these
presents selleth to the seid Thomas Lynacre and[1] to his heyres and assignes
alle and every dedes, charters, evidences, and mynuments concernyng the
seid acre and half an acre of lands with thappurtenants. And also the same
Thomas Crips covenanteth, grannteth, promytteth, and byndeth hym by
these presents that he and all and every other persone and persons havyng
any astate, title, or interesse to of or in the seid acre and half an acre of land
or to of or in any part or parcell of the same shall onthisside the ffest of the
Epiphanye of our lord Jhesu Crist nowe next comyng make or do to be made
to the seid Thomas Lynacre and to other persons such as the same Thomas
Lynacre woll name and assigne and to their heyres and assignes to the use
of the same Thomas Lynacre and of his heyres and assignes a ssure sufficient
and lawfull astate in the lawe of and in the same acre and half an acre of lands
with thappurtenants by recovere, ffyne, ffeoffament, release, or otherwyse
with warrantie of the seid Thomas Crips and of his heires, discharged of al
manere charges, arrerages of rents, former bargaynes and sales, and other
encombrannces except the cheiff rents and services of the cheiff lords therof
hereafter to be due as shalbe advysed by the lerned counceill of the seid
Thomas Lynacre of his heyres or assignes. And also that he the same Thomas
Crips shall onthisside the seid ffest of the Epiphanye of our lord Ihesu Crist
nowe next comyng delyvere or do to be delyvered to the seid Thomas to his
heires or assignes alle and every the dedes, charters, evidences, and mynuments the which the seid Thomas Crips or any other person or persons of his
delyverannce or to his knowlege have or hath or that he may come by or unto
concernyng the seid acre and half an acre of land or any part or parcell of the
same. And also that the same Thomas Lynacre, his heyres and assignes shall
peasibly have, holde, and enioye the seid acre and half an acre of lande with
thappurtenants without any lawfull expulsion or interupcion of any person
or persons. And the seid Thomas Lynacre for hym and his executors woll and
grannteth by these presents that yf the seid Thomas Crips wele and truly
performe, observe, fulfille, and kepe all and every the covenants, grannts, and
promyses aboveseid the which on his partie owen to be performed, observed,
fulfilled, and kept in manere and forme above rehersed, that than an obligacion of the date of these presents wherin the seid Thomas Crips is hold and
bound to the seid Thomas Lynacre in IIII li. sterlings shalbe voyde and had
for nought and els hit shall stond in full strenght and vertue. In witnesse
wherof the seid parties to these endentures channgeably have sett their sealls.
Yoven the XXIIIth day of Novembre the XVth yere of the reigne of kyng
Henry the VIIIth.

---

[1] 'and' inserted above the line.

APPENDIX A8. Account respecting the purchase by Thomas Linacre of land in Kent.

Merton College, Oxford. Record no. 1657. No date.

Parcells of lond bowght be Thomas att Tonge ffor IIII acres of lond and a yerd at Boddys in Northfeld otherwyse called North Halff sum tym John and Stevyn Blackettys.

The same Thomas for V yerdys of lond in Southfelde and for a acre of lond at Tylterdene layt Richard Powrys.

The same Thomas for a acre of lond in Southfeld sum tym Gilbert Thomas and Stevyn Wardys.[1]

The same Thomas for II acres and a half of lond in Wolmermersshe and for III yerdys of lond lying in Crypsyncroft otherwyse called Wolmercroft and of layt tym callyd Alys Hawe layt John and Stevyn Blacketts.

The same Thomas for a acre of lond in Southfelde layt Gylberd Warde and Robert Bolye.

The same Thomas for a acre of lond layt Stevyn Bolyes and Gylbert Warde yn Sowthfelde.

The same Thomas for I acre of lond in Wolmerfelde.

Summa III s. V d. q^a d.

APPENDIX A9. Indenture between Thomas Linacre and Thomas Cony respecting property in the parish of St. Benet, London.

St. John's College, Cambridge. Muniment Room Drawer 54, No. 32. The remains of a seal. Signed: Thomas Linacre, manu propria. 12 December 1523.

This endenture made betwene Thomas Lynacre, clerk, on that oon partie and Thomas Cony, citezein and ffletcher of London, on that other partie witnesseth that the seid Thomas Lynacre hath dymysed, grannted, and leten to ferme to the seid Thomas Cony all those his foure messuages or cotages and parcell of a yerde or voyde ground adioynyng, sett, lying, and beyng in the parisshe of Seynt Benet besides Pawlys Wharff in the warde of Castell Baynard of London betwene the newe pale sett upon the fundacion of bryke of the seid Thomas Lynacre on the est partie and the kyngs heigh wey called Adlyngstrete on the west partie and the tenements late of sir Mathewe Broun, knyght, on the north partie and the tenements perteynyng to the parisshe church of Seynt Benet besides Powles Wharff aforeseid on the south partie, to have and to holde all the seid IIII messuages or cotages with the seid yerde

---

[1] Altered from 'Wadys'.

and other the premisses to the seid Thomas Cony to his executors and assignes ffrom the ffest of the Byrth of our lord Jhesu Crist next comyng after the date of these presents unto the ende and terme of ffourescore yeres then next ensuyng and fully to be completed, yeldyng and paying therfore yerely duryng the seid terme to the seid Thomas Lynacre to his heyres or assignes ffyfty and three shelyngs and four pence sterlings at four termes of the yere in the citie of London usuely by even porcions. And yf hit fortune the seid yerely rent of LIII s. IIII d. to be behynde unpayde in part or in all by the space of a quarter of a yere overe or after any terme of payment aboveseid, than hit shalbe leefull to the seid Thomas Lynacre to his heyres and assignes into all the seid IIII messuages and other the premisses with their appur-tenants to entre and distreyne and the distresses there so taken leefully for to bere, lede, dryve, and carye awey and towards them to withholde unto the tyme that the seid rent so beyng behynde with tharrerages of the same yf any such be to them be fully contented and payde. And the seid Thomas Cony covenanteth, grannteth, promytteth and byndeth hym and his executors by these presents that he at his owne propre costs and charges in all things and by all things wele and competently shall kepe all the reparacions of all the seid IIII messuages and other the premisses duryng the seid terme of LXXX yeres. And the seid Thomas Lynacre covenanteth and grannteth by these presents that he his heyres and assignes shall pay and bere all and every cheiff and quyte rents goyng and due to be payde and borne out and for the seid IIII messuages and other the premisses with their appurtenants and therof and of every part therof shall clerely save harmeles the seid Thomas Cony and his executors and every of them duryng the seid terme of LXXX yeres. And the seid Thomas Cony covenanteth and grannteth by these presents that he his executors and assignes shall suffre all the water that shall falle or be on the est syde of the seid pale of the seid Thomas Lynacre to have his full course and renne thurgh a convenient grate to be sett in the bryke walle under the seid pale and to have free course and passage from thens thurgh the seid voyde grounde before dymysed into Adlyngstrete aforeseid at all tymes duryng the seid LXXX yeres peasibly without contradiccion, trouble, or lett of the seid Thomas Cony of his executors or assignes or of any of them. And the seid grate to be made and repayred at all tymes duryng the seid terme of LXXX yeres at the costs and charges of the seid Thomas Lynacre of his heyres and assignes. And[1] furdermore hit is condescended and agreed betwene the seid parties by this endenture that the seid Thomas Cony shall dygge and make a sufficient and partable welle under the seid pale of such stones, bryke, and tymbre as shalbe convenient concernyng the same to serve aswell the seid Thomas Cony his executors and assignes on the west partie of the seid pale as the seid Thomas Lynacre his heyres and assignes on the est partie of the seid pale there to drawe, take, and have water at all tymes duryng the seid terme of LXXX yeres at their pleasures. And that the seid Thomas Lynacre shall gyve unto the seid Thomas Cony towards the makyng of the seid welle XXXIII s. IIII d. sterlings. And furdermore hit is covenanted and agreed betwene the seid parties that after the seid welle be so made, the reparacions and clensyng of the same at all tymes duryng the seid terme of LXXX yeres

[1] There is a pointer to this entry in the margin.

shalbe atte egall costs and charges of the seid Thomas Lynacre, his heyres and assignes and of the seid Thomas Cony, his executors and assignes. And the seid Thomas Lynacre covenanteth, grannteth, promytteth, and byndeth hym and his heyres by these presents that hit shalbe leefull to the seid Thomas Cony, to his executors and assignes to make all and every such edificacions and byldyngs in and upon the seid voyde ground before dymysed and in and upon every part and parcell therof as hit shall please the seid Thomas Cony his executors and assignes at all tymes duryng the seid terme of LXXX yeres. And the seid Thomas Cony covenanteth, grannteth, promytteth, and byndeth hym by these presents that he his executors and assignes shall at their owne propre costs and charges well and sufficiently repayre susteyne and maynten all and every the seid byldyngs so by hym his executors or assignes to be made[1] in all things and by all things when and as ofte as nede shall requyre or be by all the seid terme of LXXX yeres all and every the seid byldyngs and other the premisses made[2] in the ende of the same terme of LXXX yeres well and sufficiently repayred and mayntened in all things and by all things shall leve and yelde up. And furdermore the seid Thomas Cony covenanteth and also for hym and his executors grannteth by these presents that hit shalbe leefull to the seid Thomas Lynacre to his heyres and assignes oons in every two yeres of the seid LXXX yeres into all and every the forseid tenementes and buyldyngs made and to be made and other the premisses before dymysed and into every part and parcell of the same to entre and there to serche and oversee whether the reparacions of the same and of every part of them be mayntened, repayred, and kept as they ought to be after the forme aboveseid or not, and yf they or any of them than and there at any such tyme or tymes fynde defaute of such reparacions in that behalf that than therof to gyve warnyng to the seid Thomas Cony to[3] his executors or assignes to reforme, repayre, and amend the same within two yeres next ensuyng alwey next after such warnyng so geven and that as often tymes as any such case shall fortune to falle or be duryng the seid terme of LXXX yeres. And yf hit fortune either the seid rent of LIII s. IIII d. to be behynde unpayde in part or in all by the space of a hooll yere overe or after any terme of payment therof aboveseid in which hit oweth to be payde or yf such the seid[4] defaults of reparacions so founde by the seid Thomas Lynacre his heyres or assignes be not repayred and amended within two yeres next ensuyng alwey after such warnyng therof geven to the seid Thomas Cony to his executors or assignes, that than hit shalbe lefull to the seid Thomas Lynacre to his heyres and assignes into all the seid tenementes, buyldings, and other the premisses before dymysed hoolly to reentre and the same to have ayen, receyve, and repossede as in his former astate, and the seid Thomas Cony his executors and assignes therof hoolly to expell and ammove, this present leesse or grannt in anywyse notwithstondyng. And the seid Thomas Lynacre for hym and his heyres covenanteth and grannteth by these presents that the seid Thomas

---

[1] This originally read before alteration 'so to be made by hym his executors or assignes'.
[2] 'premisses made' inserted above the line.
[3] 'Cony to' inserted above the line.
[4] 'the seid' inserted above the line.

Cony his executors and assignes for the seid yerely rent of LIII s. IIII d. and under the covenants in maner and forme above rehersed, shall peasibly and quyetly have, hold, occupye, and enioye all and every the seid tenements and other the premisses with their appurtenants duryng the seid terme[1] without any lett, trouble, vexacion, hurte, or interupcion of the seid Thomas Lynacre of his heyres or assignes or of any other person or persons. In witnesse wherof the seid parties to these endentures interchanngeably have sett their sealls. Yoven the XIIth day of Decembre, the yere of our lord M^tV^d XXIII, and the XVth yere of the reigne of kyng Henry the VIIIth.

Reverse:

Various late-sixteenth-century notes relating to the duration of the lease.

APPENDIX B I. Linacre's Will of 19 June 1524.

Transcribed from Public Record Office, Registry of the Prerogative Court of Canterbury; printed by Johnson, *Life of Linacre*, pp. 343–5, as Linacre's Last Will.

In the name of God, Amen. The XIXth day of Juyn in the yere of our lord god a thousande fyve hundred and XXIIII and the XVI yere of the reigne of kyng Henry the eight, I Thomas Lynacre, doctour of phesike, being hole of mynde and in good memory, lawde and praysyng be unto almighty god, make ordeyn and dispose this my present testament and last will in maner and fourme folowing; that is to witt, ffirst I bequeth and recommende my soule unto almighty etc. and my body to be buried within the cathedrall churche of Saint Poule of London before the rode of north dore there bitwene the longe forme and the wall directly over agaynst the said rode. And I bequeth for my buriall there to be had suche convenient summe of money as shalbe thought by the discrecions of myn executours. Item I bequeth to the high awter of Saint Benet where I am a parishen for my tithes forgotten in discharge of my soule and conscience XIII s. IIII d. Item I bequeth to the high awter of Saint Stephyns in Walbroke for my tithes there forgotten in discharge of my soule and conscience VI s. VIII d. Item I woll that suche due detts as I owe of right or of conscience to any maner persone or persones shall be wele and truely contented and paid. Item I woll that Alice, my suster, shall yerely during hir lyfe have of the londes to be bought for my lectour at Cambrige syx pounds sterlinge to be paide to hir halfe yerely. And I woll that Joane, my suster, shalhave during hir lyfe fyve pounds sterlinge of the landes to be bought for the said lectour in like maner and fourme to be paide, orells the said summes to be yerely perceyved of the profits of my londs in Kent or in London after the discrecions of my lorde of London, sir Thomas More, knyght, and maister John Stokesley, prebendary of Saint Stevyns at Westmynster. Item I bequeth to Thomas Lynacre, my brother, xl s. Item I bequeth to my two neses, Agnes

---

[1] 'duryng the seid terme' inserted above the line.

and Margaret, eche of them a bedde with all things to it complete after the discrecions of myn executours so that Margaret shalhave the better. Item I bequeth maister William Dancastre a fether bed and two Irisshe blanketts with a bolster. Item I bequeth to John Plumtre these boks: Palax, Thuchiddes with that that foloweth, Theoder and Apolones, Libanius Declamacions, Theocritas with the coment, Pynderus with the coment, the coment upon Ommer. Item I woll that my funeralls and burying shalbe doon in moderat maner after the discrecions of myn executours. Item I bequeth to Richard my servant a blak gowne of III s. a yarde and XL s. in money for the good service that he hath doon to me. Item I bequeth to eche of John Appulby and Edward Tagge, my servants, a blak gowne a pece of III s. a yarde and VI s. VIII d. a pece. And I woll that all my servants and housholde have mete and drynke for a moneth next after my decesse. Item I bequeth to my cosyn, Robert Wright of Chester, a doblet cloth of blak satyn, beyng in the keping of my suster Alice. Item I bequeth to Richard Wright a blak gowne and XX s. in money. Item I bequeth to Elizabeth, my mayde servant, a blak gown and hir wages after the rate of XXVI s. VIII d. by yere. The residue of all my goodes whatsoever they be after that my detts be paide, my funerall charges doon and these my legacies and bequests expressed in this my present testament and last wille fulfilled and perfourmed I woll shalbe solde by myn executours and the money commyng of the sale of the same to be applyed for and towards the performanns and fulfilling of this my present testament and last. And of this my present testament and last will I make and ordeyn my lord Cuthbert, bisshop of London, sir Thomas More, knyght, and maister John Stokesley, prebendary of Saint Stevyns at Westmynster, myn executours, desiring and requiring them to substitute and make som honest proctour under them to take the labours aboute the performyng of this my testament and the same proctour to be rewarded for his diligence in that behalfe with parte of my goodes after the discrecions of my said executours. Thise witnesse maister William Dancastre, clerk, William Latymer, clerk, John Wylford, notary, Richard Hardyng, John Appulby.

APPENDIX B2. Will of Thomas Linacre.

Merton College, Oxford. Roll no. 6697. 18 October 1524.

In the name of god, Amen. The XVIIIth day of October in[1] the yere of owre lord god M[lo] V[c] and XXIIII and the XVIth yere of the reigne of owre soveraigne lord Henry the VIIIth, by the grace of god of England and of Frannce kyng, defensor of the feith, and lord of Ireland, I Thomas Lynacre, doctor of phesyke and phesician to owre soveraigne lord the kyng, beyng hool of mynd and perfyte memory, lawde be therof to almyghty god, make and ordeyne this my last wyll as to the disposicion of all my maners,[2] landes, and tenementes wyche I or any other parson or parsones[3] have or hath to my use in the

---

[1] 'in' inserted above the line.　　[2] Preceded by 'lands' crossed out.
[3] Altered from 'parsons'.

countie of Kent, in the citie of London, or elswhere wyth in the realme of England as herafter folowyth.

And first I wille that alle and every persone or persones theirer heires and assignes wyche now stond and be seised of and in my maner of Tracies[1] and of and in all other my lands, tenementes, rentis, reversions, and hereditaments in Newyngton,[2] Hartlop, Halstowe, Stokebury, Upchurche, Rayneham, Tonge, and Norston wyche I late purchased and bowght of Lewes Clyfford, esquyer, and of and in alle that my mesuage callyd Frognall[3] and alle other my landis, tenementes, medowes, pastures, wodes, underwodes, rents, reversions and servises with thappurtenunces set, lyyng and beyng in the[4] parisshe of Newyngton nygh Sydyngborne wyche I late purchased of Wyllyam Blower,[5] and of and in alle other my landes and tenementes late purchased and bowght of Thomas Elmeston callyd Sevans,[6] and also of and in alle those my lands and tenementes late by me purchased and bowght of the sayd Thomas callyd Bulleslond, and of and in all my lands and tenementes in Keystrete in the parissh of Bobbyng in the sayd countie of Kent purchased of John Pothed, and of and in alle those my landes and tenementes late by me purchased and bowght of the priour of Elsyng Spytell in the cytie of London callyd the Bell and the Lanthorne in Adlyng strete in the citie of London, and of and in alle those my landes and tenementes called Stonehous in Knyght-riderstrete wyth in the seyd[7] citie of London, and of and in alle other my landes, tenementes, and other hereditaments wyth in the realme of England to thuse of me and myn hires, schall stond and be seised of and in the sayd maners, landes, tenementes, and other hereditaments wyth alle and singuler ther commodities and appurtenunces to thuse and ententes herafter in this my last wille specified, rehersyd, and declaryd, and by me hereafter to be declared and expressed and to noonother use nor entent.

And for asmoche as the[8] faculte of phesyk is right mete and expedient for thenhabitanntes in every cominaltie to the comfort of the people and remedy of many maladies contynuelly channsyng, it ys necessary ther be connyng and expert phisicions of the wiche hathe been great penury for lak of lectures and instruccions in that facultie in Oxfort and in Cambrige, and as yet ther been none certeyn substanciall nor perpetuall lectures of phisyk founded ne ordeyned in the sayd universities wyche were very necessary for the studentts of the sayd universities in the seyd facultie, therfore I, the seid Thomas Linacre, wille and by these presents ordeyne that two substanciall lectures of physyke be founded, erectyd, and stablisshed in the sayd universite of Oxford, the same lectures to begynne and to be put in execucion in as convenient tyme after my decesse as shalbe thowgth by[9] myn excecutors, to contynewe for ever, and that the seyd two lectures shalbe made and redde by two severall graduaates, masters of arte at the leest, to be assigned therunto, namyd, electyd, and apoyntyd fro[10] tyme to tyme when as oftyn as

---

[1] In the margin is written 'manerium de Tracies'.
[2] 'Newyngton' underlined.   [3] In the margin is written 'Ffrognall'.
[4] 'in the' repeated in the MS.   [5] 'Wyllyam Blower' underlined.
[6] In the margin is written 'Sevans'.   [7] 'seyd' inserted above the line.
[8] 'And for . . . the' underlined. 'Notandum' written in the margin.
[9] 'by' inserted above the line and 'convenient' crossed out.
[10] Preceded by 'by' crossed out.

necessite shall requere by the master and wardens of the company of Mercers in London and their successors,[1] and that the place tyme and howres of the seyd lectures to be made be assined, lymetyd, and appoynted by the sayd wardens and their successors.[2]

And I wylle that my feoffees and[3] recoverers, ther heiris and assiynes and suche as be[4] seased of any my maners, lands, and tenementes their heires and assignes whom I require to geve assistence unto the deu execucion of this my last wille shall yerely take the issues, revenues, and profetts of my sayd maner, lands, and tenements and other the premisses wyth the apurtenunces wyth in the sayd counte of Kent and of and in the sayd messuage callyd the Stone Howse wyth thappurtenunces wyth in the cytie of London[5] except the chapell and the chamber over the chapell wyth in my howse where I now dwell wyth in the cytie of London and the[6] same and every parcell therof, shall dymyse and lette to ferme and of parcell of the profetts, issues, and revenues therof comyng or hereafter to cum and growe over and above the rents goyng owt of the same to the chieff lord of the fee and the reperacions and other charges schall pay or cause to be payde unto oon of the sayd redars so redyng oon of the sayd lectures of physyk suche as by the sayd wardens[7] schalbe apoynted XI li. duryng the lifes of my sisters, Alice and Jonne, at the festis of Sent Mychaell therchanngell and the Anunciacion of owre lady by egall porcions to be paide, the first payment therof to begyn after the apoyntement of myne excecutors. And I will that the seid lecture be callyd the more lecture. And of the sayd issues, revenues, and profyts schall yerely pay or cause to be paide at the dayes above sayd unto the oder reder off the seconnde lecture of phisik yerely VI li. XIII s. IIII d. for there payn, dyligens, and labor in and abowte the sayd lectures, wyche sayd seconnde lecture I will shall not begyne duryng the lifes of my sayd sistors Alice and Jonne. And yf oone of them die if any overplus growe of the sayd lands the same to be bestowid by the discrecion of my sayd excecutors. And I will that the sayde lecture be clepyd and callyd the lesse lecture. And[8] I will that when so ever the roome of the persone redyng the more lecture is voide, that then the persone redyng the lesse lecture be preferryd to the redyng of the seid more lecture yeff he[9] by the sayd wardens and their successors[10] shalbe thowght most able, mete, and convenyent.

And I wylle that the sayd person apoyntyd to[11] be oon of the redars above-sayd and wyche shall have yerely the sayd XX marks schall rede every day a dowble lecture of Galyen and noon other in forme folowyng, that ys to[12] say six books of Galyen De Sanitate Tuenda for his ordynary, and for his afture

---

[1] 'the master . . . successors' added by a different hand in a space left blank. There is also a faded note in the margin.
[2] 'wardens . . . successors' added by a different hand in a space left blank.
[3] 'and' inserted above the line probably in a different hand.
[4] 'be' inserted above the line probably in a different hand.
[5] Followed by a gap in the MS. through which a line has been drawn.
[6] 'the' inserted in a different hand to replace 'this' crossed out.
[7] 'wardens' added by a different hand in a space left blank.
[8] 'Notandum' is written in the margin.
[9] 'he' inserted above the line probably in a different hand.
[10] 'wardens . . . successors' written by a different hand in a space left blank.
[11] 'to' inserted above the line.   [12] 'that ys to' underlined.

lecture three books of Galyen De Alimentis, also for his ordynary lecture XIIII books of Galyen De Methodo Medendi, and for his after lecture the V first books of Galien De Simplicibus Medicamentis.[1] And I will that the sayd persone apoyntyd and lymyted to be the other reder of the sayd II lectures, and havyng the VI li. XIII s. IIII d. for his labur, schall rede for his ordynary leccion[2] three books of Galyen De Temperamentis, three books of Galien De Naturalibus Potentiis, and six books De Morbis et Simtomatis and the II books De Differentiis Febrium, and for his aftur lecture six books of Galien De Locis Affectis, and these doon, Pronostica Hipocratis wyth Galiens comment. And I will that the tyme of the sayd redyng be not spent in tretyng of suche questions as Galien calleth logicall, but onely twoche[3] suche questions as be litterall so that they may in II yeres and a half make a yende of the sayd books or at the farthest in III yeres.

Also I will[4] that in convenyent tyme aftur lycence can be goten off the kyng owre soverayn lord or his heires and of the lords mediatt and immediate off whom the sayd maner, lands, tenementes,[5] and oder the premisses or any parcell therof be holden that the sayd maner, lands, tenements and other the premisses wyth their apurtenunces wyth in the sayd counte of Kent and the sayd Stonehowse, except before except, shalbe admortized unto the wardens off Mercers[6] for the tyme beyng and ther successors for ever[7] yeff hyt please them to accept the same. And[8] yeff they refuse to accept and take it, then I woll that it[9] be admortised to suche a corporacion or body corporat and ther successors souche as by the reverede fader in god Cuthbert, bishop of London, sir Thomas More, knyght, John Stokysley, doctor of devinite, and Willyam Shelley, sergeannt at the law and recorder of London, or by II of them over levyng schalbe lymyted and appoynted. And that the sayd wardens and there successors for ever or the sayd body corporate[10] to whom it schall happend to be admortized and ther successors shall take the issues, revenues, and profitis[11] commyng and growyng off the sayd maner, lands, and tenentes and othere the premisses wyth there apurtinunces to imploy them fro tyme to tyme in and abow3t the uses and entents above rehersed, and to no other use nor entent.

And I will that yeff the sayd reders for the tyme beyng be remysse or necligent in the redyng above rehersed, then I wille that for every soche defawte the seid redar schall forfette soche a certen soome of money as by the discrescion off the seid wardens and their successors schalbe thougth mete and convenyent.[12]

---

  [1] 'Methodo . . . Medicamentis' inserted above the line to replace crossed out 'Simplicibus Medicamentis'.
  [2] Altered from 'lecture'.   [3] MS. 'twche'.
  [4] 'Also I will' underlined, and 'notandum' and a pointer written in the margin.
  [5] 'tenementes' inserted above the line.
  [6] 'wardens off mercers' inserted above the line to replace crossed out 'wardens and masters'.
  [7] 'for ever' inserted above the line.
  [8] A faded note has been written in the margin.
  [9] 'then I woll that it' underlined.
  [10] 'corporate' inserted above the line.
  [11] In the margin a scribbled note: '. . . profyts'.
  [12] 'then I wille . . . convenyent' written by a different hand in a space left blank.

Also I wyll that all suche parsons there heiris and assignes whiche now stond and be seased off and in all those my meeses,[1] gardens, lands, and tenementes late by me purchasyd and bow3t of the prior of Elsyng Spyttyll in the citie of London called the Bell and the Lawntern in Adlingstrete with in the sayd citie, and off all those my meses and gardens, lands, and tenementes now in the holdyng of oone Thomas Cony, flecher, with all and singular ther commodites and appurtinances wyth in the sayd cytie of London when they or any of them by the reverent fader in god, Cuthbert, bishop of London, Thomas More, knygth, John Stokislay, doctor of divinite, and Wyllyam Schelley, sergeaunt at the law and recorder of the citie of London, schall resonably be desiryd or requiryd, schall make or cause to be made unto oon sooll fre man off the sayd citie of London and his heiris soche good sure and sufficient[2] estate in the law of and in the sayd mesis, gardens, lands, tenementes, and other hereditaments wythin the sayd citie of London as by the sayd reverent fader, sir Thomas More, John Stokyslay and Wyllyam Schelley schalbe resonably advisid or devisyd, wyche fre man soo beyng soole seasyd acordyng to the custome of the sayd[3] citie of London shalby his last wyll and testament gyff, assyne, and bequeth the sayd mesees, gardens, lands, and tenementes and other the premissis wyth in the sayd citie of London wyth all and singular there commodyties and apurtinnances unto the master and felowys of Seynt Johnis the Evangelst[4] Colege in the universite off Cambrigge to have and to holde to them and to there successors for ever to the use and entent her after ensuyng, that ys to say that the seyd master and felowys and ther successors for ever shall peasbly have, receve, inioy, and perseave the issues, revenues, and propfetts cumyng and growyng off the sayd meses,[5] gardeyns, londs, and tenementes and other the premissis wyth there apurtinnunces wyth in the sayd citie of London, to the entent therwyth and wyth the issues, revenues,[6] and proffetts cumyng and growyng off diverse other lands, tenementes and hereditaments wyche the seyd master and felowes of Sent Johnis Colege have covenantyd and promysyd to and wyth me, the seyd Thomas Linacur, the seid most reverent fader, Thomas More, knygth, John Stokysley, doctor of divinite, and Wyllyam Shelley to bye and purchace or cause to be bow3t and purchesed to be had to them and to there successors for and wyth the summ of CCXXI li. XIII s. IIII d. off good and lawfull money of England, of whyche money I the sayd Thomas Linacur have before hand paid and deliveryd in redi money unto the sayd master and felowys of Seynt Johnis Colege in Cambrige CCIX li. sterlyng, to the entent that they ther wyth schall founde, erecte, and stablische oon substanciall lecture of phisyk in the seid universite of Cambrige, the same lecture to begyn and be put in dew execucion at the feast off the Anunciacon of owre ladi next cumyng, the same lecture to contenew in maner and forme here after ensuyng for ever, and that the seyd lecture by made and redde by oon graduate persone off the seyd universite of Cambryge beyng a master of arte at the lest therunto to be assignyd, namyd, electyd, and apoyntyd by the seyd master off Sent Johnis

---

[1] Preceded by 'lands' crossed out.
[2] 'sure and sufficient' inserted above the line.
[3] 'sayd' inserted above the line. [4] 'the Evangelst' written in the margin.
[5] altered from 'messuage'. [6] 'revenues' inserted above the line.

College[1] and VII senors of the seyd college off Sent John the Evangelist and ther successors fro tyme to tyme for ever, and that the tyme, place, and howris off the seyd lectures to be made be assignyd, lymyttyd and appoyntyd by the seyd electors and ther successors.

And I will that of the issues revenuys and proffetts cumyng and growyng[2] or hereafter to cum and growe aswhell off the seyd meses, gardens, lands, and tenementes wyth in the citie of London wyth ther apurtinunces as off the seyd lands and tenementes by the seyd master and fellowys[3] or ther sucessors to be purchasyd as ys above seyd over and a bove the rents goyng ow3t of the same to the cheff lords off the fee or fees and the reperacions and other charges shall pay or cause to be payd unto[4] the seyd[5] reder so redyng the seyd lecture of phesyke XII li. of good and lawfull money of England at the feasts of Sent Michaell tharchangell and the Anunciacon of owre lady by egall porcions to be paide, the first payment therof to begyn at the feast of Sent Mycaell tharchangell wyche shalbe in the yere off owre lord god M[lo] V[c] XXV.

And I will that the sayd person or reder so redyng the seyd lecture in the seid universite off Cambrige shall rede every day sooche books and after suche forme as the seyde reder in Oxfort redyng the more lecture ys by me hertofore apoyntyd and assignyyd to rede and doo. And I will that the tyme of the seyd redyng be not spent in suche questionns as Gallyan callyth logycall, but onely twoche suche questionns as be litterall soo that he may in II yeeris and[6] a halfe make an ende off the sayd books or at the fethest in III yeris, and at the yend off the seyd thre yeris then to cease redyng by the space of oon half yere, and soo fro tyme to tyme affter every thre yere to cease I halff yere and then to begyn agayn.

Duryng the wyche tyme off ceasur, I wyll that the sayd reder have noo salary, stypend, ne whaiges, but that the issuis, revenewis, and profetts commyng and growyng as whell off the sayd meses,[7] gardens, lands, and tenementes with in the citie of London as of the sayd lands, tenementes, and hereditaments to be purchasid by the seyd master and felowys of Sent Johnis College and there successors duryng the seyd half yere shalbe remayn and grow3 to the seyd master and felowys of Sent Johns College and ther suc-cessors for ever to the onely use off the sayd master and felowys and there successors for ever and soo fro tyme to tyme as oftyn as hyt shall happyn the seyd III[8] yeris to be yendyd and the risidewe off the issuys, revenewys, and profetts commyng and[9] growyng or wyche herafter shall cum or growe as well off the seyd meses,[10] gardens, lands, tenementes, and other the premissis wyth in the seyd citie of London as off the seyd lands, tenementes, and other hereditaments to be purchasyd as ys above sayd over and above the seyd XII li. to be payd to the seyd redar as ys a bove seyd schall clerly remayn unto the seyd master and felowys of Sent Johns College and to ther successors

---

[1] Followed by a gap through which a line has been drawn.
[2] 'and growyng' inserted above the line.   [3] Corrected from 'college'.
[4] Corrected from 'to'.   [5] 'to the seyd' repeated in the MS.
[6] Followed by 'an' in the MS.   [7] Altered from 'messuage'.
[8] 'III' inserted above the line.   [9] Altered from 'or'.
[10] Altered from 'messuages'.

for ever to the onely use of the seyd master and felowys and ther successors for ever.[1]

Also I wyll that yff in this my last will by me before declaryd there be any omyssion[2] of matter or words sufficient for the ordenances of the lecturs above seyd to be dewly put in execucion as by me before ys rehersyd, or for any matter, words, or clause concernyng my maners, lands, and tenementes above seyd and the use of them, wyth the issuis and revenuys ther of herafter to be cumyng and growyng to be employed and bestowed in maner and forme above seyd, then I will that the seid reverent fader Cuthbert,[3] bishop of London, sir Thomas More, John Stokisley, and Willyam Schelley schall have full power and auctoryte to interpretate, expownde, adde, and augment the matters and clauses conteynyd in this my last will where they schall seme nede, and to minesh wher they shall thynk convenyent and necessary as well off the sayd lecturis as of estate of enheritannce of the seyd lands as other wise.[4] And I will that the same interpretacion, expocicion, augmentacion, and diminicion shalbe my testament and last wyll of and up on the premissis and every of them, and to be acceptyd, reputyd, and takyn and of lyke force, streynth and effecte in the law and conciens as they where specially and playnly here by me declaryd.[5]

And ferther I will and bequeth the chappell and the chamber over the chappell wyth in my howse where I now dwell wyth in the citie off London to the College of Phicicons of London and to ther successors for ever, that they shall clerly have the same to them and ther successors for ever to the entent that thei shall theder resort for to[6] treate as whell for the welth and contenuannce of the seyd college as for the examinacion of souche parsons as shall use phisyk acordyng to a estatute therof late made and ordenyd.

Item I will that mi sister Alis schall have duryng her liffe onely VI li. yerly for her fyndyng, the same to be paide to here of the profetts of my sayd lands and tenementes. And I will that my sister Jonne have also yerely for her fyndyng off the profetts off my sayd lands and tenementes V li. to be levyte by the discrecon off myne excecutors notwithstandyng any salary or poyntemet of whages by me befor to them assignid.

Witnes thes parsons Thomas Bentley, doctor in phisykke, Willyam Partryche, Willyam Latymere, John Castell, John Wylforte.

Vera copia ultime voluntatis Thome Linacri, in medicinis doctoris.

---

[1] The original will apparently continued differently, but the paper has been cut through and the following sections added to the roll.
[2] Altered from 'thyng'.
[3] MS. 'Cuthber'.
[4] 'as other wise' added above the line in a different hand.
[5] Followed by a gap in the MS. through which a line has been drawn.
[6] 'to' inserted above the line.

APPENDIX B3. **Agreement between Thomas Linacre and the Master and Fellows of St. John's College, Cambridge, respecting the Linacre Lectureship.**

St. John's College, Cambridge. Muniment Room Drawer 59, No. 74. Roll. 14 June 1524.

Articles of the aggrements hadd and made bitwen Thomas Lenacre of London, doctor of phesyke, of the one partie and Nicholas Metcalff, clerke, maister of the college of Seynt Johns in Cambrige in the name of hym and his felowes of the same college of the other partie the XIIIIth day of June in the XVIth yere of the reigne of kyng Henry the VIIIth, concernyng a free lecture of phesike contynually here after to be kypt, redde, and mayntened sufficiently and openly in the comen scoles of the seid universite of Cambrige by a sufficient and able lerned man to be named and elected by the seid maister of the seid college for the tyme beyng and his successours, with the advise and councell of the seniors masters of the collegies of   ¹ in the seid universitie for the tyme beyng and in their absens by their substitutes for the tyme being yerely, after the forme as the reders of phisik be determed and appoynted in the universitie of Oxenford, the same lecture to be kept and maynteyned by the seid master and felowes of the same college of Seynt Johns and their successours for ever.

    Where as the seid doctor Lenacre the day of the makyng and seallyng of thes present articles hath delyvered in to the hands and possession of the right reverend ffather in god Cuthbert, busshop of London, CC li. of laufull Anglysshe money to be kept by hym unto suche tyme as a sufficient suretie be made by the seid master and felowes of the seid college of Seynt Johns or their successours that the seid free lecture of phisik shalbe sufficiently mayntened, redde, and kept in the seid universite of Cambrige by suche a sufficient, able person to be therunto named and chosen by the seid maister of the seid college of Seynt Johns and his successours with the advyse and councell of the seid II other masters A. B. or one of them or ther successours at the costs and charges of the same master and felowes of the seid college of Seynt Johns and their successours for ever, the seid maister of the seid college of Seynt Johns granntith and is fully aggreed and condiscendyd in the name of hym and his felowes of the seid college that at suche tyme as the seid summe of CC li. shalbe delyvered to theym by the seid reverend ffather in godd to thentent aforeseid that ther shalbe indentures of covenannts tripartite made bytwen the seid Nicholas Metcalff, maister of the seid college, and felowes and their successours of that one partie, and the seid doctor Lenacre of the II^de partie, and the abbot and covent of   ² and their successours of the³ III^de partie accordyng to the effect, intent and true meynyng of thes articles ensuyng.

    Ffyrst that the seid maister and felowes of seid college of Seynt John or ther successours before the⁴ fest of Seynt Michell tharchanngell next

---

¹ Blank in the MS.   ² Blank in the MS.
³ Altered from 'their successours'.   ⁴ 'the' repeated in the MS.

ensuyng after the date herof with the seid CC li. shall purchas and make sure accordyng to the kyngs lawes to them and their successours for ever maners, lands, tenements, or other heredytaments of good and sure title in the countye of Lyncoln or ells wher in the reame of Englond of the clere yerly value of XII li. X s. over and above all yerly charges, to thentent that they and their successours with the issues and profits there of shall yerely kepe and mayntene the seid free lecture of phisik in the seid universitee of Cambrige in suche forme as is hereafter declared in thes articles, that is to sey that the seid maister of the seid college of Seynt Johns with the advyse and councell of the seid II other maisters of the seid colleges of A.   B.   or one of theym at the lest for the tyme beyng before the fest of Seynt Michell tharchangell next comyng shall name, elect, and chose one sufficient and able person beyng at the lest of the degre of a master or bacheler of arte of the seid universitie to redde the seid free lectoure of phisik openly in the comen scoles of the seid universitie of Cambrege yerly and daily at all conveynt days for the same and at suche convenyent houres as shalbe most convenyent for the herers of the seid lectoure.

Item that the seid maister and felowes of the seid college of Seynt Johns and their successours shall content and pay yerly to suche person or persons as shall hereafter rede the seid lecture of phisik in the seid universitie in forme aforeseid for his or their stipend or salary for the same lecture X li. of laufull money of Englond at thre termes in the yere, that is to sey at the fests of the Nativytie of our lord, the Annunciacion of our lady, the fest of the Nativitie of Seynt John Baptist and Seynt Michell tharchanngell, by evyn porcions or asmoche therof after the rate of suche tyme or tymes as any suche person or persons shall redde and exercyse the same rowme of redership of the same lector in the same universitie.

Item that yf it shall happen any suche person or persons whiche that at any tyme hereafter shalbe named, appoynted, and assigned in forme aforeseid to disces or to be put oute of the same rowme for any cause reasonable by the seid maister of the seid college of Seynt John by the advyse and councell of the seid II maisters or one of them at the lest or their successours that then the same maister of the seid college of Seynt John by the advyse and counsell of the seid II other maisters or one of them at the lest or theyr successours within one weke next after that the seid rowme shall happen so to be voide for any suche cause as is aforeseid shall chose and elect and appoynte one other sufficient and able person at the lest of lyke degree as is aforeseid to rede the same lecture of phisik in the seid universitie in lyke maner and forme and at suche dayes and houres as is before writen, and that they shall so doo as oftyn as the same rowme shall happen at any tyme here after to fall voidde for any maner of cause.

And also that the same maister and felowes of the seid college of Seynt Johns and ther successours shall content and pay yerely unto every suche person or persones that here after shall so be elected and shall exercyse and occupye the seid rowme of redership of the seid lector of phisik for suche tyme as he or they shall rede, occupie, and exercise the same rowme after the rate of X li. by the yere for his or ther salary or wages to be payd by theym and their successours in maner and forme aforeseid.

Item it is aggreed that yf it shall happen the seid maister of the seid college of Seynt John or his successours to be remyshe and neclygent in provydyng, chosyng, and namyng of the seid reder at any tyme after the seid fest of Seynt Michell tharchangell next comyng so that there be no suche sufficient and able persone by them provydyd to redde the seid lecture in the seid universitie by the space of XIIII days to gyther, that then the same maister and felowes and their successours shall forfeyte to the seid abbot and covent and their successours for every suche defaute hade or made by the space of XIIII days XL s. nomine pene. And that it shalbe then laufull to the seid abbot and covent and their successours to entre in to all the maners, lands, tenements, and other heredytaments of the seid maister and[1] felowes of the seid college of Seynt John whiche they or their successours at the tyme of suche forfeytoure shall have as in the right of ther seid college and ther to distreyn for the seid forfeyture of XL s. Et hoc tociens quociens.

Item that yf any suche person that shalbe hereafter named and appointed to the seid rowme of redership of the seid lecture by the seid maisters or theyr successours fore suche tyme as they or any of them shalbe in the same rowme to be remysse and neclygent and doo not dayly redde the seid lecture in the seid universitie at all convenyent dayes and tymes accordyng as is aforeseid without any reasonable cause, lett, or impedyment to the contrary therof be hadde, that then the seid maister and felowes of the seid college of Seynt Johns and their successours shall forfeyte to the seid abbott and covent and their successours for every day that is convenyent to have suche redyng made that any suche defaute shalbe hadde and made of the seid lecture by the seid reder XX d. nomine pene with lyke clause of distres for the same as is a foreseid. Et hoc tociens quociens.

Item that the seid maister and felowes of the seid college of Seynt Johns and ther successours shall yerly have tak and perceyve L s. residue of the seid somme of XII li. X s. to their owne use and behof for their payn and labor in true executyng of the ordre and eleccion of the seid reder for ever.

Item that the furder establysshement, rule, and ordre of the seid lecture and redership that is necessarye to be doon for the good contynuannce of the same for ever shalbe doon and made by the goode advyse and counsell of the seid reverend father in god duryng hes lyff and after hes disces by the advyse and counsell of the channceler of the seid universitie of Cambrige fro the tyme beyng from tyme to tyme as nede shall require for evermore.

---

[1] 'and' omitted in the MS.

APPENDIX B4. **Indenture between Thomas Linacre and others, and the Master and Fellows of St. John's College, Cambridge, concerning the Linacre Lectureship.**

St. John's College, Cambridge. Muniment Room Drawer 59, No. 75. Remains of 5 seals. Signed: Thomas Linacre, Cuthbert London, Ioannes Stokisley. 19 August 1524.

This indenture made the XIXth day of August the XVIth yere of the reigne of kyng Henry the VIIIth betwene Thomas Lynacre, doctor of physyke and phisycian to our soveraigne lord the kyng, Cutbert by the suffrannce of god bysshopp of London, sir Thomas More, knyght, under treasourer of England, maister John Stokesley, clerk, doctor of divinitie, and William Shelley, sergeannt att lawe and recorder of London, on that oon partie and Nicholaus Metcalfe, clerke, maister of the college of Seint John the Evangeliste in Cambridge, and the ffellowes and scolers of the same college on that other partie, witnesseth that where the seid Thomas Lynacre by his testament and last wille beryng date the seventene day of Juyn in the yere of our lord god M^lCCCCC and XXIIII and the XVIth yere of the reigne of kyng Henry the VIIIth amongest other thinges hath willed that alle his meesse, gardens, londes, and tenements with thappurtenannces whiche he purchased of the prior of Elsingspyttelle, lately called the Belle and the Lanthorne, in Adlyngstrete in the parisshe of Sent Benett besydes Baynardescastelle of London whiche oon Thomas Cony of London, ffletcher, nowe hath to fferme by indenture for certeyn termes of yeres, shalbe putt into mortmayne unto the foreseid maister, ffelowes, and scolers of the seid college of Seint John Evangelyst aboveseid and to their successours in perpetuitie forevermore, and over and besydes that the seid Thomas Lynacre the day of the date of these presentes hath geven and delyvered unto the foreseid maister, ffelowes, and scolers the somme of two hundrethe and nyne poundes of good and laufull money of England over and above the somme of nynetene markes sterlinges whiche the seid Thomas Lynacre covenanntith to pay to the seid maister, ffelowes, and scolers atte ffeest of Alle Seintes nowe next comyng for that intent and effect that the same maister, ffelowes, and scollers shalle theirwith purchase and bye unto them and to their successours in perpetuitie asmoche landes and tenementes of good and just tytle and of as good a yerely value as they convenyently may, whiche seid somme of two hundreth oone and twenty poundes thertene shillinges and foure pence the seid maister, ffelowes, and scolers covenannte and grannte by these presentes that they or their successours shalle within the space of twelve monethes next ensuyng after the date of these presentes employe oonly aboute the bying and purchasinge of the seid landes and tenementes and aboute noon other thing. Ffor and in consyderacion of alle whiche premissis the seid maister, ffellowes, and scollers covenante, grannte and them bynde unto the seid Thomas Lynacre, Cutbert, bysshop of London, sir Thomas More, John Stokesley and William Shelley by these presentes that they and their successours shalle yereley after the deceesse of the foreseid

Thomas Lynacre for evermore wele and truly content and pay or cause to be contented and payde the somme of twelve poundes sterlinges for a certeyn lecture of physike to be founded and establisshed within the universitie of Cambridge by the seid Thomas Lynacre in his lyfe tyme or by the foreseid bisshop, sir Thomas More, John Stokesley, and William Shelley, he beyng dede, or by any of them lengest levyng, that ys to sey after suche and lyke maner and fourme and in suche wyse as by them or any of them in the seid fundacion shalbe lymited, declared, and appoynted over and above alle other promosyons or advanntages off any ffelyshippes of that college or any other within the seid universitie that shalle happen to be geven to hym and that he may laufully take by the statutes of the seid college. And the reder of the seid lecture to be choseyn from tyme to tyme by the maister and the seven senyors of the foreseid college therunto sworne to electe, accepte, and take a persone moost able for the same and that the seid maister ffelowes and scolers shalle make suche assurannce and assurannces for the payment and payments of the seid twelve poundes and of every parte and parcelle thereof as by the counseille lerned of the seid Thomas Lynacre, Cutbert, bysshop of London, sir Thomas More, John Stokesley and William Shelley or of the lengest lever of them shalbe advysed, provyded alwey that yt is aggreed betwene the seid parties that the seid reder for the tyme beyng shalle in [1] every fourth yere hereafter for evermore cease his redyng by the space of halfe a yere complet, that ys to sey from the ffeest of the Annunciacion of our lady unto the ffeest of Seint Mighell tharchanngelle[2] and thadvanntage of his stypende for that halfe yere shalle hoolly be applyed and converted to the oonly use of the seid college. And the seid Thomas Lynacre, Cutbert bysshopp of London, sir Thomas More, John Stokesley, and William Shelley for them and their executors wolle and grannte by these presentes that yf the seid maister, ffelowes, and scollers and their successours on their partie wele and truly perfourme, observe, fulfille, and kepe alle and every the covenantes, granntes, aggrements, and payments aforeseid in maner and fourme as is above declared, that than an oblygacyon of the date of these presentes wherin the seid maister, ffellowes, and scolers be hold and bounde to the seid Thomas Lynacre, Cutbert bysshopp of London, sir Thomas More, John Stokeley, and William Shelley in foure hundreth poundes sterlynges shalbe voyde and had for nought, and els it shalle stande in fulle strength and effect. In witnesse wherof as welle the comon seale of the seid maister, ffelowes, and scolers as the seales of the seid Thomas Lynacre, Cutbert bysshop of London, sir Thomas More, John Stokesley, and William Shelley to these indentures interchanngeably be sett. Yoven the day and yere aboverehersed.

[1] Blank in the MS. with a line running through.
[2] 'that ys to sey . . . tharchanngelle' inserted above the line.

APPENDIX B5. Record of an indenture between Thomas Linacre and others, and St. John's College, Cambridge, respecting a benefaction to the College.

St. John's College, Cambridge. The Thin Red Book, fol. 51ᵛ. 19 August 1524.

Noverint universi per presentes nos Nicholaum Metcalf, clericum, magistrum collegii Sancti Iohannis Evangeliste in Cantebrigia, ac socios et scolares eiusdem collegii teneri et firmiter obligari Thome Lynacre, in medicinis doctori ac phisico domini regis, necnon Cuthberto, permissione divina Londonensi episcopo, Thome More, militi, subthesaurario Anglie, Iohanni Stokesley, sacre theologie professori, et Willelmo Shelley, servienti ad legem ac recordatori civitatis Londonensis, in quadringentis libris sterlingorum solvendis eiisdem Thome Lynacre, Cutberto Londonensi episcopo, Thome More, Iohanni Stokesley et Willelmo Shelley aut eorum uni sive eorum certo attornato vel executoribus suis in festo Omnium Sanctorum proximo futuro post datum presencium. Ad quam quidem solucionem bene et fideliter faciendam obligamus nos et successores nostros per presentes sigillo nostro comune sigillatas. Datum decimo nono die Augusti anno regni regis Henrici octavi sexto decimo.

The condicion of this obligacion is suche that if the within bounden maister, ffelowes, and scolers and theire successourers on their partie well and truly performe, observe, and kepe all and singler articles, covenants, grannts, and agrements specified in a pare of indentures bering day of the date within writen, made betwene the within named Thomas Lynacre, doctor of phisik and phisicion to ouer soverayne lorde the king, Cutbete, by the sufferance of god busshop London', Thomas More, knight, undertresorer of Englonde, maister John Stokesley, clerke, doctor of devinite, and William Shelley, sargeannte at the lawe and recorder of London, opon the on partie and forsaide maister, felowes, and scolars opon that other partie, that this present obligacion to be voyde and had for nought or ellis it shall stande in full strenghte and effecte.

APPENDIX B6. Agreement between Thomas Linacre and the Master and Fellows of St. John's College, Cambridge, respecting the terms of the Linacre Lectureship.

St. John's College, Cambridge. The Thin Red Book, fol. 220. 18 October 1524.

Noverint universi per presentes nos, Nicholaum Metcalf, sacre theologie professorem, magistrum collegii Sancti Iohannis Evangeliste in Cantibrigia, et socios eiusdem collegii recepisse et habuisse die confectionis presencium de Thoma Linacre, in medicinis doctore et medico domini nostri regis, ducentas

viginti et unam libras, tresdecem solidos, et quattuor denarios sterlingorum
nobis ex conventione in plenam solucionem solutas pro fundacione lecture in
medicinis in universitate Cantabrigie predicta, sic ut in indenturis de data
decimi none diei mensis Augusti anno regni regis Henrici octavi decimo sexto
inter prefatum Thomam et nos factis plenius continetur. De qua quidem
summa ducentarum viginti et unius librarum, tresdecim solidorum, et quattuor denariorum, nos prefati Nicholaus, magister, et socii collegii predicti
dictum Thomam et eius heredes et executores liberamus et acquietamus ac
liberatos et quietos esse fatemur per presentes. In cuius rei testimonium nos
prefati magister et socii collegii predicti sigillum nostrum commune presentibus apposuimus. Datum Cantabrigie in collegio¹ nostro predicto decimo
octavo die mensis Octobris anno regni regis Henrici octavi sextodecimo.

APPENDIX B7. Record by William Hebelthewayte, servant of Cuthbert Tunstal, of the income and expenditure
of the manors of Traces and Frognall for the year 1543–4.

Merton College, Oxford. In envelope E.2. 28a. 1543–4.

Anno XXXVᵒ H. 8.

The yerly ferme rent of the maner of Tracis		X li.
Wherof payd for reparacions and owt rents:		
Item payd to thacher and his man for XIIII dayes thatchyng, mete, drynke and wages	XIIII s. ⎫	
Item for gatheryng of VI honderyth of rodds	VI d. ⎭	XIIII s. VId.

Owt rents:

Item payd to the kyngs rent	IIII s. ⎫	
Item payd to the lordship of Austens for rent	X s. ⎪	
Item payd to Lucis for rent	VIII d. ⎪	
Item payd for the howse att Kaystrete for rent and sute	VIII d. ⎬	XXIII s.
Item payd to the borow sylver	XII d. ⎪	
Item payd to the fyffetene	VI s. VIII d. ⎭	

Summa payd   XXXVII s. VI d.

Anno XXXVᵒ H. 8.

The yerly ferme rent of the maner of Frognall		VIII li. VI s. VIII d.
Wherof payde for reparacions and owt rents:		
Item payd to a thatcher and his man for IIII dayes mete, dryng and wages	IIII s. ⎫	
Item payd for oon bondell of lathes	VI d. ⎬	IIII s. X d.
Item for V hondrith of spregg	IIII d. ⎭	

¹ 'in collegio' inserted above the line.

Owte rents:

Item payd to the kyngs rent	VII s. VII d.	
Item payd to the yocke of Chesteley for II acres and di' of woods callyd Bersteddyll III d. a yere, behynd VII yeris,	XXI d.	Xs. VIII d.
Item payd to Norwood for rent of II acres of land lying at Goldehorde VIII d. and II hennes	XVI d.	

Summa payd   XV s. VI d.

The hole yere rent of the saide two fermes endyd at Michelmas in the XXXVth yere of the rigne of kyng Henry the VIIIth	XVIII li. VI s. VIII d.
Wherof payd by the saide John Lyford as ys above saide	LIII s.
So remayneth dew by the same John Lyford	XV li. XIII s. VIII d.
The ferme rents of the maner of Tracis for II yeris endyd at Michelmas in the XXXIIIIth yere of the reigne of our soverayne lorde kyng Henry the VIIIth the som	XX li.
The ferme rent of the maner of Ffrognall for oon yere endyd at the saide Michelmas anno 34 H. 8	VIII li. VI s. VIII d.

Summa totalis   XXVIII li. VI s. VIII d.

Wherof payd by John Lyford fermer of the saide fermes in the saide II yeris for reparacions and owte rents and payments as aperythe by a byll of the parcells therof	XIX li. VII s. X d.[1]
So restith dew by the said John Lyford of the same fermes	VIII li. XVIII s. X d.
Recevyd of the saide John Lyford by me William Hebylthwayte	VIII li. XVIII s. X d.

Wherof payd by me William Hebylthwayte:

In primis payd for my costs to Newyngton when I recevyd the saide money of the saide John Lyford	II s. V d.
Item payd for the copy of a recovery of the maner of Tracis to master Rewle	III s. IIII d.
Item payd for my costs to Newyngton and Richard Hardyngs to se the lands and wood ther	III s. VI d.
Item payd to master Lynager syster at Ester	L s.
Item payd for costs in suyng a ple in the Exchequior to stope the shryve for mercements for the maner of Tracis	LVIII s. IIII d.
Item payd to master Lynager syster for her annuite dew at Michelmas anno XXXV° H. 8	L s.

[1] Corrected from 'XXV li. XVI s. VIII d.'.

Item payd for my costs and Richard Hardyngs to
   Neyngton the Xth day of December   VI s. VIII d. ob.
     Summa totalis payd by me William Hebyl-
       thwayte   VIII li. XIIII s. III d. ob.
     So remayneth de by me William Hebyl-
       thwayte   IIII s. VI d. ob.

APPENDIX B8. **Indenture between Cuthbert Tunstal and the Principal and Scholars of Brasenose College, Oxford, and the Warden and Fellows of All Souls College, Oxford, respecting the foundation of lectureships.**

Merton College, Oxford. Roll no. 6696. 6 May 1540.

This indenture trypartyte made the VI day of May in the XXXIIth yere of the reign of our soveraign lord Henry the eight, kyng of Englond and of Ffrannce, defendor of the fayth, lord of Irelond and in erth supreme hed of the churche of Englond, betwene the reverend father in god Cutbert, bysshop of Duresme, executor of the last will and testament of Thomas Lynacre, doctor of phesyk, deceased, on the one partie and Mathew Smyth, pryncipall of the kings hall and college of Brasinose in Oxford and scolers of the same place on the second partie and   ¹ wardeyn of All Sowle Colledge in Oxford afor-said and the felows of the same colledge on the thirde partie, witnesseth that where as the said Thomas Lynacre infeoffed the said reverend father Cutbert, bysshop of Duresme, and other of and in his maner of Tracis and of and in all other his lands, tenements, rents, revercions, and hereditaments in Newyngton in the countie of Kent whiche he the said Thomas Lynacre pur-chased and bowght of Lewes Clyfford, esquier, and of and in all that his mesuage called Ffrognall and all other his londs, tenements, medowes, pas-tures, woods, underwoods, rents, revercions, and services with the appur-tenances set, lying, and being in the parisshe of Newyngton nygh Sydenburne which he late purchased of William Blowere, and of and in all other his lands and tenements which he late purchased and bought of Thomas Elmeston called Sevans, and also of and in all those his lands and tenements late pur-chased of the said Thomas called Bulles lands, and also and in all those his lands and tenements late by hym purchased and bowght of John Potehed lying in Keys Strete in the parishe of Bobyng in the said countie of Kent, and of and in all those his lands and tenements called the Stone Hows in Knyght Ryders Strete within the citie of London, to have and to hold to the said re-verend father Cutbert, bysshop of Duresme and his cofeoffes and their heires to the use of the said Thomas Lynacre and his heires by force of whiche feffe-ment the said reverend father Cutbert, bysshop of Duresme, and other his co-feoffes were therof seased in their demeane as of fee to the use of the said

¹ Blank in the MS.

Thomas Lynacre and his heires and to the performance of his last will and testament, and they so beyng therof seased the said Thomas Lynacre by his last will and testament bering date the XVII day of October in the yere of our lord god M¹ Vᶜ XXIIII wylled that all and every persone and persones their heires and assignes whiche then dyd stand and were seased of and in the said maner of Tracis and other the premisses sholde fromthensfurth stande and be seased of and in the same maners, lands, and tenementes and other the premisses to the only uses, intents, and purposes herafter in theis indentures specifyed and declared. And where also forasmoche as the same Thomas thought the facultie of phesyk to be mete and expedient for the enhabitannts in every comynaltie to be to the comfort of the people and remedy of many maladyes contynually channsyng[1] moche covetyng and desiryng for the better lernyng of the said facultie to be had in both the unyversities Oxford and Cambrydge entended to fownde and ordeyn certeyn substanciall and perpetual lectures of phesyk whiche be very necessary for the students of the said unyversities in the said facultie, the said[2] Thomas therfore willed and declared by his said last will and testament that two substanciall lectures of phesyk shulde be fownde, erected, and establysshed by his said executors in the said universitie of Oxford after the will and testament of the seid Thomas Lynacre, and ordeyned and named to be his executors the said reverend father and John Stokesley, doctor in divinatie, whiche after that was bysshop of London and other and before the said lectures or any of them were establisshed all the executors of the said Thomas Lynacre except the seid reverend father Cutbert, bysshop of Duresme, dyed, so that the hole trust for the performannce of the last will of the seid Thomas Lynacre resteth and remayneth only in the seid reverend father Cutbert, bysshop of Duresme, whiche in and for the accomplysshement and establishement of the seid last will and testament of the seid Thomas Lynacre, now by theis presents doth gyve and grannte unto the seid Mathew Smythe, principall of the kings hall and colledge of Brasynose in Oxford, and scolars of the same and their successors to the fyrme and suer stablisshyng of the seid II lectures, the said maner called Tracyes with the appurtenances and also all the londs and tenements, medowes, leasues, and pastures with thappurtenances called Sevans set, lying, and being in the said countie of Kent, and also all those lands and tenements called Bulles lands, and also the said mesuage with thappurtenances called Ffrognalls lyings in the said countie of Kent, and also the said Stone Hows with the appurtenances in Knyght Ryders Strete in London, except the hall within the seid Stone Hows and a certeyn chamber over the seid hall whiche the said Thomas Lynacre hath willed to be reserved for the colledge of the phesycians in London to their use for them to kepe their counsells in, and also the said lands and tenements set, lying, and being in Kays Strete in the parysshe of Bobbyng in the countie of Kent, and all other the said lands tenements and other the premisses except before except, to have and to hold the said maner called Tracys and all other the said lands tenements and other the premisses with all and singuler their appurtenances except before except to the said Mathew Smythe, pryncipall of the kynges hall and colledge of Brasnose in Oxford and scolars of the same, and to their successors for ever more. And the

---

[1] 'channsyng' inserted above the line.   [2] 'said' repeated in the MS.

said reverend father Cutbert, bysshop of Duresme, covenantith and granntith by theis presents that the seid maner, lands, tenements and other the premisses with their appurtenances be at the day of makyng of this present indenture of the clere yerely value of XXIIII li. X s. over and above all charges and repryses and that at this present day they may so be letten to ferme. And the said pryncipall of the kings hall and colledge of Brasynose in Oxford and scolars of the same covenante and grannte to and with the said reverend father Cutbert, bysshop of Duresme[1] and to and with the said wardeyn and felows of Alle Sowle Colledge and their successors in maner and forme folowyng, that is to sey that the seid principall of the kings hall and colledge of Brasynose in Oxford and scolars of the same and their successors as long as they may have and enjoy the said maner, londs, tenements and other the premisses except before except for ever more shall kepe and mayntene two honest and substanciall lerned and expert men in the seid facultie and sciens of phesyk, whiche shalbe at the lest maisters of arte, wherof the one to be called the reder of the more lecture and the other to be called the reder of the les lecture, and fyrst that the reder of the les lecture shall begyn to rede his lecture every day within the terme herafter to be appoynted at IX of the clok in the mornyng and so to contynue till X of the clok, and so to rede every day one howre at the lest. And the seid pryncipall of the kings hall and colledge of Brasynose in Oxford and scolars of the same for them and their successors covenante and grannte by theis presents that the seid reder, called the reder of the les lecture, shall have yerely during the tyme that he shalbe reder in the seid colledge of Brasynose for his salary and stypend fyve pounds of good and laufull mony of Englond to be paid yerely at there termes of the yere, that is to sey at Cristmas, the Annunciacion of our lady, and the Nativitie of Seint John Baptist. And further the seid principall and scolars of Brasinose aforsaid for them and their successors covenante and grannte by theis presents that the said reder of the les lecture shall rede theis books folowing in order and non other, that is to sey III boks of Galyen De Temporamentis, three boks of Galyen De Naturalibus Potenciis, and six boks of Galyan De Morbis et Sintomatis, and II boks of De Differenciis Febrium, and VI boks of Galyan De Locis Affectis; and this done Pronestica Hipocratis with Galyens coment. And also that the seid reder shall in no wise spend the tyme in treating of suche questions as Galyan calleth logycall, but only suche questions as be litterall so that the seid reder may in II yeres and a half make an ende of the said boks or at the furthest in III yeres. And further the seid principall and scolars of Brasinose aforsaid for them and their successors covenante and grannte by theis presents to and with the seid bisshop of Duresme and wardeyn and felowes and their successors that the reder of the more lecture shall have yerely for his salary and stypend during suche tyme as he shalbe reder the somm of ten pounds of good and laufull mony of Englond by the yere quarterly to be paid as is aforsaid, and that the said reder of the more lecture shall rede theis boks folowing and non other, that is to say six boks of Galyan De Sanitate Tuenda, and III boks of Galyen De Alimentis, and XIIII boks of Galyan De Methodo Medendi, and the V first boks of Galyen De Simplicibus Medicamentis, and not to spende the tyme

[1] Corrected from 'London'.

in such questions as Galien calleth logicall but only towche such questions as be litterall. And it is further agreed betwene the seid parties that the seid reders shall contynew the reding of their lectures but the space of III quarters of a yere in every yere, that is to say every yere fro the fest of Seint Mighell tharchanngell untill the fest of the Nativitie of Seint John Baptist from tyme to tyme for ever, to this purpose and intent that is to sey that the seid reders may take recreacion and prepare for their lectures ageinst the fest of Seint Mighell tharchanngell then next folowyng and the scolars to conferre their lernyng togyder and prepare them selfs more apte to receyve lernyng. And it is further agreed betwene the said parties that the reders before rehersed, their rowmes being voide, shalbe elect and chosen after this maner and forme folowing, that is to say the rowme of the reder of the les lecture being voyde, that then the principall of Brasynose aforsaid for the tyme being togider with the wardeyns of Alle Sowle College for the tyme beyng, or in his absens the vyce wardeyn, with thadvyse and counsell of hym whiche redeth the more lecture shall nominate two men well lerned in phisik, maisters of arte at the lest, and those so nominate to be taken the one owt of Brasinose Colledge and the other out of Alsowse Colledge, yf any suche there may be founde mete therunto, yf non suche may be found mete therunto to take then of the most apte and mete for the said purpose owt of any other colledge or hall within the said universite, and those so nominate to be presented unto the seid reverend father in god Cutbert, byshop of Duresme, yf he be so nere the universite as London, and he the said reverend father to electe and chose one of the two so nominate to rede the seid lecture whiche shalbe accept and taken of the seid colledge of Brasinose for the seid reder. And yf so be the seid reverend father be absent in the north contrey, orels where, orels departyd owt of this worlde, that then the two nominate to the seid lectures shalbe within one day after they be so nominate presented unto the commysarie of the seid universitie of Oxford, or to his deputie in his absens, the which commyssary or his deputie in his absens, calling to hym suche doctors of phisyk and divinitie as then shalbe there present or askyng of them cownsell, shall electe one of the seid two to rede the seid lecture, and then the seid colledge of Brasinose shall receyve the reder[1] so electe to be the reder there, and shall entertayn and take hym as the reder so long as he shalbe disposed to rede, so that the seid reder be of good and honest conversacion and apply his lecture according to the will and ordinance of the seid doctor Lynacre. And also it is agreed betwene the seid parties that when the rowme of the reder of the more lecture shalbe voyde, that then the reder of the les lecture shalbe therunto elect and taken yf he be the principall of the seid colledge of Brasinose and wardeyn of All Sowle Colledge with the advise of suche as be doctors of phisyk be founde so mete, and then a reder for the seid les lecture to be chosen as is abovesaid. And yf the said reder of the les lecture woll not take the redyng of the more lecture when it is or shalbe so voyde, that then one to be nominate and elect to the reding of the said more lecture as is above said, that is to say in the eleccion and chosyng of the reder of the les lecture as is above rehersed and in no other wise save only for the absens of the reder of the more lecture, whiche then cannot be present because there

---

[1] MS. 'rede'.

is non suche. And it is further agreed betwene the seid parties that the seid principall and felows of Brasinose aforsaid and their successors for evermore ones in the yere upon the same day that the reders shall begyn to rede in Mighelmas terme shall kepe a dirige at nyght and masse on the morow, at the whiche dirige and masse all the felows and scolars being then at home in the said colledge of Brasinose shalbe present and pray for the sowle of the said Thomas Lynacre after their devocions. And further that the seid reders at the redyng tyme before the said dirige shall gyve warnyng to all their audiens of their devocion to be present with the seid reders at the said dirige and masse to pray for the sowle of the seid master Lynacre and all Christen sowles. It is also agreed betwene the seid parties that every yere at the day of the said dirige monicion shalbe gyven by the said pryncipall of the kings hall and college of Brasynose in Oxford or by the vyse pryncipall, the pryncipall being absent, unto the wardeyn of All Sowle Colledge, and in his absens unto the vyce wardeyn of All Sowle College, that it may pleas the one of them to be present at the anniversary and masse don for the seid doctor Lynacre, and there to offer I d. and receyve III s. IIII d. of the said principall of Brasinose aforsaid, and further that day to dyne with the said principall, and dyner ended to comen togiders in the presens of the seniors of the seid colledge of Brasynose concernyng the fulfillyng of the covenants or agreaments before expressed. And yf any defawte be founde in the said principall and felowes of Brasynose aforsaid in not fulfyllyng of the covenants or articles aforsaid on their partie to be observed, then the wardeyn of Alle Sowle Colledge for the tyme being to gyve admonicion and warnyng that the seid defawts may be with diligens amended to the intent that the reding of the seid lectures may with dyligens procede and go forward according to the covenants or agreaments above said, and according to the last will and testament of the seid master doctor Lynacre. And if it shall fortune the seid principall and scolars of the kings hall and colledge of Brasinose for the tyme being not to regarde the monicion so to them gyven by the seid wardeyn or vyce wardeyn of Alle Sowle College aforsaid, but doth suffer suche covenants as be tofore here expressed necligently to be kept or regarded and the said lectures not to be red and observed as is aforsaid, that then the said wardeyn for the tyme being with IIII[or] or VI of the seniors of the said Alsowle Colledge and that within one quarter of a yere then next folowing shall admonyshe and warne the principall and scolars of the kings hall and colledge of Brasinose for the tyme being that they with all diligens amend or se to be amendyd all such defawts as be founde or shalbe by them founde concernyng the covenants or articles before expressed to the entent the said lectures with every thing within the said covenants within this present indenture comprehended on the partie of the seid principall and scolars of the kings hall and college of Brasinose aforsaid for the tyme being may truly and substancially be doon with effecte, and that within one quarter of a yere then next folowing. And if it than so fortune, as god forbyd it shulde, that the seid principall and scolars for the tyme being of Brasinose[1] aforsaid do neclecte and not regard the defawts so founde by the said wardein or vyse wardein of Alsowle College aforsaid, that then it shalbe laufull to the seid wardeyn or vyse wardeyn and felowes for the tyme being

---

[1] MS. 'Basinose'.

of Alsowle College aforsaid to entre into all and every the forsaid maners, lands, tenements, rents, revercions, and services and other the premisses with all and their appurtenances, and the same to have and hold and possede to them and their successors forever, they kepyng all suche covenants and grannts as the seid president and felows of Brasinose aforsaid were bounde to kepe, and that then the said principall of Brasynose aforsaid for the tyme being to have lyke auctoritie as the wardeyn of All Sowle Colledge aforsaid by this indenture had to se that the seid wardeyn and felowes of Alsowle College and their successors do well truly and substancially kepe all suche articles,[1] covenants, and grannts specified within this present indenture in the same maner and forme as the seid principall and felowes of Brasinose aforsaid were bound to do. And that if there be any defawte or defawts in fulfyllyng or executyng of the seid covenants and the seid wardeyn and felows of All Sowle Colledge aforsaid having like monyshions and warnyng to redresse and amend the same fawte or fawts of the seid principall of Brasinose aforsaid[2] for the tyme being as the seid principall of Brasinose aforsaid had of the said wardeyn and vice wardeyn of Alsowle Colledge aforesaid, and the seid wardeyn and felowes of Allsowle Colledge aforsaid not to regard the same warnyng so gyven by the principall of Brasinose nor yet to amend the same fawte or fawts so that the said lectures be not red nor yet the covenants abovesaid performed, that then it shalbe leefull and laufull to and for the seid principall and scolars of Brasynose aforsaid for the tyme beyng and for their successours to reentre ageyn into the seid maners, lands, tenements, and other the premisses with all and singuler their appurtenances, and the same to have, holde, and possede ageyn to them and their successors forever as in their former estate, they kepyng the covenants aforsaid this indenture notwithstandyng, provided alweys and it is agreed betwene the seid parties that the seid principall and scolers of the kings hall and colledge of Brasynose in Oxford or any of their successors shall not herafter at any tyme or tymes be any further charged with the fyndyng of the said reders or any other of them or of any other charges before rehersed or concernyng the seid lands and tenementes or any parcell therof or concernyng the sutes of the same or by any maner of meanes otherwyse, then they may conveniently susteyn and kepe with the rents, yssues, and profyttes of the seid maner, londs, tenements, and hereditaments having alweys allowed unto them yerely to their owne profytts over and above all charges nyne pounds III s. IIII d. of good and lefull mony of Englond, goyng out of the seid lands and tenements.

1 MS. 'arcles'.
2 MS. 'aforsad'.

APPENDIX B9. **Indenture between Cuthbert Tunstal and the Warden and Scholars of Merton College, Oxford, respecting the foundation of lectureships.**

Merton College, Oxford. Roll in envelope E.2. 28a. 10 December 1549.

This indenture made the Xth day of December[1] in the thirde yere of the reigne of our sovereigne lord Edward the syxth, by the grace of god etc., betwene the right reverend father in god, Cuthbert bisshop of Dureham, executor of the last will and testament of Thomas Lynacre, doctor of phisic and sometime phisycion to the late king of England of famous memory, Henry the VIIIth,[2] of thon parte and the warden and scolers of the howse of scolers of Merton called Merton Hall in Oxford of the other part, where the seid[3] Thomas Lynacre[4] by his last will and testament touching the dysposicion of his maners, lands, and tenements bering date the XVIII^{ths} day of October in the XVIth yere of the reigne of the said late kyng willed[6] that all and every person or persons, theyre heyres and assignes which then stode and were seased of and in his maner of Traces and of and in all other his lands, tenements, rents, reversyons, and heredytaments in Newyngton, Hertlopp, Hallstone, Stokebury, Uppchurch Rayneham, Tong, and Worston which[7] he the said Thomas Lynacre purchesed and bought of on Lewys Clyfford, esquyer, and of and yn all that his mesuage called Ffrognall, and all other his lands, tenements, medowe, pastures, wodds, underwodds, rents, reversions, and services sett, lying, and being in the paryshe of Newyngton nyghe Sytyngborne which he purchesed of William Blower, and of and in all other his lands and tenements called Sevans whiche byn in the countie of Kent,[8] and of and in all thos his lands and tenements called Stonehousse in the city of[9] London in Knyght Ryder Strete, except the parler[10] there and the chambre over the same parler,[11] shuld stand and be seased of and in the seid maner, lands, tenements, and other the premisses to thuse and intents in his same last will specified and rehersedd, and where the seid Thomas Lynacre by the same last will declared and rehersed in maner and forme folowyng, that is to wytt ffor as moch as the facultie of phisik was right mete and expedyent for

---

[1] Altered from 'Septembre'.
[2] 'executor . . . VIIIth' inserted above the line.
[3] And the warden . . . seid' altered from 'and Thomas Reynolds, clerke, warden of Merten College in Oxford and the scolers of the same of thother parte where the seid'.
[4] Followed by 'doctor of phisik and sometyme phisicion to the late kyng of England of famous memory, Henry the VIIIth' crossed out.
[5] Altered from 'XX'.
[6] Preceded by 'made and ordeynyd his last will and testament' crossed out.
[7] Preceded by 'and of and in' crossed out.
[8] 'whiche . . . Kent' inserted above the line.
[9] 'the city of' inserted above the line. [10] Altered from 'chapell'.
[11] 'parler' altered from 'chapell'. 'except . . . parler' inserted above the line.

the inhabytants in every commynaltie to the comfort of the people and remedy of many maladyes contynually channsing, he thought necessary there shuld be connyng and expert phisicions of which hath byn grete penury for lack of lectures and instruccions in that faculty in Oxford and in Cambrige, and as then there were no[1] certen substancyall nor perpetuall lectures of phisyk founded nor ordeynyd in the seid unyversites which were very necessary for the students of the seid unyversites in the seid facultie, therfore the seid Thomas Lynacre willed by the seid will that two substancyall lectures of phisyk shuld be founded, erected, and stablished in the seid unyversite of Oxford, the same lectures to begynn and to be putt in execucion in as convenyent tyme after the deceas of the seid Thomas Linacre as shuld be thought by his executors to contynue for ever, and that the seid two lectures shuld be made and reade by two severall graduates, masters of arte at the lest, to be assigned therunto, namyd, elected, and apoynted from tyme to tyme when and as often as necessytie shuld requyre, and ferther willed by the said will as aperyth among other things that the feoffees and receverrers of the said Thomas Lynacre theyr heyres and assignes of his maners, lands, and tenements shuld yerely take the issues, revenues, and profeits of the seid maners, lands, and tenements and other the premisses with thappertenants within the seid county of Kent and of and in the seid mesage called the Stone House within the seid city of London, and the same and every parcell therof shuld demyse and lett to ferme and of parcell of the[2] profeits, issues, and revenues therof comyng over and above the rents going owt of the same to the chif lordes and the reparacions and other charges, shuld pay or cause to be paid unto on of the seid reders so redyng on of the said lectures of phisyk XI li. duryng the liffe of Alice and Johanne, systers of the seid Thomas Lynacre, which Alice and Johane now att the present be desceassed, and now from hensforth to have XII li. by yere to be payd[3] att the feasts of Saynt Mychell and Thanunciacion of our ladye by evyn portions.[4] And the same Thomas Lynacre ferther willed that the seid lecture shulde be called the more lecture, and of the seid issues, revenues, and profeits shuld yerely pay or cause to be paid att the days aboveseid unto the other reder of the seconde lecture of phisyk yerely VI li.[5] for theyre paynes, dylygens, and labers yn and about the seid lectures, which seid second lecture the seid Thomas Lynacre willed shuld not begyn duryng the liffe of his seid systers Alice and Johan which be now desceassed, as ys above rehersed, and the seid Thomas Lynacre willed that the seid lecture shuld be clypped and called the lesse lecture, and also willed that what so ever the rome of the person reding the more lecture shuld be voyde, that then the person reading the lesse lecture shuld be preferred to the reding of the seid more[6] lecture, if the seid person shuld be thought most hable and convenyent for the same, and willed ferther that the seid person apoynted to be on of the reders aboveseid and which shuld have yerely the

---

[1] 'no' inserted above the line. [2] 'the' inserted above the line.
[3] 'and now . . . payd' inserted above the line.
[4] Followed by 'to be paid, the first payment therof to begyn after the poyntement of thexecutors of the seid Thomas Lynacre', crossed out.
[5] Followed by 'XIII s. IV d.'(?) crossed out.
[6] Corrected by addition from 'to reding the more'.

XX marks[1] shuld rede every day a doble lecture of Galyen and none other yn forme folowyng, that is to say syx boks of Galyen De Sanitate Tuenda for his ordynary and for his after lecture III boks of Galyen De Alimentis, also for his ordynary lecture XIIII boks of Galyen De Methodo Medendi, and for his after lecture the V fyrst boks of Galyen De Simplicibus Medicamentis, and willed that the seid person apoynted and lymytted to be thother reder of the seid two lectures and having the VI li.[2] for his laber shuld rede for his ordynary lectyre III boks of Galyen De Temperamentis, III boks of Galyen De Naturalibus[3] Potentiis and VI boks De Morbis et Simtomatis and the II boks De Differentiis Febrium, and for his after lecture VI boks of Galyen De Locis Affectis and this don Pronostica Hipocratis with Galyen is Coment, and willed that the tyme of the seid reading shuld not be spent in treating of such questyons as Galyen called logycall but only toch such questions as shuld be litterall so that they might in II yeres and a halff make an ende of the seid boks or att the ferthest in thre yeres, and wylled that in convenyent tyme after lycens could be gotten of the seid late kyng or his heyres that the seid maners, lands, tenements, and other the premisses with theyr appertenants in the seid county of Kent and the seid mesuage called the Stone House, except before excepted, shuld be amortized to such a corporation for refusell of the Mercers of London, which have refused, as by the seid reverent father in god Cuthbert, now bysshop of Dureham, sir Thomas More knight, John Stokeley, then doctor of dyvynytie, and William Shelley sergeant at the law and then recorder of London, or by two of them overlyvyng, shuld be lymyted and apoynted, and after the seid sir Thomas More and[4] John Stokeley dyed and the seid Cuthbert, now bishopp of Dureham, and William Shelley then overlyvyd and apoynted the premisses to be amortized and assuryd for thentents and purposes above rehersed unto the seid warden and scolers of Merton College and to theyr successors for ever for thentents specifyed in the seid will. And ferther yt is conteyned in the seid will that the body corporatt to whom the premisses shuld happen to be amortized and theyre successors shuld take the issues, revenues, and profetts commyng and growing of the seid maner, lands, tenements and other the premisses with theyr appertenants to ymploy them from tyme to tyme in and about the uses and intents above rehersed and to none other use nor entent, and the seid Thomas Lynacre willed by the seid will that if the seid readers for the tyme beyng shuld be remysse or neglygent in the reading above rehersed, than he willed that for every such defalt the seid reder shuld forfete such a certen sum of money as by the dyscretion of the seid body polytique or corporate[5] shuld be thought mete and convenyent which things here expressed, being parcell of the seid will, amongs other things att lenghe now largely appere in the

---

[1] In the margin: 'Notandum XX marks'. Inserted at this point is the following: 'and now appoynted to be XII li. bycause the revenues of [MS. 'if'] the premysses besides the reprises, charges, and repereiens of the same may not convenyently extend otherwyse'.

[2] Inserted at this point: 'now appoynted for the consyderation aforeseid', and followed by 'XIII s. IIII d.' crossed out.

[3] MS. 'naturabus'.

[4] 'sir . . . and' inserted above the line.

[5] 'or corporate' inserted above the line.

same will, where also the seid Cuthbert, bisshop of Dureham,[1] being the last survyvor and overlyver of the feoffees and receverers of the seid Thomas Lynacre and also executor of the last will and testament of the same Thomas Lynacre, after the lycence of the said late kyng had and opteyned for the amortizyng of the premisses unto the seid wardens and scolers, as by generall words in the seid licence now playnely doth apere, in fulfillyng and performance of the seid will by his dede hath gevyn and grannted and by the same dede hath consynd unto Thomas Reynolds, clerke, now warden of the seid howse or college of Merton, and the scolers of the same all and singler the premisses lymyted and apoynted in the seid will for the foundacion, meynetenance, and contynuance of the seid two lectures and two readers to have and to hold all and syngler the premisses with thappertenants unto the seid warden and scolers and theyre successors for ever to the use and behof of the seid warden and scolers and theyre successors for ever as by a dede of feoffement therof made by the seid byshop unto the seid warden and scolers bering date the fyrst day of Decembre in the thyrde yere of the reigne of our seid soveregne lord kyng Edward the syxt[2] particulerly and more playnly doth apere,[3] wyttnesseth that the seid warden and scolers for them and theyre successors do covenant, promyse, and grant to and with the seid Cuthbert busshop of Dureham, his heyres and executors[4] in maner and forme folowyng, that is to wytt that they the seid warden and scolers and theyre successors for ever shall contynually meyneteyne and fynde with the revenues, issues, and profetts of the premisses to them gevyn by the seid Cuthbert as well the seid two reders as also the seid two lectures of phisyk to be readd in the seid universytie of Oxford after the forme, tenor, true meanyng, and effect of the seid Thomas Lynacre in maner and forme and with all the cyrcumstans as ys conteyned in the seid will for that purpose which is above rehersed, except it be in suche thyngs and articles as shalbe herafter alteryd for good consideracions by the assent of the seid bysshope,[5] without any breach therof by any negligens, fraude or collusion and as they the seid warden and scolers and theyr successors,[6] be syde theyre present covenant promyse and grant, shall answer afore almightie god, and also the seid warden and scolers shall within the space of on yere next after the date herof ordeyne, constytute, and make by the assent of the seid bysshope[7] within theyr seid college certen statutes and ordynances for the contynuall meyntenance as well of the seid two readers as for the payment of theyre contynuall stypende and wages to be contynuyng for ever in forme now above lymyted[8] after such forme and maner as other statutes and ordynances byn made or have byn made within the seid universytie of Oxford for the meyneteynance and contynuance of other lectures in such sorte and as the best devyse that the seid warden and scolers can order and provyde the same, provyded alweys that att all tymes herafter

---

[1] Followed by 'in fulfillyng and performance of the seid will' crossed out.
[2] 'bering . . . syxt' inserted above the line.
[3] Followed by 'which dede' crossed out.
[4] Followed by 'and successors' crossed out.
[5] 'except . . . bysshope' inserted above the line.
[6] 'and theyr successors' inserted above the line.
[7] 'by the assent . . . bysshope' inserted above the line.
[8] 'in forme . . . lymyted' inserted above the line.

during the natural lif of the seid byshop yt shalbe lefull for the seid byshop to apoynte the said two readers, any thing in thes presents to the contrary notwithstanding. In wyttnes wherof the parties aforeseid to thes presentes enterchangeably have putt theyr seales. Yoven the day and yere fyrst above wrytten.

APPENDIX C: Calendar of Documents.

NO. I

Merton College, Oxford. Record no. 1348. 14 January 1515.

Thomas Linacre grants to Thomas More, gentleman, John Davy, John Babham son of John Babham, and Richard Hardyng property in the parishes of 'Ffeversham et Boughton subtus Le Blee' in Kent acquired from Thomas Bevercotes of 'Wollatton iuxta Notingham', gentleman, and Anna his wife, daughter and heiress of Richard Pratte, son and heir of William Pratte, citizen and mercer of London, for the purpose of implementing his last will. William Bylbroke and William Carkeke, junior, are appointed Linacre's attorneys.

The remains of a seal. Latin.

NO. 2

Merton College, Oxford. Record no. 1432. 21 September 1519.

Lewis Clyfford binds himself to pay to Thomas Linacre £300 on Christmas day next following. Beneath the obligation is the name Carkeke and, roughly written: 'Be mee Lewys Clyfford'.

The remains of a seal. Latin.

On the reverse is a note in English that the obligation is to be void if Clyfford carries out his agreement with Linacre.

NO. 3

Merton College, Oxford. Record no. 1449. 8 January 1523.

Richard Hyll of London, gentleman, and Thomas Gale of London, 'haberdassher', grant to Linacre, Tunstal, Richard Pace, Roger Drewe, John Chambre, Roger Denton, John Stokesley, clerks, Thomas More, knight, William Shelley, sergeant at law, Franciscus Poyntz, and John Clement, gentlemen, the Stone House and its adjoining garden, in the parish of St. Benedict, London, in Knight Rider Street. The property is stated to lie between land belonging to St. Paul's, London, on the east and south, and the property of William Gysnam, gentleman, once inhabited by Thomas Waren and William Lewes, and that of the hospital or priory of 'beate Marie Elsyng London' on the west, with Knight Rider Street on the north. The house and garden were previously inhabited by William Lytton, squire, and came to Hyll and Gale by grant from William Gysnam. Hyll promises to defend Linacre and his colleagues against John, abbot of St. Peter's monastery, Westminster. Hyll and Gale appoint William Carkeke and Thomas Maskall as their attorneys. Beneath the grant is the name Carkeke.

The remains of 2 seals. Latin.

On the reverse is a note in Latin that William Carkeke delivered possession of the property to Linacre on 11 March 1523, in the presence of William Pertryche, 'coteler', Edward Lake, William Robynson, Richard Hardyng, and Gilbert Patryk.

NO. 4

Merton College, Oxford. Record no. 1519. 4 February 1523.

Thomas Elmeston of 'Reynham', Thomas Dryland, 'generosus', Ralph Heyman, and Thomas Darland grant to Linacre, Tunstal, Pace, Roger Drewe, Chambre, Denton, Stokesley, clerks, More, knight, Shelley, sergeant at law, Poyntz, Clement, gentlemen, and Hardyng, 'yoman', lands in the parishes of 'Newenton iuxta Sydyngborne, Hertlep, Stokbery, Bobbyng et Halstowe' amounting to ninety-six acres. This property came to Elmeston's use by grant from William Scott, knight, John Scott, knight, and Vincent Ffynche of 'Sandherst' in Kent, gentleman, on 15 March 1521. William Woode alias William Taillor, William Fflawne alias William Essex are appointed attorneys. Beneath the grant is the name Carkeke.

The remains of 4 seals, signed by the four grantors. Latin.

On the reverse is a note in Latin that possession was delivered to Richard Hardyng on 10 February 1523 in the presence of William Blakborne, John Treules, Thomas Pope, Ralph Lorell, John Lyford, William Goodwyn, John Kyngeswoode, John Redyssh, John Potett, and many others.

NO. 5

Merton College, Oxford. Record no. 1522. 4 February 1523.

John Norton, knight, Henry Ffynche, gentleman, and Thomas Elmeston grant to Linacre, Tunstal, Pace, Roger Drewe, Chambre, Denton, Stokesley, clerks, More, knight, Shelley, sergeant at law, Poyntz, Clement, gentlemen, Hardyng, 'yoman', six acres of land known as 'Skrewles' in the parish of 'Newenton' in Kent, with the land of Richard Lee, squire and heir of Robert Barrey to the north, the king's highway between 'Newenton' and 'Chesteley' to the east, the land of John Dyggis, gentleman, to the south, and the land of William Blakborne to the west. The land was assigned to the use of Thomas Elmeston by Richard Bulle of 'Hothfeld' in Kent, 'clothman', son and heir of Anne Bulle, daughter and heiress of William Harryes of 'Newenton', on 12 May 1518. The appointed attorneys are the same as in document no. 4. Carkeke's name appears at the foot of the grant.

The remains of 3 seals, signed by the three grantors. Latin.

On the reverse is a note in Latin that possession was delivered to Richard Hardyng on 10 February 1523 in the presence of the same witnesses as in document no. 4.

NO. 6

Merton College, Oxford. Record no. 1359. 5 February 1523.

Receipt by John Norton, knight, for £80 'for landes caulyd Sevans', £6. 13s. 4d.

'for repracyon and other charges', and £11 'for landdes callyd Screles somtyme Rychard Bulles' for the use of Thomas Elmeston from Linacre.

The remains of a seal, signed by Norton. English.

NO. 7

Merton College, Oxford. Record no. 1524. 20 August 1523.

William Bloor of 'Reynham' in Kent, gentleman, grants to Linacre, Tunstal, Pace, More, Shelley, and Hardyng the property of 'Ffrognall', and all lands in the parish of 'Newenton iuxta Sydyngborne' in Kent acquired from Thomas Draper of 'Erithe' in Kent, gentleman. Also he grants the same two acres of land in the parish of 'Hertlep' in Kent at 'Goldhord' acquired from Thomas Draper. John Treules, Thomas Stretes, and William Fflawne alias William Essex 'yomen' are appointed attorneys.

The remains of a seal, signed by Bloor. Latin.

On the reverse is a note in Latin that possession was delivered to Richard Hardyng on 24 August 1523 in the presence of Thomas Elmeston, Robert Lyfford, John Godfrey, Thomas Crype, Reginald Bratt, Henry Teryndon, John Lyfford, Thomas Bratt, John Bawse, William Bartey, and many others, also a note in Latin of the enrolment of the transaction.

NO. 8

Merton College, Oxford. Record no. 1364. 5 November 1523.

William Bloor releases to the same persons as in document no. 7 his rights in property in 'Ffrognall', 'Newenton', and 'Hertlep'. Carkeke's name appears at the foot of the document.

The remains of a seal, signed by Bloor. Latin.

On the reverse a note in Latin of the enrolment of the transaction.

NO. 9

Merton College, Oxford. Record no. 1363. 23 November 1523.

Thomas Crips of 'Newenton iuxta Sydyngborne' Kent binds himself to pay Linacre £4 on Christmas day next following. Beneath the obligation is the name Carkeke.

The remains of a seal. Latin.

NO. 10

Merton College, Oxford. Record no. 1360. 20 September 1523.

'Thomas Cryps' acknowledges the receipt from Linacre of seven nobles as payment for two acres of land in the parish of 'Newynton bysyde Sydyngborn lying by Wurdall gate'.

The remains of a seal. English.

NO. 11

Merton College, Oxford. Documents both numbered under 6700 (two identical copies, one probably a first rough draft). Michaelmas term, 1520.

Linacre, Pace, Tunstal, More, Shelley, John Drewe, and Clement seek through their attorney, John Mountagne, to recover the manor of Traces with its named appurtenances from John Halys, after Nicholas Hunt has 'disseised' them of the property. John Halys, Lewis Clyfford, Nicholas Clyfford, and Thomas Fysh appear as witnesses. On adjournment Fysh fails to appear. Judgement is granted to Linacre etc.

Latin.

NO. 12

Merton College, Oxford. Record no. 1435. 2 December 1520.

Linacre, Pace, Tunstal, More, Shelley, John Drewe, and Clement appoint John Ascott, 'generosus', and Richard Hardyng as their attorneys to recover against John Halys, squire, the manor of 'Traceys' and its appurtenances; and two properties of 160 acres of land, 10 acres of meadow, 20 acres of pasture, 20 acres of woodland, and 100 shillings of revenue with their appurtenances in 'Newyngton iuxta Sythyngbourne, Hertlepp, Stokberye, Reyneham, Bacchyld, Tong, Beney, Rodmarsham, Sythyngbourne, Eschurche, et Wardon in insula de Scapeia' in Kent from the sheriff of Kent, by virtue of a royal writ.

The remains of 6 seals, 1 missing, signed by Linacre, More, and Shelley. Latin.

On the reverse in English a note that Mecott the deputy (? the document is damaged here) sheriff of Kent delivered possession to the attorneys in the presence of John Trynlas, John Towne, Thomas Baily, William Sybley(?), and others.

NO. 13

Merton College, Oxford. Document no. 6695. Date uncertain.

Linacre, Pace, Tunstal, More, Shelley, John Drewe, and Clement conduct a law suit concerning the manor of 'Tracies' before the royal justices at Westminster. The exact dating and interpretation of this document cannot be given here as it consists of a large number of unnumbered pages which have been totally disarranged. It is probable, however, that it refers to the case mentioned in documents numbered 11 and 12 in this Calendar.

Latin.

NO. 14

Merton College, Oxford. In envelope E.2.28a. No date.

Richard Hyll writes to Linacre concerning the Stone House. William Litton has lived in the Stone House without having documents of possession, thinking William Gysnam would never claim it since he had previously assisted him. Litton had not, so far as Hyll knows, passed on the property to anyone. Litton should have granted Hyll certain property for money paid to Litton; instead on his deathbed he passed on the Stone House to Hyll. Gage and servants of Litton informed Hyll of this and stated that if Hyll did not require the house, Litton's executors would sell it and pay Hyll his money. Hyll entered the house and enfeoffed William Tyler and others and was in possession for more than a year. Then Gysnam's wife and others entered the Stone

H

House by force. Hyll proceeded by law against her and finally obtained a ruling by masters Wyndesore, Baudwyn, and Cholmeley. He sends the award to Linacre and requests him to keep the matter secret. Signed: Hyll.

English.

NO. 15

Merton College, Oxford. In envelope E.2.28a (two identical copies, one probably a first rough draft). No date.

A refutation of the claims of William Litton to have had ownership of the Stone House. Litton has been executor of Henry Gysnam's will and was expected to be a 'good master' to Gysnam's nephew William Gysnam. After Henry Gysnam's death, William Gysnam for 40*s.* per year leased the Stone House to Litton before Laurence Gobder and others. Litton then wrongfully took the income from property in Stratford belonging to William Gysnam's inheritance from his uncle and allowed the estate to decay. Litton made a loan of twenty marks to William Gysnam which was duly repaid. Litton then offered Gysnam a loan of forty marks to be repaid by a reduction of payments of rent for the Stone House. Gysnam accepted and allowed Litton to live rent free in the Stone House for life. Finally five reasons are noted to show that Litton had never purchased the Stone House, but only leased it.

English.

NO. 16

Merton College, Oxford. Record no. 1448. 15 October 1522.

An indenture between William Gysnam, alias William Guysnam, gentleman, relation and heir of Henry Gysnam, late of London, gentleman, that is the son of William Gysnam, brother of Henry Gysnam, and Richard Hyll of London, gentleman, and Thomas Gale of London, 'haberdassher', notes that William Gysnam has sold for forty marks to Hyll and Gale the Stone House and its adjacent garden. The boundaries of the property are given. Excepted are a chimney, 'caminus', and a 'pentice' belonging to William Gysnam's property, Warens House. William Gysnam and his heirs reserve the right to enter the Stone House to repair their chimney and 'pentice' when necessary. Gysnam appoints John Davy and William Carkeke as his attorneys. Signed: Per me Willelmum Gisnam. Beneath the document is the name Carkeke.

The remains of a seal. Latin.

On the reverse is a note in Latin that possession of the property was delivered by Carkeke to Richard Hyll on 5 December 1522, in the presence of John Iverye, Richard Hardyng, Thomas Tayllor, Edward Lake, Edmund Toursey, Thomas Martyn, William Robynson, Elias Russell, and others.

NO. 17

Merton College, Oxford. Record no. 1451. 12 August 1523.

William Gysnam, alias William Guysnam etc. (as in the previous document) and his wife Christiana release to Linacre, William Dancastre, clerks, and John Davy, 'yoman', their heirs and assignees, all their rights in the Stone House,

its adjacent garden, and another piece of land in Knight Rider Street purchased by Linacre from Gysnam. The boundaries of the properties are given.
Gysnam and his wife promise to support Linacre against the abbot of Westminster.

The remaines of 2 seals. Latin. Beneath the fold at the foot of the document
is written: 'Per me Iohannem Rudstone(?)'. There is also a faded and badly
creased note of the examination of the document on 18(?) January 1524. The
names of William Guysnam, Christiana, William Shelley, John Rudstan(?)
'aldreman'(?), John Ritwes(?) 'magistrum scole sancti Paulle(?)', and Richard
Hardyng are recorded.

On the reverse is a note in Latin that this document was read and enrolled
'in hustengo London' on 18 January 1524. The note is signed: Paber W.

NO. 18
Merton College, Oxford. Record no. 1439. 21 August 1523.
The advice of William Shelley and Roger Cholmeley 'lerned councell' of
Linacre concerning land in 'Ffrognall', 'Newton' and 'Hertlep' purchased from
William Bloor. First, Bloor is to make a deed of enfeoffment dated 20 August
1523 to Linacre and others as feoffees for the use of Linacre. Second, Bloor is
to make a grant to these feoffees and deliver possession to Hardyng. Third,
Bloor is to make a deed of release and deliver it to Hardyng. Finally, Bloor
before 28 August is to appear before the Chancery court and have the deeds
enrolled by John Taylor, clerk.
English.

NO. 19
Merton College, Oxford. Record no. 1355. Wednesday after St. Bartholomew.
No date.
William Bloor writes to Linacre in London from 'Raynham'. He would have
come to London, but sir Thomas Cheyny has sent for him. He promises to
come at the beginning of the next term and have his deeds enrolled. If
Linacre insists, he will come immediately. Signed: Wylliam Bloor.
The remains of a seal. English.

NO. 20
Merton College, Oxford. Record no. 1361. 12 September 1523.
Linacre sells by an indenture to 'Rauff Symonds, citezein and ffysshmonger of
London' property in the parish of 'Ffeversham and Boughton under the Blee
otherwyse called the Blene' in Kent, once the property of William Pratte,
citizen and mercer of London, purchased by Linacre from Thomas Bevercotes
of Wollatton near Nottingham, gentleman, and from Anne, his wife, daughter
and heiress of Richard Pratte, son and heir of William Pratte, for the sum of
£85. Arrangements are made for the transfer of deeds, the grant of the
property to persons for the use of Symonds, and the completion of any legal
documentation required. Linacre gives assurances that the lands bring in
annually £4. 5s. 0d. over and above all chief and quit rents.
The remains of a seal, signed by Symonds. English.

NO. 21

Merton College, Oxford. Record no. 1452. 1 May 1524.
Linacre sells to William Mortymer, 'citezein and brawderer' of London, for
£30, property purchased by Linacre from William Guysnam, cousin and heir
of Henry Gysnam, late of London, gentleman, where Thomas Waren once
lived and William Lewes recently lived. The property is in Knight Rider
Street in the parish of St. Benet in the ward of Castle Baynard in London,
between the Stone House to the east, lands previously belonging to the prior
and convent of Elsyng and now to Linacre with part of the Stone House to
the south, property of Mathewe Browne, knight, to the west, and Knight
Rider Street to the north. Linacre promises to grant to a chosen group this
property for Mortymer's use before the coming feast of the birth of St. John
the Baptist.
    The remains of a seal. English.

NO. 22

Merton College, Oxford. Roll in envelope E.2.28a. 1 December 1549.
Tunstal grants to the Warden and scholars of Merton College the lands left
by Linacre for the establishment of the Oxford lectureships. He appoints
Thomas Carpenter as his attorney.
    From the untidy appearance of the document, with many alterations and
crossings-out, probably a first draft. Latin.

NO. 23

Merton College, Oxford. Document no. 1453. 5 December 1549.
The Warden and scholars of Merton College appoint Edward Bell as their
attorney to receive from Tunstal Linacre's lands.
    The remains of a seal. Latin. What is apparently a first draft of this docu-
ment also survives as a Merton College roll in envelope E.2.28a.

NO. 24

Merton College, Oxford. Document no. 1525. 2 January 1550.
Tunstal appoints the Warden and scholars of Merton College as his proctors
to receive any arrears of rent etc. connected with Linacre's lands.
    The remains of a seal, signed by Tunstal. Latin.
    On the reverse is a note in Latin and another in English summarizing the
contents of the document.

NO. 25

Merton College, Oxford. Liber Statutorum, p. 31. 25 July 1550.
The Warden and scholars of Merton College bind themselves to observe the
terms of the indenture made between them and Tunstal on 10 December
1549. They promise to enter the indenture in their statute book so that it
will be publicly read three times yearly when the other statutes are read.
    Latin.

NO. 26

Merton College, Oxford. Document no. 1454. 28 December 1549.
The Warden and scholars of Merton College grant to 'Edmond Cryspyne' of London, gentleman, a lease of twenty-one years for the Stone House, for an annual rent of £4 to be paid in two equal amounts, with the usual safeguards. The college agrees to repair the property within two years, after which time Crispin shall be responsible for its maintenance.

The remains of a seal. English. At the foot of the document is written: Per me Edwardum Bell eius verum atturnatum ut patet litore.

On the reverse is a Latin note describing the contents of the document.

Thomas Linacre and the Foundation of the College of Physicians

CHARLES WEBSTER*

THERE CAN BE NO DOUBT THAT ONE OF LINACRE'S most enduring achievements was the establishment of the College of Physicians of London. From its foundation in 1518 the College superintended the organization of medicine in London; ultimately it came to exercise a wider national function as the Royal College of Physicians. Linacre is accordingly important for our understanding of a crucial development in the evolution of the medical profession in England.

Although direct evidence about the early history of the College of Physicians is distressingly slight, few would disagree with the characterization of Linacre's role given by the pioneer medical historian John Freind.[1] According to Freind, Linacre was alarmed by the low status of the London medical profession, 'engros'd by illiterate Monks and Empiricks' who were ineffectively controlled by the ecclesiastical authorities. Linacre, 'using his interest at Court', gained through services to such notable personages as Henry VIII and Cardinal Wolsey, was able to give 'encouragement to men of Reputation and Learning' by securing the power of medical licensing for a 'corporate Society of Physicians in this City'. Under the terms of the establishment of the College, Linacre secured the rights of its members to 'make such Statutes and Ordinances as they, from time to time, shou'd think most expedient for the publick Service'.

* Reader in the History of Medicine and Director, Wellcome Unit for the History of Medicine, Oxford University.

[1] John Freind, *The History of Physick from the Time of Galen to the Beginning of the Sixteenth Century*, 2 vols., London, 1725–6, ii. 410–15.

From the time of Linacre they constructed a body of statutes framed 'with regard to their own dignity, the good of the people, and in particular to the honour of the Universities'. Upon the foundation of the College, Linacre became its first President and retained this office until his death in 1524. Furthermore, the corporate meetings were held at his home, the Stone House, in Knight Rider Street. As a result of Linacre's generosity this house became the permanent headquarters of the College in the sixteenth century. In summary:

> His scheme without doubt, was not only to create a good understanding and unanimity among his own Profession, which itself was an excellent thought, but to make them more useful to the publick: and he imagin'd that by separating them from the vulgar *Empiricks*, and setting them upon such a reputable foot of distinction, there wou'd always arise a spirit of emulation among men liberally educated which wou'd animate them in pursuing their inquiries into the *Nature of Diseases* and the *Methods of Cure*, for the benefit of mankind.[1]

Providing allowance is made for Freind's unswerving loyalty to the much-maligned College, his tendency to attribute Newtonian qualities to the humanists of the previous age, and his errors in small matters of fact, the above outline account of the origins of the College of Physicians resembles in major respects the authoritative and fully documented history compiled recently by Sir George Clark.[2] After drawing together the fragmentary records relating to the early College, Clark was able to conclude that 'the most remarkable achievement of [Linacre's] whole life was the founding of the College of Physicians'. It is true that its legal status was guaranteed by more powerful authorities and that within the association Linacre enjoyed the co-operation of notable fellow physicians, but his name alone is relevant to almost every facet of the affairs associated with the foundation of the College.[3]

The essential details of the chronology of the founding years of

[1] Ibid. ii. 414. For a similar sentiment see Sir Norman Moore, *History of the Study of Medicine in the British Isles*, London, 1908, pp. 55–6.

[2] *A History of the Royal College of Physicians of London*, 2 vols., Oxford, 1964–6, i. 37–67. See also J. N. Johnson, *The Life of Thomas Linacre*, London, 1835, pp. 277–95. For a survey of the general state of medicine in England in the sixteenth century, see R. S. Roberts, 'The Personnel and Practice of Medicine in Tudor and Stuart England: Part I', *Medical History*, vi, 1962, 363–82; Part II, viii, 1964, 217–34.

[3] Clark, op. cit. ii. 51–2. Johnson (op. cit.) described the College as 'the last and most magnificent' of Linacre's designs (p. 277).

the College are well established, but it is less well understood why in 1518 Linacre was successful in persuading the authorities to abandon the unrestricted practice of medicine and to accept rigid organization of the London medical profession. It is also not clear what factors influenced Linacre and his successors in framing the elaborate collegiate organization which is known from the earliest statutes. As Freind suggests, one factor in the explanation is Linacre's creative genius, which enabled him to convince contemporaries that a learned and well-regulated medical profession would be a more effective agency for the welfare of the commonwealth. Linacre was a characteristic advocate of the civic humanism of the More circle, and his classical learning, cosmopolitan associations, and active involvement in London affairs provided a range of experience which was essential for the success of his plan. He was able to pursue his objectives at an ideal moment, drawing upon detailed knowledge of professional organization which could be judiciously applied to the London situation. Linacre's foundation of the College of Physicians should therefore not be regarded as a spontaneous instance of individual initiative, but as a development intimately influenced by social conditions in Tudor London, as well as by the evolution of medical organization elsewhere in Europe.

It is not possible to consider the establishment of the College of Physicians without some reference to the general process of incorporation, which was one of the most conspicuous features of urban development in the fifteenth century. While it has been customary to consider the evolution of the medical profession in a self-contained manner, there is no doubt that medical practitioners were influenced by the example of corporate development in other vocational groups. Indeed, in the relatively flexible structure of late medieval medicine, the medical arts were not sharply distinguished from associated crafts and trades. Barbers, grocers, and spicers dominated important aspects of medicine and undoubtedly displayed a propensity to extend their activities into general practice. These groups of medically oriented tradesmen became both numerous and prosperous. University-trained physicians represented merely one facet of the medical profession and in London their services would have been utilized by only the small upper-class section of the community. They enjoyed no corporate identity in the fifteenth century, while increasing numbers of other vocational groups were seeking and obtaining Royal Charters. Grants of incorporation carried specific privileges and commercial advantages, but also conferred on companies an immortal collective personality which provided the key to enhanced social status.[1] The charters granted in the fifteenth century had basic common characteristics. A fellowship was permitted to enjoy a perpetual commonality; it could hold lands in mortmain, frequently to the value of about £20, and possess a common seal. In addition each company was given powers of regulation, usually within the city of London and its immediate environs. Once established, a company supervised the activities of its members, regulated standards of manufacture, and exercised powers of inspection and prosecution of unqualified practitioners and aliens. Companies established in this manner flourished commercially and invested considerable energies in the development of their corporate identity. As resources increased the companies acquired substantial halls and expensive plate, furnishings, and decorations; secular and religious ceremonial functions provided an aristocratic façade for their commercial activities. Charitable functions were taken on and chaplains maintained. Hence merchants or yeomen discovered that their companies were the means to dignity and social prestige as well as to commercial profit.

Within the companies there rapidly developed a rigidly hierarchical form of government. Power increasingly passed from the freemen into the hands of the Court of Assistants, an executive consisting of Masters and Wardens which recruited new members by co-option. Rigid divisions came to exist between the senior and junior members, giving rise to internal dissension in the company.

The first wave of incorporation occurred in the decade before 1400 and the success of the pioneer companies provided the impetus for a continuous stream of similar developments which persisted until the second decade of the sixteenth century. 'Incorporation thus became the established rule amongst the great mysteries, and an object of legitimate ambition to all the rest.'[2] By 1500, most of the traditional London trades had become organized into a tightly inter-

---

[1] G. Unwin, *The Guilds and Companies of London*, 4th edn. with an introduction by W. K. Kahl, London, 1963; W. Herbert, *The History of the Twelve Great Livery Companies*, 2 vols., London, 1837; S. L. Thrupp, *The Merchant Class of Medieval London, 1300–1500*, London, 1948. For a history of a typical company, see C. Welch, *History of the Worshipful Company of Pewterers*, 2 vols., London, 1902.

[2] Unwin, op. cit., p. 161.

locking network of company organizations. The highest level of this structure was represented by such bodies as the Mercers and Gold-smiths, whose wealthy companies had been established before 1400. By the later fifteenth century company organization had extended to the more modest Barbers (1462), Ironmongers (1463), and Pewterers (1468). In the final phase of development, 1500–18, charters were obtained by the Poulterers (1504), Bakers (1509), Innholders (1515), and Physicians (1518). After this there was a long break before the grant of a charter to the Stationers' Company (1554), the leading representative of the new trades of London. Thus the physicians' charter marked the completion of a long epoch of corporation development among the traditional trades of London.[1] Physicians, having witnessed this mechanism infiltrate into every facet of the social fabric, could not avoid noticing its contingent advantages. It was therefore inevitable that the medical profession should follow their continental counterparts by seeking integration into this system of company organization.

Physicians may not have felt any strong identity of interest with the merchants and tradesmen of London. But like tradesmen, they were obliged to enter into competition, for the privilege of tending the sick. Accordingly there was an inducement to follow the precedent of the commercial classes by introducing a division of labour to coincide with the interests of the dominant emergent groups within the medical profession.

It is important not to exaggerate the social gulf between the physicians and members of the city companies. Owing to the subordination of the yeomanry, the élite Court of Assistants was often not fully representative of the interests of the company. Freedom of the Mercers' Company was obtained by merchants with various trading interests who sought a prestigious social position and a basis for political influence within the City. It was common for families to have some members involved in the livery companies and others in the universities, Church, or medicine.[2] Hence it is not surprising to find that the humanists in Linacre's circle had close merchant associations. Near relatives of Thomas More and John Colet were

[1] Unwin, op. cit., p. 243. The Stationers, like the Physicians, had strong humanist associations; see C. Blogden, *The Stationers' Company: A History, 1403–1959*, London, 1960, pp. 19–38.

[2] It will be remembered that William Harvey's six brothers were active members of the London merchant community.

members of the Mercers' Company and More himself became a free-man of the Company in 1509, soon after undertaking legal work on behalf of the Mercers. Colet entrusted the management of St. Paul's School to the Mercers' Company, and Linacre placed the endow-ments of the Linacre lectures in the same hands.[1] Accordingly, the Mercers were to administer one part of the Stone House, while the College of Physicians was in possession of the rest. These examples indicate the importance of the major companies as media-tors of financial transactions, but they also demonstrate common feeling between leading humanists and merchants. On Colet's motives for placing St. Paul's under merchant control, Erasmus commented: 'over the revenues he set neither priests, nor the bishop, nor the chapter (as they call it), nor noblemen; but some married citizens of established reputation. And when asked the reason, he said that though there was nothing certain in human affairs, he yet found the least corruption in them.'[2] Not surprisingly the humanists took an interest in the charitable organizations asso-ciated with the Mercers' Company. As McConica has shown, humanist influence can be detected in the revival of both the Hospital of St. Thomas Acon and Whittington College.[3] Such foundations, housing aspiring humanist scholars and divines, would have reinforced Linacre's belief in the value of collegiate institutions as a means to the advancement of the humanist interest.

The reasons for the delay in establishing corporate organizations within the medical profession are not difficult to find. In spite of its numerical strength, the medical profession in London lacked any sense of unity, since the practitioners were drawn from diverse educational and social backgrounds. Some were essentially grocers, others barbers, displaying loyalty to guilds with long-established codes of practice. Educated physicians were often deflected into a clerical career, or their security was jeopardized by competition

[1] R. Ames, *Citizen Thomas More and his Utopia*, Princeton, 1949, pp. 40–57; J. K. McConica, *English Humanists and Reformation Politics under Henry VIII and Edward VI*, Oxford, 1965, pp. 48–51, 102; J. H. Lupton, *A Life of Dean Colet, D.D.*, London, 1909, pp. 7–18. See above, John M. Fletcher, 'Linacre's Lands and Lectureships', pp. 107–97.

[2] Letter from Erasmus to Justus Jonas, 13 June 1521, *Opus Epistolarum Des. Erasmi Roterodami*, ed. P. S. Allen, 12 vols., Oxford, 1906–58, iv. 518; Lupton, op. cit., pp. 166–7. See also J. Simon, *Education and Society in Tudor England*, Cambridge, 1967, pp. 73–80, 93–6.

[3] McConica, op. cit., pp. 100–5.

from immigrant practitioners or the wide spectrum of indigenous empirics. The English universities gave medical degrees, but their medical schools were insufficiently well developed to provide a basis for a lay medical profession possessing a unified set of values.[1] Nevertheless, there was some attempt in the fifteenth century to initiate associations within the medical profession, in line with the corporate bodies which were springing up in other social groups. At this embryonic stage, alignments were tentative and ephemeral, sometimes anticipating later developments, but often not reflecting the ultimate lines of settlement. The most imaginative proposal for the organization of the higher grades of the medical profession came from three London physicians and two surgeons, who in 1423 proposed a 'Communaltie' to control all physicians and surgeons practising in the capital. One of the petitioners, Gilbert Kymer, described as Doctor of Medicine and Rector of Medicine, was to be the 'president and Reader' of this association.[2] The court of this company, consisting entirely of medical graduates, aimed to appoint surveyors who would enforce apprenticeship regulations in the craft of surgery and demand academic qualifications from intending physicians. The association of the 'Rector and Surveyors of Physicians and the Masters of Surgery' of the type successfully established on the Continent, after a brief period of activity proved unsuccessful in London.[3] Thereafter the 'Faculty' of Surgeons retained their identity as a minority group of specialists until they associated with the more numerous Barbers' Company in the sixteenth century.[4] In response to the petition of 1423, the barbers successfully defended their rights to practise surgery and this responsibility was written into their charter of incorporation in 1462. This established the mystery as 'unum Corpus et una Communitas perpetua' under the control of two masters, a barber-surgeon and a barber alternating

[1] V. L. Bullough, 'Medical Study at Mediaeval Oxford', *Speculum*, xxxvi, 1961, 600–12; idem, 'The Mediaeval Medical School at Cambridge', *Mediaeval Studies*, xxiv, 1962, 162–8.

[2] R. R. Sharpe, ed., *Calendar of Letter-Books Preserved among the Archives of the City of London at the Guildhall. Letter Book K*, London, 1911, p. 11; J. F. South, *Memorials of the Craft of Surgery in England*, ed. D'Arcy Power, London, 1886, pp. 299–306; C. H. Talbot and E. A. Hammond, *The Medical Practitioners in Medieval England*, London, 1965, pp. 60–3. This association is often referred to as a 'college', but that term was not used in the original document.

[3] *Letter Book K*, pp. 14–15, 29–31, 36, 41.

[4] Ibid., pp. 97–9, 143–4, 222.

as the senior partner. The charter followed traditional lines: authority resided with the masters and a court of twelve senior members
(*principales*); a common seal was granted; the company could acquire
and possess lands to the value of five marks; they could plead and
be impleaded in courts and assemble to make statutes and ordinances governing 'all Surgeons, exercising the Mystery of Barbers'.[1]

By the end of the fifteenth century the Barbers had entered into
a 'Composition' with their associates, the Surgeons, and accumulated sufficient resources to establish a Hall at Monkwell Street.
Thus by 1500 the barbers were firmly established in the hierarchy
of London companies, having formed an association with the surgeons which naturally evolved into a full partnership in 1540.[2]

The incorporation of surgeons and their increasing wealth and
social prestige must have been of little comfort to the disorganized
ranks of the physicians. The indignity of their position must have
seemed particularly great to the increasing number of physicians
equipped with medical degrees from Italian universities. This class
believed that they possessed a professionally valuable qualification;
furthermore their education led to the absorption of the spirit of
confidence and self-esteem of the Italian humanists. It is therefore
not surprising that Linacre, the most effective exponent of medical
humanism, should play the leading role in the attempt to secure a
position of esteem for his fellow physicians who were academically
qualified.

The success of Linacre's operation was undoubtedly assisted by
the conditions prevailing during the early years of the reign of
Henry VIII. The King was initially favourable both to the confirma-
tion of company charters and to proposals for new corporations.
Furthermore, Henry and his political aides Wolsey and Fox were
inclined to become patrons of enterprises having a humanistic bias.
With specific reference to Queen Katherine, Linacre, Tunstal, More,
Pace, Colet, and Stokesley, Erasmus praised the learning of the
English Court and epitomized it as a humanistic museum (μουσειν).[3]

It was probably out of a desire to extend sympathy for humanistic
medicine that Linacre was prompted to publish his first Galen trans-

[1] S. Young, *The Annals of the Barber Surgeons of London*, London, 1890,
pp. 52–5.
[2] The Company of Barber Surgeons was established by Act of Parliament
(32 Henry VIII, c. 42) in 1540; Young, op. cit., pp. 78–80.
[3] Letter from Erasmus to Paul Bombasius, 26 July 1518, Allen, iii. 356–7.

lation, *De sanitate tuenda*, in 1518. Linacre, ever reticent over matters of publication, had prepared his translation by 1515;[1] in late 1516 it was reported that Lupset would supervise the printing in Paris.[2] Thereafter Linacre's friends enthusiastically awaited the text, which eventually appeared in the summer of 1517.[3] Linacre addressed his beautifully printed folio to potentially powerful patrons of the humanistic physicians. The printed dedication, dated 16 June 1517, was addressed to Henry VIII; in addition copies with separate hand-written letters of dedication were presented to Wolsey and Fox. The former was assured of Linacre's highest regard for the main-tenance of his health; Fox was recommended to follow the precepts of Galen in order to ensure the continuing health needed for the accomplishment of his great design—undoubtedly a reference to the establishment of Corpus Christi College, Oxford, in 1517.[4] Linacre probably hoped to persuade the Court that it was desirable to estab-lish a collegiate organization of humanist physicians charged with reforming London medicine. They would complement the group of scholars introduced by Fox into Oxford to inject humanistic stan-dards into higher education.

A crucial factor in inducing receptivity to Linacre's ideas was public concern over the serious threats to health in the capital. The chroniclers noted that the sixteenth century opened with a 'great pestilence' throughout England, 'but speciallie and most of all in the citie of London'.[5] Thereafter, during the first two decades of the century, almost every year was punctuated by epidemic outbreaks

---

[1] Letter from Thomas More to Martin Dorp, 21 October 1515: More, *Lucubrationes*, Basle, 1563, p. 416; E. F. Rogers, ed., *The Correspondence of Sir Thomas More*, Princeton, 1947, p. 65.

[2] Letter from More to Erasmus, 15 December 1516, Allen, ii. 420. 'Linacer protinus a Natali quae vertit e Galeno mittet Luteciam excudendo, comite Lupseto qui calcographis castigator aderit.' For Lupset's role, see J. A. Gee, *The Life and Works of Thomas Lupset*, New Haven, 1928, pp. 59–63.

[3] *De sanitate tuenda* was issued from the press of Rubé on 22 August 1517. See below, pp. 218–19; Johnson, op. cit., pp. 208–14.

[4] The copy of *De sanitate tuenda* addressed to Wolsey is preserved in the British Museum, C.19.e.15. The copy addressed to Fox is in the library of the Royal College of Physicians. For the letter to Fox, of September 1517, see P. S. Allen and H. M. Allen, eds., *Letters of Richard Fox 1486–1527*, Oxford, 1929, pp. 109–10. See also below, G. Barber, 'Thomas Linacre: A Biblio-graphical Survey of his Works', pp. 296–7.

[5] R. Holinshed, *Chronicles of England, Scotland and Ireland*, 6 vols., London, 1807–8, ii. 1454.

of some kind. It is not possible to know precisely what disease was involved in each epidemic. Bubonic plague was one of the regular contributing factors. Also involved were influenza, typhus, small-pox, and measles.[1] Rivalling plague as a cause of mortality during this period was the 'new disease', sweating-sickness. The first major outbreak of this disease occurred in 1485, the second in 1508, and the third in 1517.[2] Often the population was ravaged by more than one epidemic at a time. In September 1517 the Venetian ambassador reported the difficulty of avoiding both the plague and sweating-sickness, while in the following year Pace noted that 'they do die in these parts in every place, not only of the small pokkes and mesils, but also of the great sickness'.[3] Sweating-sickness was par-ticularly alarming since, unlike plague, which was regarded prima-rily as *morbus pauperum*, the new disease, *Sudor anglicus*, seemed most prevalent among the upper classes. Erasmus was suffering from sweating-sickness upon his arrival at Cambridge in 1511, and ill health continued to affect him throughout his English visit, fre-quently preventing communication with friends in London.[4] Per-haps the most celebrated figure to be claimed by the sweat was Andreas Ammonius, the Latin Secretary to the King, whose death was reported by More to Erasmus on 19 August 1517.[5] The 1517 outbreak of sweat was the most destructive of the five recorded outbreaks; Fox, Wolsey, and the King were affected and many members of their households died. Reports from London indicate the severity of its effect on the daily life of the capital and in both 1517 and 1518 there were complaints that public business was dis-rupted through the enforced absence of the Court.[6] The constant threat of illness created deep anxieties within the Court and high officials were constantly searching for places of safety for the King and his family. In this crisis situation, officials were induced to

---

[1] C. Creighton, *A History of Epidemics in Britain*, 2nd edn., with additional material by D. E. C. Eversley, E. A. Underwood, and L. Ovenall, 2 vols., London, 1968; J. F. D. Shrewsbury, *A History of Bubonic Plague in the British Isles*, Cambridge, 1971.

[2] Creighton, op. cit. i. 237–81; M. B. Shaw, 'A Short History of the Sweating Sickness', *Annals of Medical History*, v, 1933, 246–73.

[3] *Letters and Papers, Henry VIII*, vol. ii, part 2, 1864, documents 3697, 4320.

[4] Letter from Erasmus to Andreas Ammonius, 25 August 1511, Allen, ii. 466; see also D. F. S. Thomson and H. C. Porter, *Erasmus and Cambridge*, Toronto, 1963, pp. 78–83.

[5] Allen, iii. 47.   [6] Creighton, op. cit. i. 245–50.

examine continental precedent and to pay attention to preventive measures. This context may be relevant to the apparently spontaneous decision to introduce medical licensing in 1511. Under the new regulations, clearly designed to limit the activities of dangerous empirics, the control of surgeons and physicians in London and the surrounding area was placed in the hands of the Bishop of London (Robert Fitz-James) and the Dean of St. Paul's (John Colet).[1] This measure would offer some protection to the public from adventurers intent on profiting from the epidemic conditions. Wolsey was responsible for the first Royal Proclamation on the Plague in January 1518. This ordered the marking for forty days of the doors of infected houses, the inhabitants being obliged to carry four-foot-long white rods when walking in the streets.[2] More incurred some unpopularity through enforcing this order in Oxford in the spring of 1518.[3] In this context it is notable that Linacre in translating Galen concentrated on practical texts which might be relevant to epidemic situations, and as further evidence of serious concern over this problem among humanist physicians, John Caius wrote both Latin and vernacular tracts on sweating-sickness.[4]

The proposals of Linacre and his associates for the establishment of a medical organization capable of more expert regulation of the profession, and sufficiently responsible to accept obligations on matters of public health, were entirely appropriate to this situation. The King responded by granting, on 23 September 1518, Letters Patent incorporating the President and College of Physicians of London.[5] The Charter acknowledged a petition received from three

[1] Clark, *A History of the Royal College of Physicians*, i. 54–5.

[2] F. P. Wilson, *The Plague in Shakespeare's London*, Oxford, 1927, pp. 56–7.

[3] *Letters and Papers, Henry VIII*, document 4125, John Clerk to Wolsey, 28 April 1518. More insisted 'that the inhabitants of those houses that be and shall be infected shall keep in, put out wispes and bear white rods, according as your Grace devised for Londoners'.

[4] *A boke or conseill against the disease called the Sweate*, London, 1552; *De ephemera Britannica*, London, 1555; C. G. Gruner, *Scriptores de sudore anglico*, Jena, 1847. For Caius, see *The Works of John Caius*, ed. E. S. Roberts, with a biographical introduction by J. Venn, Cambridge, 1912; C. E. Raven, *English Naturalists from Neckam to Ray*, Cambridge, 1947, pp. 138–47.

[5] Clark, op. cit. i. 58. The Charter is given in full in W. Munk, *Roll of the Royal College of Physicians*, 3 vols., London, 1878, i. 2–6. Roberts rightly stresses the importance of the College in 'a general but tardy attempt to deal with public health problems' in London: 'The Personnel and Practice . . .', part II, p. 222.

royal physicians, John Chambre, Thomas Linacre, and Ferdinand de Victoria, three other physicians, Nicholas Halswell, John Francis, and Robert Yaxley, and finally one layman, Cardinal Wolsey. The latter had experienced the sweat and as Lord Chancellor had been responsible for the protection of the King and the introduction of rudimentary public health measures. He was therefore fully aware of the medical problems of London and Linacre, as his personal physician, would probably have been consulted as his expert adviser. At this time Wolsey's influence at Court was supreme, and his support was invaluable for the success of the physicians' petition.

With the Charter of 1518 the physicians attained full recognition as a professional group and their College joined the ranks of the London companies. Apart from minor verbal peculiarities, the Charter followed the traditional pattern outlined above. The petitioners and their colleagues in London were established as *unum corpus et communitas perpetua sive Collegium perpetuum*, having perpetual succession, the right to a common seal and to the possession of lands to the value of £12. The College was permitted to hold regular meetings and to frame appropriate statutes and ordinances. Four senior representatives would be responsible for the inspection and control of all physicians within the city and the surrounding districts, up to a seven-mile limit. Like members of other companies the physicians were granted exemptions from jury service and inquisitions.[1] Under the presidency of Linacre, the academic physicians assumed a position of authority within their profession. Once they were incorporated their history repeated the pattern of other companies. Their rights were vigorously defended and attempts were made to extend their influence over all groups involved in London medicine. New civic privileges were sought and obtained. A corporate spirit was successfully cultivated and the College quickly evolved a complex body of ordinances and statutes designed to elevate the perpetual association into a place of dignity and honour.

During the years immediately following the 1518 Charter, the College effectively established its identity and laid the foundations for a professional organization distinct in character from other London companies. Apart from such terms as 'college' and 'president', there was little sign of this differentiation in 1518. However, in 1523, just over a year before Linacre's death, the Charter was

[1] Munk, op. cit. i. 2–6.

ratified by an Act of Parliament. This repeated the provisions of the Charter, but added certain remarks about organization which provided a foretaste of the complex rules later embodied in the statutes. The six senior members of the College were to combine with two others to form a body of eight 'Elects'. This self-appointing group, from which the president was selected annually, was the physicians' equivalent of the Court of Assistants. The President and three Elects were now given authority to govern medical practice throughout England. Some companies such as the Pewterers successfully exercised national responsibilities, but this clause was completely premature with respect to the medical profession.[1]

It is important to appreciate that in spite of its dreams of national jurisdiction, the College operated at an extremely modest level between 1518 and October 1524, when Linacre died. The six original members (*collegae*) had been joined by six others by the end of 1523, after which the pace of expansion slowed down; a membership of eighteen was recorded in 1537.[2]

Linacre was by far the most impressive figure in the early College. Erasmus came to address him, not only as 'royal physician', but as 'Sereniss. Anglorum Regis medico primario'. In whatever terms the estimate is made—academic qualifications, professional status, accumulation of ecclesiastical preferments, literary productivity, or social connections—Linacre was superior to his colleagues. Of the other pre-1524 members of the College, John Chambre most closely resembled Linacre, having identical academic qualifications, a miscellany of ecclesiastical preferments, and an established position as a court physician. Ultimately as Warden of Merton he helped to secure the Linacre lectureships for his College. In the early College of Physicians, Oxford and Padua M.D.s were preponderant; there were no Cambridge graduates or M.D.s. Linacre's colleagues had acceptable medical credentials and most were probably competent physicians serving the upper classes of London; but they appear to have had few scholarly pretensions. It was not until the election of John Clement and Edward Wotton in February 1528 that the College recruited humanist physicians of the calibre of Linacre. Had it not been for this injection of talent drawn from the younger generation of Oxford humanists, the College would certainly have fallen short of the ambitious intellectual goals framed by Linacre.

[1] 14 and 15 Henry VIII, c. 5; Munk, op. cit. i. 7–10.
[2] Clark, op. cit. i. 70–1; Munk, op. cit. i. 10–29.

The only record of the affairs of the College during these years comes from the Annals begun by John Caius in 1555, the first year of his presidency. In compiling a brief sketch of events prior to this date he relied on oral testimony and documents which have not survived. Caius rescued little information about the period before the 1523 Act. The members were enjoined by their original charter to hold regular meetings, or *congregationes*, but it is not known how frequently, or where they met. In all probability their proceedings were not regularized for some time.

A crucial stage was reached when Linacre made part of the Stone House, Knight Rider Street, available for the meetings of the College. It has generally been assumed that Linacre was already in possession of the Stone House in 1518, but the documents calendared by Fletcher in this volume make it clear that the house was not acquired until four years later. It was not until after the conclusion of complex legal negotiations, lasting from August 1522 to January 1523, that Linacre became the undisputed owner of the Stone House, together with its garden and outbuildings.[1] It was probably not before March 1523, at about the date of the parliamentary confirmation of the 1518 Charter, that the College began to hold meetings at Linacre's house. It was at this time that the first new members were recruited, and the complement of Elects established. Caius must accordingly have been referring to 1523, not 1518, when he described Linacre's gift of part of his house to form the first site for the *comitia* and library of the College.[2] Only at this stage was it appropriate for the Annals to record an attempt to enforce regular attendance at the *comitia*.[3] Under the terms of Linacre's Will, the Stone House, its garden, court, and stable passed to Merton College, while the more modest 'parlour adioyning to the sayd house and a chamber over the same adioyning to the stret' were bequeathed to the College of Physicians.[4] It is likely that the

---

[1] See above, pp. 151–2 (Appendix A2); and pp. 191 and 193–5 (Appendix C: Calendar of Documents, nos. 3 and 14–17). I am grateful to Dr. John Fletcher for allowing me to use his transcripts of Linacre documents.

[2] 'Is dono dedit Collegio primam faciem seu partem aedium suarum in locum Comitiorum et Bibliothecae.' London, Royal College of Physicians Library, [John Caius], MS. Annals [unfoliated]. Annals for 1518 [*sic*].

[3] Ibid. Annals for 1523.

[4] For Linacre's Will, see above, pp. 165–71 (Appendix B2), where the College is granted 'the chappell and the chamber over the chappell . . . that they shall clerly have the same to them and their successors for ever to the entent that

upper room was used for the library, and the parlour (sometimes called the chapel, or the hall) for meetings. Under Linacre's arrangement the members of the College were obliged to coexist with the tenants of Merton College. This was not altogether convenient, but their only recorded attempt to attain greater privacy, by building a partition wall and moving a doorway, ended in failure.[1]

The compilation of statutes was a first priority for Linacre and his small body of colleagues. It is probable that Linacre left the statutes in an incomplete state; the earliest preserved date from the presidency of John Caius. However, Caius fully acknowledged Linacre's role in a preamble.[2] Thus although the original statutes carry the imprint of Caius, they probably bear a close relationship to the version originally compiled by Linacre.[3] These statutes appear to have been framed during the early years of the College, according to a plan which, with minor modifications, endured for an extremely long period.

In view of the importance of these statutes in determining the identity of the College of Physicians, it is imperative to establish whether they were original or alternatively whether they were derived from an earlier model. In either case Linacre may be regarded as the prime architect of the statutes handed down to Caius.

While the College of Physicians followed the general lines of company organization, its statutes have little in common with counterparts produced by other London companies. But the College statutes were not entirely original. Although they have certain distinctive elements, in major respects they resemble the statutes governing similar medical organizations on the Continent. By 1518 colleges of

thei shall theder resort for to treate as whell for the welth and contenuance of the seyd college as for the examinacion of souche parsons as shall use phisyk acordyng to a estatute therof late made and ordenyd'. The slightly fuller description of the property given above is taken from the indenture between the Warden of Merton College and Edmond Cryspyne (described above, p. 197, Calendar No. 26.)

[1] Annals for 1552.

[2] 'Statuta Collegii Medicorum Londini per clarissimum virum Thomam Linacrum et Collegium predictum regia authoritate incepta atque edita anno Domini 1520. Et per Joannem Caium presidentem in ordinem redacta aucta et absoluta eadem authoritate Collegio, anno domini 1555.' Bodleian Library, MS. Ashmole 1826, f. 9ʳ.

[3] The earliest preserved version of the statutes, 'Statuta Collegii Medicorum Londini', MS. Ashmole 1826, is given in full by Clark, op. cit. i. 376–92.

the type established in London were to be found in various parts of Europe but they were most numerous and highly organized in Italy, and during his prolonged visit, Linacre would undoubtedly have become familiar with the highly organized state of the medical profession in Italian cities. This would have provided valuable experience which could be applied to the English situation when the opportunity was presented of establishing a new college in London. Significantly, the opening section of the 1518 charter cited Italy as the major precedent for the establishment of the college: 'Itaque partim bene institutarum civitatum in Italia, et aliis multis nationibus exemplum imitati'.[1] Colleges of Physicians were an integral aspect of civic order in Italian cities and it was regarded as a sign of maturity for this practice to be imitated elsewhere.

By the time of Linacre's arrival in Italy, virtually every city had framed statutes governing all guilds, including the various branches of the medical profession.[2] From our point of view, particular interest is attached to those cities which permitted the formation of colleges. Like the London foundation these were primarily controlled by physicians, but often surgeons were also included. The colleges were given extensive powers of regulation and their responsibilities extended to many aspects of medicine, including public health, hospital organization, and relief of the sick poor. Most of the Italian colleges were long-established institutions and by 1500 their statutes had been revised and improved on many occasions. Each college developed peculiarities appropriate to its situation, but there were two main categories. The first type was found in such ancient university towns as Bologna, Padua, Pavia, and Parma. The college here was primarily a corporation of Doctors of Arts and Medicine operating as the executive body of one of the higher studies faculties of a university. In addition to controlling teaching and admission to degrees, these colleges increasingly assumed control of medical practice within their region.[3]

---

[1] Munk, op. cit. i. 2.

[2] G. Gonetta, *Bibliografia statutaria delle Corporazioni d'Arte e Mestieri d'Italia con saggio di Bibliografia estera*, Rome, 1891. For typical statutes not involving collegiate organization in medicine, see R. Ciasca, *Statuti dell'Arte dei medici e speziali*, Florence, 1922.

[3] C. Malagola, *Statuti delle Università e dei collegi dello Studio Bolognese*, Bologna, 1888; *Statuta Dominorum Artistarum Achademiae Patavinae* [Venice, c. 1496]; *Statuta almae Universitatis D. Artistarum et Medicorum patavini Gymnasii*, Venice, 1589; *Statuti e ordinamenti della Università di Pavia dell'anno 1361 al 1859*,

The second type of college was a chartered corporation of local physicians not associated with an institution of higher education, but controlling the practice of medicine in the locality. This form of college recruited medical graduates from universities elsewhere. Colleges in this category were in a position very like the College of Physicians in London, which required medical degrees for admission, but was not directly associated with a university. An important representative of this category is the College of Physicians of Milan, which, like so many other examples can be traced back to the thirteenth century. Its earliest preserved statutes date from 1396; a revised version was ratified by Galeazzo Maria Sforza in 1470 and this version was published in 1517, the year before the formation of Linacre's college.[1] Just as Bologna influenced the structure of medical faculties elsewhere, so the Milan college was used as a model by the physicians of Lodi and Cremona.[2] Colleges of a similar type were established at such towns as Turin, Brescia, Bergamo, and Siena, before Linacre's visit.[3] This pattern of organization gradually ex-

---

Pavia, 1925, pp. 119–29; V. Cordero di Montezemolo and U. Gualazzini, 'Statuta Collegii Doctorum Artium et Medicinae' in U. Gualazzini, ed., *Corpus Statutorum Almi Studii Parmensis*, Milan, 1946, pp. 43–68; R. Bettica-Giovannini, *La Medicina Vercellese nel Mediono e nel Rinascimento*, Turin, 1964. The medical schools at Bologna and Padua were established in the thirteenth century and those at Pisa, Pavia, and Parma in the mid-fourteenth. For a general survey of the medieval universities, see H. Rashdall, *The Universities of Europe in the Middle Ages*, revised and edited by F. M. Powicke and A. B. Emden, 3 vols., Oxford, 1936. For an account of the organization of colleges at Padua, see G. Whitteridge, *William Harvey and the Circulation of the Blood*, London, 1971, chapter 1. For a brief survey of the medieval medical schools, see V. L. Bullough, *The Development of Medicine as a Profession: The Contribution of the Medieval University to Modern Medicine*, Basle/New York, 1966.

[1] A. Bottero, 'I più antichi Statuti del Collegio dei Medici di Milano', *Archivio storico Lombardo*, N.S. viii, 1943, 72–112. *Statuta et Ordinationes Dominorum Physicorum Collegii Mediolanensis*, Milan, 1517. See also B. Corte, *Notizie istoriche intorno a' medici scrittori milanesi*, Milan, 1718; L. Belloni, 'Storia della medicina a Milano', in *Storia di Milano*, vol. xi, Milan, 1958, 595–696.

[2] V. Maragioglio, 'Gli Statuti del Collegio dei Medici di Lodi in un codice del XV° secolo', *Archivio storico per la città e comuni del territorio e dalla diocesi di Lodi*, lxix, 1950, 67–84; lxx, 1951, 40–9; L. Belloni, 'Gli Statuti del Collegio dei Fisici di Cremona', *Bollettino storico Cremonese*, xx, 1955–7, 5–46. The Lodi statutes date from 1471 and those of Cremona from 1495.

[3] F. A. Duboin, *Statuta Collegii Philosophorum et Medicorum civitate Taurini an. 1448*, Turin, 1847; P. da Ponte, *Statuta Collegii Medicorum Brixiae saeculi XVI, Cenni e notizie*, Brescia, 1876; A. Pinetti, *Ricerche storiche sulla sanità*

tended to other parts of Europe, but colleges were not widespread by 1500. Hence in France colleges had been established at Nîmes (1397) and Bordeaux (1411), but they admitted physicians on the basis of local apprenticeship and only rudimentary formal education. Most French colleges were founded after 1600.[1] As in Italy, the French medical faculties took on licensing functions, but their qualifications were often little regarded by local colleges.[2] Whatever the precise form of college adopted in Italy and France, their social role was similar. Delaunay's characterization of a continental college of physicians could well apply to the London situation.

Ce monopole engendre l'esprit de corps et le formalisme: formalisme intérieur, qui règle les droits respectifs des membres de la corporation; formalisme extérieur, à l'égard des intrus ou autres corps, contre lesquels il faut parfois défendre les prérogatives et préséances de la communauté.[3]

It is instructive to note the major features of the statutes of the London and Italian colleges. In view of the general uniformity of the Italian statutes, the following remarks will be made with specific reference to Milan, which like London was a major non-university town. In form and organization the London and the Italian statutes were strikingly similar, consisting of a series of brief chapters, dealing in turn with the officers and their duties, rules of membership and the form of admission, medical ethics, and finally relations with other sections of the medical profession. The London statutes were divided into twenty-six chapters; the Italian ranged between Lodi, with twenty-three chapters, and Milan, with forty-one. There was little variation in the word-length of the various statutes, but the

---

pubblica in Bergamo, Bergamo, 1900; A. Garosi, 'Medici, speziali, cerusici e medicastri nei libri dei protomedicato senese', *Bollettino senese di Storia Patria*, N.S. vi, 1935, 1–27; idem, 'I Protomedici del Collegio di Siena dal 1562 al 1808', *Bollettino senese di Storia Patria*, N.S. ix, 1938, 173–81; F. Gabotto, 'Sulla condizione della medicina pubblica e privata in Piedmonte del 1500', *Archivio per le scienza mediche*, xxi, 1897, 365–93.

[1] Paul Delaunay, *La Vie médicale aux XVIe, XVIIe et XVIIIe siècles*, Paris, 1935, pp. 289–91.

[2] For a general survey of the French medical faculties, see P. Huard, 'L'Enseignement médico-chirurgical' in *Enseignement et diffusion des sciences au XVIIIe siècle*, ed. R. Taton, Paris, 1946, pp. 171–236. For a study of a local situation see A. Boquel, *La Faculté de médecine de l'Université d'Angers (1432–1792)*, Angers, 1951.

[3] Delaunay, op. cit., p. 296.

Bologna and Padua colleges, with their complex academic responsibilities, developed extremely long statutes.

The members of the London College consisted of a group of eight Elects (*electores*), who were obliged to be of English nationality and doctors of medicine.[1] From this group was elected a President, and his deputy was the Pro-President. Outside this self-appointing élite was the general membership of the College, which it was not necessary to limit at first; when numbers increased in the reign of Elizabeth, the size of the College was limited to twenty, and this was raised to thirty in 1590. But in the early years of the College its fellowship only slightly exceeded the number of Elects. This arrangement resembled that in Turin, where power within the college resided in the hands of eight '*numerarii*'; beneath them were fifteen '*supranumerarii*'. At Parma there were twelve *numerarii* and an unspecified number of *supranumerarii*. In Cremona and Milan there were fifteen or more members of the college, from whom were selected the Rector and his deputy.[2] Italian colleges called their senior officer the *rector* or *prior*, although in Siena the title *protomedico* was preferred. Full membership was restricted to doctors of medicine with proven family connections with the city.[3] Indeed most Italian colleges went further by insisting on adherence to the Roman Catholic Church and legitimate birth. The celebrated

---

[1] 'Volumus igitur et statuimus ut e numero collegarum electores octo . . . doctoratusque gradu insigniantur, et natione Angli sint.' Clark, *A History of the Royal College of Physicians*, i. 377. Later the term *electi* was used for the eight senior members. In Italian colleges this term was frequently used for either elected senior officials, or full members of the college. See Cremona Statutes, cap. I, *De electione rectorum et eorum officio . . .*: '. . . Et post electionem acceptationemque, electus, aut electi noviter, statim iurare teneantur in manibus processorum'. *Statuti del Collegio di Cremona*, op. cit., p. 11.

[2] Clark, op. cit. i. 132. For Turin, see Gabotto, op. cit., p. 373; Parma illustrates the degree to which power resided with the *numerarii*: 'supranumerarii non habent voces in dictis collegiis, nec auctoritatem approbandi vel reprobandi in examinibus publicis vel privatis, nec recipiant salarium . . .', *Corpus Statutorum Almi Studi Parmensis*, p. 48. *Antichi Statuti di Milano*, p. 92; *Statuti di Cremona*, p. 11.

[3] In Parma, the *numerarii* were restricted to 'doctores oriundi civitatis Parme aut de eius districtu vel episcopatu'. *Corpus Statutorum Almi Studi Parmensis*, p. 48. In Bologna, none were admitted 'nisi fuerit et sit verus civis civitatis bona ratione originis proprie et paterne vel proprie et avite, vel proprie et proavite'. *Statuti . . . Bolognese*, pp. 498–500. The early statutes of Milan and Cremona placed only minor restrictions on foreign practitioners, but the Milan statutes published in 1517 were much less lenient.

natural philosopher Cardano was excluded from the Milan college on the grounds of illegitimacy.[1]

Each college appointed a group of officers, the most important being the *consiliarii*, who acted as the main advisers to the President. Both Milan and London appointed two *consiliarii*. In addition colleges appointed various minor officials such as Bedells. Particularly active in London were the four Censors, who were responsible for inspection. This function was exercised by the senior members (usually the rector and *consiliarii*) of Italian colleges. Every college devoted a considerable amount of space in the statutes to penal clauses outlining fines for members, candidates, and offending outsiders. Foreign physicians were permitted to associate with the colleges, but only upon payment of fines. Great attention was given to the process of examination and admission. The London statutes were particularly explicit over the form and scope of examinations. Extensive formal knowledge of and acquaintance with basic texts of Galen was required. Applicants were obliged to have obtained an M.D. before taking the college examination and to serve as a candidate for four years before becoming a full member. Later, fines were imposed on doctors with foreign degrees and eventually full membership of the college was restricted to physicians possessing an M.D. from Oxford or Cambridge.[2] At Milan and similar Italian colleges, the prescribed texts for examination were not indicated in great detail, but it was assumed that the candidate had studied for at least four years in the *Studium Generale* and had received an M.D. or other approved qualification.[3] In Italian and French colleges it

---

[1] D. Bianchi, 'Gerolamo Cardano e il Collegio dei Fisici di Milano', *Archivio storico Lombardo*, Series 4, xviii, 1912, 283–9. In accordance with the eleventh statute the Milanese college required candidates to be 'legiptime natus et quod non sufficiat quod sit per subsequens matrimonium legiptimatus'. The revised Milan statutes insisted that members should come from Milan or the surrounding principality, be of families of proven gentle birth for at least 120 years and of legitimate birth. In Bergamo it was necessary for members to be of the Catholic faith and from families resident in the city for at least seventy years.   [2] Clark, op. cit. i. 385–8, 133–4.

[3] The 1517 Milan statutes required candidates to have studied logic, philosophy, and medicine for seven years at an approved university: Bottero, op. cit., p. 90. The topics and texts listed in London statutes are given in detail comparable with the Bologna statutes: Malagola, op. cit., pp. 274–6. Students were not accepted for an M.D. examination in the college at Bologna unless they were over twenty years old and had studied medicine for five years, after obtaining an education in the liberal arts.

was necessary for the candidate to serve for a probationary period in the neighbourhood before becoming a full member.

An Italian physician would have found the statutes of the London College completely congenial. In essence, the London and Italian colleges were constructed according to a similar pattern. They consisted of small élites of academically qualified physicians; their statutes conferred advantages on local men and local academic qualifications, and discrimination was exercised to varying degrees against foreigners and foreign qualifications. Rigid rules controlled the activities of members and stringent authority was exercised over ancillary sections of the medical profession. Within the colleges a hierarchical structure prevailed, and complex rules governed the election to key offices. Allowing for adaptation to local conditions and the gradual process of evolution, the London College was clearly generically related to prototypes in major Italian cities.

Nevertheless there are certain minor peculiarities about the organization of the London College which require explanation. In particular it is noticeable that the head of the English College was known as 'president', a term which is not used in any of the Italian colleges. Furthermore the Presidency was a permanent appointment, whereas in Italy rectors usually served for one year only. The abortive proposal for an association with the surgeons in 1423 also used the term president, but the more likely source for Linacre's title was Corpus Christi College, Oxford, which received its Letters Patent in 1517. Like the London College, Corpus was headed by a President, Vice-President, and *censores* responsible for discipline. Corpus Christi College was described as a 'Collegium perpetuum eruditionis scientiarum sacrae theologiae et philosophiae, ac bonarum artium, de uno Praesidente et triginta scholaribus graduatis et non graduatis'.[1] It will be remembered that in 1517 Linacre inscribed a copy of *De sanitate tuenda* to the founder of Corpus, Richard Fox, writing enthusiastically about the new foundation and meetings of scholars at the founder's home. The new college represented a self-conscious attempt to introduce humanistic studies into Oxford.[2] Greek occupied

---

[1] *Statutes of the Colleges of Oxford*, 3 vols., Oxford, 1853, ii, *Corpus Christi College*, p. iv. For a general account of the early history, see T. Fowler, *The History of Corpus Christi College*, Oxford Historical Society, xxv, Oxford, 1893.

[2] Fowler, op. cit., pp. 37–46; P. S. Allen, 'The Trilingual Colleges of the Early Sixteenth Century' in *Erasmus: Lectures and Wayfaring Sketches*, Oxford, 1934, pp. 138–63; McConica, op. cit., pp. 80–4.

a particularly important role and Corpus appointed the first public reader in Greek ever established in the University. There is some evidence that the first Greek lectures (1518–20) were given by John Clement and Thomas Lupset. Both were friends of Linacre and prominent in humanist circles. Lupset had supervised the printing of Linacre's *De sanitate tuenda*. David Edwards was the first officially attested *lector publicus* in Greek (1521). He was followed in 1524 by Edward Wotton, a Padua M.D. and student of natural history, who became President of the College of Physicians (1541–3). He was succeeded in the latter office by John Clement.[1] Acknowledgement was made to Clement, Lupset, and Edwards for their assistance in the preparation of the Aldine *editio princeps* of Galen in 1525.[2] I suspect that the early Greek lecturers at Corpus were directly influenced by Linacre's interest in Greek medicine. In addition, separate medical lectures were given at Corpus by Thomas Moscroffe.[3] Finally, Linacre was directly in touch with the first President of the College who, before taking up his appointment, was encouraged by Linacre to make Oxford a secure home for the study of Greek.[4]

In view of his varied associations with Corpus Christi College, it is not surprising that Linacre organized the College of Physicians in such a way as to suggest an affinity between the academic and professional bodies. It was correctly recognized that a professional association could only demand high standards for entry if the universities developed their faculties of medicine along humanistic lines. Accordingly, Linacre cemented the connection between the universities and the College of Physicians by establishing the Linacre lectures to teach the Galenic corpus which was required for admission to the College.

[1] Fowler, op. cit., pp. 85–9, 369. P. S. Allen, 'Early Corpus Readerships', *The Pelican Record*, vii, 1905, 155–9; J. A. Gee, *Life and Works of Lupset*, pp. 96–101. C. E. Raven, *English Naturalists from Neckam to Ray*, pp. 39–42, 68–70. E. Wenkebach, *John Clement, ein englischer Humanist und Arzt des sechzehnten Jahrhunderts*, Studien zur Geschichte der Medizin, xiv, Leipzig, 1925.

[2] The five volumes of this edition appeared between April and August 1525. In the preface to the final volume it is acknowledged that the main medical editor Opizzoni was aided by four Englishmen, the three named above and 'Roseus', as well as the German, Georg Agricola: N. Mani, 'Die Griechische Editio princeps des Galenos (1525), ihre Entstehung und ihre Wirkung', *Gesnerus*, xiii, 1956, 29–52.

[3] Fowler, op. cit., p. 87.

[4] Allen, *Erasmus: Lectures and Wayfaring Sketches*, pp. 153–4.

The foregoing remarks have attempted to throw greater light on one of Linacre's most celebrated enterprises, the establishment of the College of Physicians of London. Attention to the accelerating process of company development in England and recognition that the statutes of the Italian colleges determined the structure of the London College may appear to diminish Linacre's achievement. Instead of being regarded as a major pioneering venture with European significance, the College of Physicians could be seen as a very late imitation of a pattern of organization developed elsewhere. The appearance of the London College in 1518 might simply reflect the backwardness of English institutions compared with their Italian counterparts.

But, although the creation of the College of Physicians seems unremarkable in European terms, Linacre's achievement remains considerable when viewed in an English context. When Linacre left England in 1487 as a young graduate with a taste for classical studies, the English medical profession was in a totally disorganized state. The barbers were sufficiently numerous and active to join the ranks of incorporated companies and to lay claim to a considerable area of the craft of surgery. Medicines were dispensed by a variety of shopkeepers. The more specialist and formally trained surgeons had failed to establish a viable company, but they maintained some kind of informal association. Physicians, elsewhere the dominant element in the medical profession, were wholly unco-ordinated, without the support of strong English medical schools and largely at the mercy of empirics and aliens.

Linacre returned to England as a humanist scholar, specializing in the difficult area of Greek medicine. Furthermore he had obtained an M.D. at one of the leading medical schools of Europe and had witnessed the manner in which physicians had risen to a position of considerable social prestige in Italy. Italian physicians enjoyed both prosperity and parity with the highest ranks of the educated élite. Their colleges and university medical schools provided the foundation for this elevated position.

Linacre quickly established himself as a leading figure in the English circle of humanist scholars. Individually he was highly successful, becoming intimate with both influential members of the court and important ecclesiastical and lay officials. This position was used to promote a transformation in the organization of London medicine. Taking advantage of crisis induced by an endless succession of epidemics, Linacre drew attention to the merits of the humanist physicians by pressing forward with his translations of prophylactic and general medical works by Galen. As a scholar and personal physician, Linacre was in an ideal position to influence the King and his major adviser Cardinal Wolsey, as well as numerous more minor officials. Thus, perhaps with a little assistance from other physicians, Linacre was able to engineer in 1518 the establishment of a permanent corporate organization for his colleagues. Thereafter the embryo College was rapidly guided towards maturity under his supervision. London physicians had hitherto been a most heterogeneous group. Linacre recognized that the introduction of the Galenic corpus into the medical schools provided the basis for the standardization and improvement of medical training. Therefore graduates of Bologna, Padua, or Oxford could be expected to share a common educational experience, and their degrees could be regarded as the standard qualification for admission to the College of Physicians. As in Italy the creation of a professional college working in association with reformed medical schools could be expected to revitalize the medical profession and secure a place of dominance for the physicians. Linacre himself became the model for physicians aspiring to this new order, and his College provided a focus for the dissemination of the humanistic medical ideal. Since Linacre was personally involved in every facet of the foundation and early history of the College, this institution can rightly be regarded as his permanent monument.

From the point of view of the evolution of the medical profession in England, Linacre's foundation was of fundamental importance. If the College was not able to bring about a substantial improvement in the health of the citizens of London, it created an élite corps of physicians, pledged to support a rigorous code of medical ethics. During Linacre's presidency the College recruited a small group of new members who were willing to subscribe to these standards. After Linacre's death, Edward Wotton, John Clement, and John Caius maintained the humanistic tradition. From the point of view of the public it was reasonable to give monopolistic privileges to a group which was pledged, by the standards of the sixteenth century, to guarantee more consistent and improved services. This was precisely the balance of public service and self-interest which was involved in the creation and perpetuation of other London companies. But as the system matured there was a tendency for this delicate equilibrium to be disturbed in the interests of combinations of avaricious adventurers, until monopolies became the source of a great national grievance. More's *Utopia*, published two years before the foundation of the College of Physicians, perceptively described both the advantages of social planning and the dangers of rapacious sectional interest.

Linacre's College was not able to resist the common trend.[1] The flexible structure of the early College was replaced by a more rigid and hierarchical organization, which adopted an increasingly aggressive and domineering attitude to other branches of the medical profession. Restrictions placed full membership of the College beyond the reach of many fully qualified physicians; eligible candidates were obliged to wait long periods before election, and junior Fellows of the College exercised little authority.

These changes were made possible by the introduction of a succession of subtle modifications to the original statutes. The effect was to produce a reorientation which diminished the capacity of the College to become a national medical qualifying association, the goal first expressed in the Act of Parliament passed in the year before Linacre's death.

[1] For the later trends in the College of Physicians and reaction to its monopolistic position see Clark, op. cit. i, *passim*; Roberts, 'The Personnel and Practice . . .'; P. M. Rattansi, 'The Helmontian–Galenist Controversy in Restoration England', *Ambix*, xii, 1964, 1–23; C. Webster, 'English Medical Reformers of the Puritan Revolution: A Background to the "Society of Chymical Physitians"', *Ambix*, xiv, 1967, 16–41.

The Linacre Lectureships Subsequent to their Foundation

R. G. LEWIS*

'THE LINACRE LECTURES HAD LITTLE INFLUENCE upon medical education.'[1] At Oxford 'only a few men of distinction have held the lectureship. . . . There is only too much truth in what B. W. Henderson says in his history of the college [Merton]: "The happy inheritor of the Linacre bequest received his money gladly and made no pretence of work."'[2] 'The Cambridge bequest was mismanaged and the stipends were regarded as nothing more than a welcome addition to the income of the fellow, who treated the appointment more or less as a sinecure.'[3]

What a damning indictment this is, what a gloomy picture: an educational reform which failed, an endowment administered with cynicism and neglect. Has the history of the Linacre lectureships really been so sad a story from Linacre's own day right up to the nineteenth century?

The evidence available in college and university records, in the collections of antiquarians like Anthony Wood and Thomas Baker, and in the surviving letters and publications of Linacre lecturers themselves, suggests that it has not. Not, at least, until about 1690. True, Linacre's attempt to reform medical education in Oxford and Cambridge did not succeed precisely as he would have hoped; true, some watering-down of the requirements was *de facto* accepted from

---

* Fellow of St. Anne's College, Oxford.

[1] Sir W. Osler, *Thomas Linacre*, Cambridge, 1908, p. 52.

[2] Ibid., pp. 54–5.

[3] Sir Humphrey Davy Rolleston, *The Cambridge Medical School, a Biographical History*, Cambridge, 1932, p. 17.

an early stage; true, some of the lecturers have left little sign of medical learning; true, in the eighteenth century, these posts, like so many other medieval and Renaissance pedagogic improvements, survived as mere sinecures—*rector theologiae, examinator rhetoricae, praelector physicae*—decorating the lists of college offices like empty cartridge cases from some bygone shoot. But the later 'scandals' were not the cause of the earlier failure: how could they be? They, and the failure itself, were each the outcome of the long unchanging pressures upon collegiate universities established in small provincial towns; and of that conservative respect for property and for tradition which administers an endowment more or less according to the letter, when a bold interpretation of the spirit would call for new duties, augmented stipends, and an active quest for new endowments to stand alongside and help fulfil the intentions of the old. The failure is sharp, when it is set against Linacre's high hopes, his rigorous scholarly standards, and his longer aims. But the standards and criteria of classical medical scholarship in the 1520s had only ever been part of what was needed in medical education; by 1600 they seemed already dated, and to some extent irrelevant. Even so, the administrators of the Linacre bequests had not yet fallen into idleness or cynicism. Between 1560 and 1690 the lectureships, according to the eclectic, widely read, practical, and far from insular standards of English medicine of the day, were a useful institution, held by a variety of able men. It is not too much to say that the heyday of the lectureships lasted (if patchily) for 130 years. Merton and St. John's continued to administer the bequests with thought and with care. Few of the incumbents were absentee, or obviously unsuitable; most, probably, performed some version of their duties with reasonable regularity, or at the least made themselves available to medical students for consultation and advice. If many of them fell short of what Osler regarded as distinction, few were really obscure; and among the apparently mediocre, there are several worthy of closer and more sympathetic attention.

The Early History of the Lectureships, 1524–c. 1560

From the outset, there was a gap between Linacre's intentions and the likelihood of their achievement. It was precisely because of the difficulty of establishing regular lectures in medicine at Oxford and Cambridge that Linacre set out to do so. But his endowments were not, even when they were followed in 1540 by the establishment of the better-paid Regius chairs of physic, enough to break out of the vicious circle of no patrons in the locality, no incentive for a doctor of medicine to stay on, no regular lectures by qualified persons, no incentive to embark on medicine rather than theology after the M.A. If his lectureships succeeded, they would weaken all these disincentives and difficulties at one blow, and they would provide at least some medical teaching in Oxford and Cambridge of a rigour, regularity, intensity, and humanist exactness then quite strange to medicine at the English universities. Accordingly, the requirements he set out were strict.

The Linacre lecturer at St. John's College, Cambridge, was to be a Master of Arts, well versed in the works of Aristotle. He was to lecture daily in term on Galen's *De sanitate tuenda*, *Methodus medendi*, *De alimentis*, and *De simplicibus*, using Linacre's own editions. He was to refrain from private practice while holding the lectureship.[1]

The arrangements at Oxford were rather more complicated, and a number of changes were made between their first version in Linacre's own will and the version accepted by the Warden and Fellows of Merton in 1549.[2] The only significant change (apart from the fact that the lectureships were to be College not University appointments, with a consequent loss in status and perhaps in usefulness) was that the lecturers, instead of lecturing twice daily, as Linacre had intended they should, were required to lecture only once each day, for a full hour. This reduction may well have been already a serious departure from Linacre's reforming intention. A respectable education in the arts and sciences depended, according to the traditional view (powerfully reinforced by the high linguistic standards demanded by Linacre and all his generation of humanist scholars), upon an intimate acquaintance with the texts, for the purpose of detailed commentary and the extraction of difficult points worthy of debate. Linacre had himself worked hard to establish reliable versions of the medical classics, precisely in order that generations of medical students should be able to acquire such familiarity with Galen's very words. This would mean for the student hard and unremitting reading over a number of years, much of it under the guidance of a more seasoned scholar. The Linacre

---

[1] J. E. B. Mayor, *Early Statutes of the College of St. John the Evangelist in the University of Cambridge*, Cambridge, 1859, pp. 171, 253.

[2] See above, J. M. Fletcher, 'Linacre's Lands and Lectureships', pp. 107–97.

lecturers were to be such seasoned scholars, expected to sit, day in, day out, morning and afternoon, with an attentive audience, going minutely over the details of Galenic texts. The courses were to be planned by the lecturers to last three full academic years, and the emphasis was almost entirely upon pathology and therapeutics; anatomy and botany as such do not figure there, as they would certainly have done had the bequest been made twenty years later; the emphasis throughout is on the diagnosis and treatment of disease. The lectures are intended not primarily as a contribution to *philosophia naturalis*, but rather as a course of basic training for the learned practitioner, very much in accordance with Linacre's intentions in the founding of the College of Physicians of London.

But this scheme needed the presence of Masters of Arts not only 'well versed in the works of Aristotle' but also already familiar themselves with Galen and Hippocrates. Ideally, too, the lecturers should have had some opportunity actually to practise medicine, so that their understanding of the texts would not be purely a philosophical or a philological one. After all, Galen himself had been a practising physician, as well as a medical philosopher. In short, what was needed was a seasoned M.D., of impeccable learning and shrewd clinical sense.

Where were such paragons to be found? Even the larger medical faculties of Europe found it difficult to keep the abler physicians in academic employment. Practice at Court, in a great city, or in the household of nobleman or prelate was almost always more tempting. Padua had gone some way towards solving the problem by attracting handsome endowments for professorial chairs, and by keeping up a minimum number of medical students at any one time to provide the possibility of a good livelihood from students' private fees. Montpellier, hitherto vulnerable because of the small size of the faculty, and its reliance upon the chance residence of regent masters, had recently acquired from the French Crown four well-paid professorial chairs, or readerships. While Padua was near enough to Venice to secure for her doctors a ready supply of rich patients, Montpellier, altogether more remote, found that she could keep her professors to their duties for only half the year at most; the rest of the time they were away at the courts of France or Navarre, or in private service, which paid them better, and worked them less hard.

The situation was more difficult still in England, as Linacre clearly understood. Not only were the two universities hampered by their distance from London and from the Court, they were situated in small towns offering scope to no more than a handful of medical practitioners. They also lacked, in 1524, any endowed provision for medical teaching; they relied entirely on the chance of there being regent masters able and willing to teach. One or two colleges had, by convention, or more rarely by statute, provision for a medical fellow.[1] But the real problem was one of incentive: why should the M.A., even if he was interested in medicine, stay for another six or twelve years, and go through the elaborate and expensive business of supplicating for a medical degree, with all the formal disputations this involved? Only, one would expect, if a medical degree was going to be a helpful qualification in his intended career. But the interest of a powerful patron was, and long continued to be, far more useful. This was true also in the Church, where preferment long depended as much upon one's friends as upon one's capacities; but here the B.D. and the D.D. had, in addition, come to be regarded as necessary qualifications—or at least conventional ones—for substantial benefices.

The founding of the College of Physicians of London, and the endowment of the Linacre lectureships, can be seen as two facets of the same policy. Just as the College was intended to set and to safeguard a standard for clinical practice, so the lectureships were intended to establish, and to begin to provide, a higher standard of medical teaching in the universities. In view of the social and institutional pressures against the likelihood of a race of resident and learned M.D.s flourishing in two small market towns in the Thames valley and the Fens, this was, perhaps, too tall an order; but there was no harm in trying.

St. John's College, Cambridge, took up without delay the challenge of finding a competent Latinist willing to take on the formidable task of lecturing, in the modern philological way, on the prescribed Galenic books. It was, perhaps, the college most likely at this juncture to be able to do so. Its recent statutes, drawn up in part by Bishop Fisher, provided for *lectores* and examiners in grammar, logic, rhetoric, dialectic, and mathematics, like those of other colleges, and also in Greek and Hebrew.[2] Like Linacre's endowment,

---

[1] These included Merton and Magdalen at Oxford; Trinity, King's, Gonville and Caius, Peterhouse, and Clare at Cambridge.

[2] St. John's College Register, 'Admissiones Lectorum', has their names from 1546 to 1611.

these statutes represented a hope as much as an actuality, but the College was, in the 1520s, a self-consciously *avant-garde* establishment.

The 'first that held the Linacre lecture' was, according to Thomas Baker, late-seventeenth-century antiquary and historian of the College, one *George Daye*, later D.D., Master of the College, and Bishop of Chichester.[1] John Caius, writing in 1555, compliments Daye on his medical learning: 'Quem Cantabrigiae ex multis annis medicinae studiosum fuisse, et medicinae praeceptis aeque delectari novi atque oratoriae artis (quam tum profitebaris) aut aliarum scientiarum liberalium, in quibus es egregius.'[2] From Caius this was serious praise, even in the complimentary context of a dedicatory letter. Daye was evidently a worthy first incumbent for Linacre's lectureship.

Did he in fact lecture? We have no certain evidence that he did; but then we have no evidence that any of the other college *lectors* at this time performed their duties either. It would be dangerous, indeed perverse, to argue from the silence of the records that they did not. The whole tone of the surviving registers and letters from St. John's in the 1520s and 1530s suggests that it was a busy teaching college in these years;[3] almost certainly negligence would have been remarked upon.

When Caius wrote his dedicatory letter in 1555, he was writing about the Bishop of Chichester and his early interest in medicine; from the point of view of Linacre's hopes, this is both revealing and sad: the promising young medical scholar had, like so many others, deserted medicine for theology, and sought preferment in the Church.

Christopher Jackson, allegedly also an early Linacre lecturer, has left little trace. Fellow in 1525, M.A. in 1527, he can have been little more than a beginner in medical studies when he died in 1528.[4]

The College records preserve no reference to a Linacre lecturer in the years 1528 to 1546; but it would be unsafe to argue from this that there was a prolonged vacancy. It is rather a question of a gap in the evidence.[5] It is hardly likely that all the College lectorships

[1] T. Baker, *History of the College of St. John the Evangelist, Cambridge*, ed. J. E. B. Mayor, 2 vols., Cambridge, 1869, i. 112.

[2] Ibid., n. 4.   [3] Ibid., *passim*.

[4] On Daye and Jackson see above, Fletcher, op. cit., p. 136. See Plate III.

[5] The 'Admissiones Lectorum' register had not yet been started; the 'Liber Thesaurarum' for these years preserves no reference to a Linacre lecturer.

lapsed simultaneously, although the beneficent Mastership of Daye did give place to seven turbulent years under John Tayler, a stranger to the College, whose election had been unpopular with some of the Fellows, and whose period in office was punctuated by quarrels, culminating in a Visitation by the Bishop of Ely and the imposition of new statutes on the College in 1544.

In 1546 calm returned with the election as Master of *William Bill*, a friend of Cheke and brother to Thomas Bill, physician to the King. William Bill appears also in the *Admissiones Lectorum* for 1546 as Linacre lecturer; it seems likely that he had been elected two or three years earlier. Unlike his elder brother Thomas, who held a Paduan doctorate in medicine and who had been a Fellow of the College of Physicians of London since 1543, William Bill never took a medical degree; instead, like George Daye, he became a learned divine. However, he had long been regarded in the University as a competent medical scholar. In 1537/8 he acted, with Dr. Wendye and another, as examiner to decide whether or not one John Edwards was qualified to become Bachelor of Medicine, and to be licensed to practise surgery and physic.[1] If Bill was ever an active Linacre lecturer it was probably between 1545 and 1547, rather than between 1547 and 1550, for in 1548/9 he was both Master of St. John's and Vice-Chancellor; he must have been much too busy to lecture daily. Baker, indeed, was puzzled to notice that Bill kept his Linacre lectureship, and concluded that he must have been short of money.[2]

It was during Bill's Vice-Chancellorship and tenure of the Linacre lectureship that an opportunity was lost to transform medical teaching at Cambridge. In 1548/9 the University experienced a Visitation of Royal Commissioners, including Bill's old colleague, Dr. Thomas Wendye; among the plans discussed was one whereby a single College would be devoted entirely to the study of medicine: medical fellows from other colleges would be encouraged to migrate there, and non-medical fellows to move away. But the plan came to nothing, in spite of the presence of William Bill, and in spite of the fact that the Regius Professor of Physic, John Blyth (1540–54), was a Doctor of Ferrara with some experience, like Linacre earlier, of continental medical schools and how they made their teaching arrangements.

[1] *Grace Book* Γ, ed. W. G. Searle, Cambridge, 1908, p. 326.
[2] Baker, op. cit. i. 128.

The next named Linacre lecturer at St. John's was *Henry Ayland*, or *Eland*, elected in 1550, but dead by the end of the following year. There is no evidence about his medical interests.

Between 1551 and 1555 no lecturer is recorded; but again, this may indicate merely an interruption in the recording of College business, not necessarily a breakdown in the business itself, nor a gap in this particular office. Under Thomas Lever, Thomas Watson, and George Bullock the College suffered (as did the University as a whole) from the political and religious upheavals of Edward VI's last years, and of Mary's reign; the College was visited more than once, while the University underwent the painstaking inquiry in 1556/7 of the Commissioners of Cardinal Pole.

By that time there was once more a Linacre lecturer, *Edward Raven* (1555–7), a friend and correspondent of Roger Ascham. He is the first to leave any evidence that he intended to go on to a medical career proper; in 1557 he obtained his licence to practise,[1] but in 1558 he died, the third Linacre lecturer out of five to die young. *Peter Foster* (1557–60), his successor, may have been the fourth; at any rate he disappears from sight in 1560.

These were active years for medicine in Cambridge. In 1557 the statutes drawn up by John Caius for Gonville Hall made provision for two medical fellowships, and stipulated that two bodies should be dissected each year in the presence of the medical students. There is evidence of considerable interest in medicine in other colleges at this time. The number of medical graduates (itself always no more than a partial indication of the numbers actively studying medicine) increased from eight between 1501 to 1520, to twenty-one between 1521 and 1540; between 1541 and 1560 it was again twenty-one. Thirteen of these latter, nearly twice the number of the two decades before, were Doctors of Medicine. There were in addition seven M.D.s by incorporation—that is, doctors of other universities, returning to Cambridge armed with qualifications to fit them

---

[1] J. and J. A. Venn, *Alumni Cantabrigienses*, 4 vols., Cambridge, 1922–7, iii. 423. Where dates of degrees are given without specific reference, the information has been taken from Venn (for Cambridge) and J. Foster, *Alumni Oxonienses*, 4 vols., Oxford, 1891–2; *Register of the University of Oxford*, i, 1449–63; 1505–71, ed. C. W. Boase, Oxford Historical Society, i, Oxford, 1885; ii, parts 1–4, 1571–1622, ed. A. Clark, Oxford Historical Society, x–xii, xiv, Oxford, 1887–9; and G. C. Brodrick, *Memorials of Merton College*, Oxford Historical Society, iv, Oxford, 1885. Specific reference is given below only where one or other of these sources has been found to be inaccurate.

for the M.D. there as well. The most striking increase, however, between 1541 and 1560 was in the number of licences to practise medicine or surgery, or both.[1] This curious boom deserves further investigation; it is tempting to speculate that it may have had something to do with the encouragement of John Blyth and of others who had experience of Italian universities. In this respect, St. John's, although it was producing its few medical graduates in each year, was not in the forefront; none of the Linacre lecturers so far had been to an Italian medical school.

Meanwhile, what of Oxford? Here the endowment had failed to get off to so good a start. Perhaps Tunstal's agreement to Merton's nominees had been difficult to obtain during this stormy part of his political career; or perhaps they had not put forward any names. Tunstal was by now an old man; but he lived long enough to give his approval to the election in November 1559 of *George James*.[2] James had been a Fellow of Merton for nine years, M.A. for eight; he supplicated for his M.B. on 6 July 1560, resigned his lectureship in December, and then is heard of no more.

During the 1540s, a great effort had been made to bring the Merton library up to date; more than 200 volumes in all kinds of subjects were purchased. They included the 1543 edition of the *De fabrica humani corporis* of Vesalius, and the botanical works of Ruel and of Fuchs.[3]

[1] A. H. T. Robb-Smith, 'Medical Education in Cambridge before 1600', *Cambridge and Its Contribution to Medicine*, ed. A. Rook, London, 1971, p. 11. Robb-Smith emphasizes a feature characteristic of the Oxford and Cambridge medical schools right up to 1800—their small size and the informal and personal nature of their teaching. It was, he says, 'partly by apprenticeship, partly by tutorial instruction and though [there] were formal lectures they were, for the most part as they should be, a relatively unimportant part of medical education, in striking contrast to the mass of impersonal lectures that characterized the continental schools' (p. 24). A. Rook, 'Medical Education at Cambridge 1600-1800', ibid., pp. 60-1, argues that in the later part of this period also responsibility for medical teaching was left to the colleges, and adds in 'Medicine at Cambridge, 1660-1760', *Medical History*, 13, 1969, 119, that 'The suggestion that medical teaching in our period must be evaluated primarily in terms of what each college offered and that university and private lectures merely supplemented college teaching, must obviously be supported by a detailed study of each college as a medical teaching unit.' He is engaged upon such a study.

[2] See above, Fletcher, op. cit., p. 146.

[3] N. Ker, 'Oxford College Libraries in the Sixteenth Century', *Bodleian Library Record*, vi, 1957-61, 483.

Among the students who must have benefited from this book-buying programme was *Robert Barnes*, appointed to the senior, or 'superior' Linacre lectureship, according to Anthony Wood, in 1558. Fellow in 1538, M.A. in 1541, Barnes had already taken his M.B. in 1547; he had relinquished his fellowship on his marriage, but had settled down as a medical practitioner in Oxford. When the Queen visited Oxford in 1566, Barnes (hastily made M.D.) was one of those selected by the University to conduct the formal physic disputation before her. Barnes held the senior Linacre lectureship for upwards of forty-five years, until his death in 1604. It seems unlikely that he was allowed entirely to neglect his duties, especially for the first few years. Every time a young Merton man expressed an interest in studying medicine, he was no doubt sent to see Dr. Barnes. But it is probably unlikely also that he can have lectured daily, or even weekly, year in, year out, on the same texts, without having left some trace in the registers or in the reminiscences of pupils. In the last few years he was in any case a very old man. The fact that he was a practitioner was not in itself an abuse of the terms of the endowment. The Merton agreement, unlike the St. John's arrangement, had expressly stipulated that the lecturer might practise physic during his tenure, provided he also lectured.[1] This suggests that the problem of creating incentives for Bachelors and Doctors of Medicine to stay on in Oxford had not been solved in the 1550s, and that the Fellows of Merton recognized that their best hope of finding a suitable senior lecturer lay in looking for him among the handful of graduate physicians who practised in Oxford.

Robert Barnes may perhaps have held the job too long. But he was by no means a negligible candidate for it. Anthony Wood records that he had been a friend of Henry Billingsley, the celebrated translator of Euclid,[2] and of one Whytehead, an Austin friar and notable mathematician, who bequeathed to Billingsley all his manuscript notes on Euclid's elements. Wood's information came from the notebooks of Brian Twyne, who had it from Thomas Allen of Gloucester Hall, who had it in turn from Barnes himself.[3] Barnes

---

[1] See above, Fletcher, op. cit., p. 144.

[2] *The Elements of Geometrie of . . . Euclide . . . now first translated into the Englishe toung, by H. Billingsley . . .Whereunto are annexed certaine . . . annotations . . . of the best Mathematiciens . . . With a . . . preface . . . by M. J. Dee . . .*, London, 1570.

[3] Anthony Wood, *Athenae Oxonienses*, ed. P. Bliss, 4 vols., Oxford, 1813–20, i.762.

had a considerable library, including a copy of the famous 1538 Basle edition of the complete works of Galen in Greek. Could he read it? There seems to be no means of knowing. The book, in three volumes, has an Oxford binding of the early 1540s, and may have been purchased by Barnes when he was a student; he gave it in 1596 to the library of St. John's College, Oxford.[1] He also possessed a copy of the *De revolutionibus orbium cœlestium* of Copernicus (1543), which he gave to Merton in 1597, together with Galen, *De compositione pharmacorum localium*, Basle, Cornarius, 1537; Rhazes, *Liber Elhavy*, Brescia, 1486; Montagnana, *Consilia*, Lyons, 1525; Walter Burley, *Expositio in Physica Aristotelis*, Venice, 1482; and Jacobus Hollerius, *De materia chirurgica*, Paris, 1552.[2]

How, then, had the Linacre lectureships fared between the framing of Linacre's will in 1524, and 1559 or 1560? In Cambridge they were now well established; St. John's was regularly appointing a lecturer from among its Fellows. By sheer misfortune, no less than four of these had died young, during or just after their tenure. The others, although apparently learned in medicine as in other branches of *literae humaniores*, had gone on to become not physicians, but divines. In Oxford, at last, the tradition had begun: the first junior lecturer a Fellow of the college, the first senior one an Oxford physician of scholarly tastes. Both Merton and St. John's had started in more or less the way they were for many years to go on.

The Long Heyday, 1560–c. 1690

For about 130 years the Fellows of Merton and St. John's elected from among themselves[3] Linacre lecturers nearly all of whom were either graduates in medicine already, or took their M.D. towards the end of their period of tenure. In most cases the tenure lasted for single or multiple terms of three years in Oxford, four years in Cambridge. There were examples of the same man holding a lectureship for considerably longer than two or three such terms consecutively, but such situations were the exception rather than

[1] Ker, op. cit., p. 512.

[2] Oxford, Merton College Library, (MS.) card-index of donors.

[3] Invariably, at St. John's, until Paget in the nineteenth century, it was a Fellow of the College who was elected; at Merton the practice early developed of appointing an Oxford practitioner who might or might not be a Fellow of any college, not necessarily an old Merton man, to the senior post. But many of the senior lecturers and nearly all the junior ones were Fellows of Merton throughout the history of the lectureships.

the rule. Merton renewed its lecturers with more formality than
St. John's, at triennial intervals; regularity in such renewals, or in
recording them, is patchy, but occurs often enough over the whole
period to suggest that when Merton lectureships were held for a
long time, this was deliberate policy on the College's part, rather
than the accidental by-product of inertia or neglect.

From the 1640s on it becomes the pattern at Merton, more often
than not, for the junior lectureship to be held 'in expectancy' as it
were of the senior one. This may reflect some change in the attitude
of the Fellows towards the office. Perhaps it was now beginning to
be regarded as a useful perquisite for a medical Fellow, rather than
as a post carrying with it an obligation to give regular and frequent
lectures. But the appointments continued to be respectable ones;
most of the men appointed would have been competent to contribute to medicine in the University, and we know that several of
them in fact did so.

It is, unfortunately, impossible to state categorically that any of
the lecturers in this long period did lecture regularly either at
Merton in Oxford, or at St. John's in Cambridge, let alone that they
lectured daily as prescribed upon the set Galenic texts. The probability of the latter's having been the case recedes rapidly from the
early seventeenth century on. Medical lecturers, where we have
evidence about them from other universities, had mostly by this
time ceased to use Galen's writings as anything more than a starting-
point for the discussion of a wide variety of questions in anatomy,
physiology, pathology, and therapeutics. But the probability is that
some kind of regular medical tuition, even formal lectures, for Merton and St. John's men was provided by the Linacre lecturers, at any
rate between 1560 and about 1640, and intermittently thereafter
until the 1680s or 1690. Certainly the possibility should not be
ruled out simply because the College records are silent on the
matter. After all, they are silent too about the actual occurrence of
teaching in other subjects within the College, apart from the occasional reference to someone's being dispensed from lecturing, or
from attendance at lectures, mostly for reasons of health; and yet
we know from students' notebooks, and from reminiscences, and
from the steady stream of graduates in arts (and for that matter in
medicine) that such teaching did occur.[1] Our difficulty is much the

---

[1] Examples are cited in M. Curtis, *Oxford and Cambridge in Transition 1558–*

same with the University records; we have only occasional references to dispensation from lecturing, or to penalties exacted for non-performance of duties; this may equally mean either that penalties were too rarely imposed, or that non-performance was rare. Our only recourse is to use what little direct evidence we have, and to interpret it in the light of what we may safely infer from the general tone and regularity, and content and emphases of the records for the relevant period of time.

The picture we can piece together in this way is, by and large, a reassuring one for Merton and St. John's alike.

Merton, 1562–1636

In June 1562 a meeting of the Warden and Fellows of Merton listened to a letter from their Visitor, the Archbishop of Canterbury, Matthew Parker, written at the request of *Roger Gifford*, Linacre lecturer since October 1561, and Fellow of the College until his resignation earlier in 1562. Gifford sought reinstatement in his Fellowship, but even if he failed to secure that, he wanted to establish that he was still entitled to the stipend of the Linacre lectureship, for the lectures already performed, and in future until his term of office expired. He argued that he had been 'redinge that lecture so diligentlye as dothe appertayne' and pointed out that 'one other' (probably Barnes) 'relinquishing his felowship by yor benevolence dothe yet enioye a stipende for . . . redinge'. The College agreed that Gifford should get his stipend for the year past, but did not re-elect him to a Fellowship, and went on to discuss further the question of whether or not the Linacre lectureship should remain in the hands of an incumbent for three years invariably. They looked carefully again at the Indenture of 1549, copied out several provisions of it into their Register for June 1562, and resolved that their action a few days earlier, in re-electing to the junior Linacre lectureship *Henry Atwood*, Gifford's predecessor, had been correct.[1] However, in October 1562 they yielded to Gifford's insistence that he (and not Atwood) should be regarded as Linacre lecturer.[2] In 1563 Gifford was elected a Fellow of All Souls, and ceased to trouble Merton; he readily relinquished the lectureship, went on to obtain

1642, Oxford, 1959, pp. 239–41, and R. T. Gunther, *Early Science in Cambridge*, Oxford, 1937, pp. 222, 279–81 (William Stukeley's Journal).

[1] Oxford, Merton College MSS., Reg. 1. 2, 'Registrum Collegii Mertonensis 1521–67', fol. 330.   [2] Ibid., fol. 332.

his licence to practise medicine, took his M.D. in 1566 at the same time as Robert Barnes, disputed formally before the Queen on her state visit, and became well known in Oxford as a physician. He later moved to London, where he became Fellow and later President of the Royal College of Physicians, and M.P. for Old Sarum. In the long run he bore Merton no ill will, for he left them about forty medical books. As a small medical library, collected mostly, from the publication dates, in the 1560s and 1570s, it is compact, consistent, and impressively up to date; it includes a good deal of botany, anatomy, and medical *consilia*, the *Epistolae medicinales* of Giovanni Manardi, Antonius Musa on Hippocrates, Thomas Erastus, *De occultis pharmacorum potestatibus*, Girolamo Cardano, *Contradicentium medicorum libri duo*, as well as several commentaries on Avicenna, Mesue, and Rhazes.[1] If Gifford did indeed lecture 'diligentlye' between 1560 and 1563, the medical students of Merton were probably fortunate, and were receiving a diet which may or may not have been precisely what Linacre ordered, but which was probably well worth having.

Gifford's successor *John Handcocke* has left less trace. He did borrow medical books from the library in 1563–4, presumably so that his lectures should be 'substancyallye studied for before'. The books borrowed suggest that he may have been little more than a beginner in his medical studies—'Themistium super Phisicam Aristotelis et alterum librum medicine . . . Opera Constantini Africani medici',[2] and Linacre might well have found this rather an old-fashioned approach. At the same time one Magister Pott, also a Fellow, was borrowing the works of Avicenna.[3] In any case, plague interrupted the business of the College and dispersed its students for much of the summer of 1564, and Handcocke was dispensed from his lectures in January 1565. In April, 'magister Hanncocke admissus est ad studium sacrae theologiae'.[4] Medicine, apparently, had never really been to his taste. Nevertheless, we have it on Anthony Wood's testimony that he 'was esteemed by the academians to be a person of an acute judgement in philosophy, an excellent Grecian and Hebrician. Afterwards he was a godly and sincere preacher of the word of God.'[5]

---

[1] Merton College Library, card-index of donors.
[2] 'Registrum Collegii Mertonensis 1521–67', fol. 337^v.
[3] Ibid.   [4] Ibid., fol. 340^v.
[5] Wood, *Fasti Oxonienses*, i, col. 162, in idem, *Athenae*, ii.

His successor, *Thomas Jessop*, elected in April 1565, was given permission by the College just after his election to the lectureship to be admitted 'ad studium medicinae';[1] possibly the lectureship was here being used for a purpose rather more modest than the intended one, but still useful—namely to give a young M.A. an opportunity to embark seriously on medical study. Jessop certainly profited from the occasion, whether or not his lecture audiences did also. He went on to take his M.B. and licence to practise in 1566, his M.D. in 1569. He became a Fellow of the College of Physicians, and left to Merton a Basle, 1533–5, Aetius, which had belonged to his predecessor Henry Atwood; a Venice, 1521, *Practica* of Bernard of Gordon; Fuchs's edition of Galen's *De temperamentis*, Paris, 1554; Galen, *Opera*, Basle, 1561–2; J. B. Montanus, *Consultationes*, Basle, 1565; and the great *Historia generalis plantarum*, Lyons, 1587.[2] It would be interesting to know where he bought the clutch of books published in the 1550s and 1560s; did he perhaps travel abroad shortly after his tenure of the lectureship?

Next came *Thomas Wanton*, elected 1568, having already taken his M.B. and licence to practise. He took his M.D. in 1573, just after the end of his tenure of the lectureship, and then is heard of no more. He had been elected specifically to read 'sub ijs conditionibus quae exprimuntur in Ordinatione Linacre hoc negotium concernente'.[3] The job was still no sinecure.

In March 1572 the College elected *James Whitehead*, already M.B. and licentiate. His tenure was renewed for a further three years in 1575, but he died in 1576. The next holder was *John Chamber* (not, it seems, a kinsman of the John Chamber, or Chambre, Warden of Merton, who had been so closely associated with Linacre in the founding of the College of Physicians). He held the post for seven years, having been Greek lecturer earlier. According to Anthony Wood he was 'much respected as a scholar, and is said to have instructed Sir Henry Savile in mathematics'.[4] He left the College £100 for two Eton postmasterships (or scholarships) but took no medical degree.

His successor, *John Norris*, held the lectureship for almost ten years, from 1583, and this in spite of the fact that he had ceased to

---

[1] 'Registrum Collegii Mertonensis 1521–67', fol. 340.
[2] Merton College Library, card-index of donors.
[3] Merton College MSS., Reg. 1. 3, 'Registrum Collegii Mertonensis 1567–1730', p. 5.   [4] Wood, *Fasti*, i, col. 193.

be a Fellow in 1586; he was formally renewed as Linacre lecturer in 1589, but immediately afterwards dispensed 'urgentibus negotiis ab academia advocato pro suis ordinariis proxime termino omittendis'.[1] If he failed to give some of his lectures, at least he secured a dispensation.

The next incumbent, *Benjamin Bentham*, may have taken this as an encouragement for slackness, for at the triennial renewal of his lectureship in 1596 it was expressly laid down that no fewer than twenty lectures were to be given in the first year, and no fewer than thirty in the second.[2] Whether or not this does suggest that Bentham had been neglecting his duties already, it is clear that the College was prepared to accept from him a very much watered-down version of Linacre's original requirements. There is no means of knowing whether this stipulation represented merely a temporary concession for Bentham, or whether it is an indication of the amount of work which by this time it had become conventional to expect of the lecturers. Certainly it is unlikely that Robert Barnes, by now aged eighty-two, had been lecturing daily for some years past, if indeed he had ever done so.

Bentham fades from the Oxford scene after having been suspended from his fellowship for insubordination in 1598. There may well have been a gap of two or three years in the effective or even formal tenure of the lectureship. There is no mention in the register of a successor until August 1602, when the name of *Thomas Dochen* appears briefly, to reappear as senior lecturer after the death of Barnes in October 1604.[3] But Dochen himself died in January 1605, and his tenure is worth noticing mainly because he was the first of a succession of non-Merton men, nearly all of them Fellows of Magdalen, and all of them practitioners in Oxford, who held the lectureship early in the seventeenth century. They were *Henry Bust* (1605–17), *Bartholomew Warner* (1617–*c.* 1619), and *Edward Lapworth* (*c.* 1619–36). Each of these was a respectable enough appointment in itself, and the principle of choosing a respected Oxford practitioner perhaps had its merits, but it is nevertheless surprising that there was no senior medical fellow of Merton anxious on any of these occasions to take up the post, or, if there was, that Merton did not elect him. Clearly, no solution had yet been found at Merton to the old problem of keeping enough M.D.s, or even M.B.s, in Oxford to

---

[1] 'Registrum Collegii Mertonensis 1567–1730', p. 136.
[2] Ibid., p. 177.   [3] Ibid., pp. 208, 213.

establish a College medical school which was big enough always to be a going concern.

Thomas Dochen himself had taken his M.B. over twenty years before, in 1580, but it took a royal visit to Oxford (as in the case of Barnes) to prompt him into taking his M.D. The fact that Dochen, a local practitioner but not then a Doctor of Medicine, was chosen to deputize for Dr. John Case at the formal physics disputation staged for the Queen in 1593 suggests that Oxford was as short of resident M.D.s then as it had been nearly thirty years earlier.

Henry Bust was also a Magdalen man, Fellow there in the 1570s, but by 1582 married and with a house in the town. His M.B. and licence to practise had been obtained in 1572, his M.D. in 1579. In January 1597, when the City of London wrote to the University asking for nominations for the professorial chairs (or readerships) in the newly established Gresham College, his was one of the two names put forward for the readership in physic, although the appointment went, in fact, to the other nominee, Dr. Matthew Gwinne.[1] Anthony Wood reports of Bust that 'he practised his faculty many years in Oxford with great repute'.[2] Of his assiduity as Linacre lecturer it is hard to speak; but the College, after allowing his appointment to continue without recording its renewal in 1608 or in 1611, did renew it formally in 1614 for a further three years.

Bartholomew Warner, elected in 1617 for three years, seems at first sight to be quite out of the ordinary pattern. He had already held the Regius Chair of Medicine, between 1597 and 1612. But the Regius Chair at this time, far from attracting medical men of distinction back to Oxford from the outside world, had almost always been given (like the senior Linacre lectureship) to reputable learned men who had stayed on as practitioners in the locality. The same was the case in Cambridge. Warner was a bird of the same feather as Drs. Barnes, Bust, and Dochen, the only surprising feature being that he was so old when he was elected. He was originally a Lincoln College man, who had migrated to St. John's when he took his M.B. in 1585. Earlier that year he had been allowed to moderate for another M.B. candidate, since there was neither a Doctor nor even a Bachelor of Medicine available in Oxford at the time;[3] admittedly

---

[1] Clark, *Register*, i. 232–3.   [2] Wood, *Fasti*, i, col. 210.
[3] Clark, *Register*, i. 129. The questions upheld by Warner at the public disputation held on the occasion of the Queen's visit in 1594 are reproduced by Clark (ibid. i. 190).

it was July, so they may all have been elsewhere engaged upon practice, but July was the time of the year when many degrees were taken, and the absence of anyone senior to Warner reminds one again of the very small numbers involved in Oxford academic medicine at any one time in this period. Warner took his M.D. in 1594. Whether or not he lectured between 1617 and 1621 seems doubtful; he was already nearly sixty. The appointment looks more like a small honour for a local physician than a conscientious attempt on Merton's part to secure teaching for their students. And yet, he might have been very useful to such students.

Edward Lapworth, the last of the senior Linacre lecturers to be elected during the Wardenship of Henry Savile, was a member of a long-established medical family, most of whom had been educated at Oxford.[1] He was never a Fellow of Merton, but took his medical degrees as a member of Magdalen, having matriculated originally at St. Alban Hall. Between 1598 and 1610 he had been Master of Magdalen College School; he supplicated for his M.B. in March 1603, and obtained the licence to practise in 1605. At the visit of James I in 1605 Lapworth was respondent in natural philosophy, but he seems then to have been away from Oxford until about 1611, when he returned briefly to take the M.B. supplicated for earlier, together with the M.D. Between 1611 and 1618 he was away again, in practice, probably in Kent. In 1618 he was appointed first Sedleian Reader in Natural Philosophy, returning to Oxford in 1621 when Sedley's Will took effect. On his return, he was promptly elected senior Linacre reader by Merton, and settled down in Oxford as a teacher and practitioner. From then until his death in 1636 Lapworth resided part of the year in Oxford, part in Bath. He wrote a number of celebratory verses, including some in Edward Jorden's treatise, *Discourse of Naturall Bathes and Minerall Waters*, 1631, and he left some medical notes on a monstrous birth in Oxford in 1633.[2] The records of College and University preserve no evidence on the question of his assiduity in fulfilling the duties either of Linacre lecturer or of Sedleian reader, but it seems unlikely that he would have chosen to live in Oxford during so much of the year unless he had been willing to provide some sort of academic tuition.

The junior Linacre lecturers during the same period of years were

[1] In particular Michael Lapworth, Fellow of All Souls, 1562, M.B. and licence to practise medicine, 1573. Foster, op. cit., p. 882.

[2] Oxford, Queen's College, MS. 121, fol. 29.

a remarkable group of men, *Theodore Gulston* (1604–11), *William Simonson* (1611–22), *Richard Hawley* (1622–8), *Peter Turner* (1628–31), and *John Bainbridge* (1631–6).

Theodore Gulston, or Goulston, later famous as the founder of the Gulstonian lectures at the College of Physicians, took simultaneously his M.B., his M.D., and his licence to practise in April 1610, during his tenure of the lectureship. He was allowed to take all his degrees at once in spite of the statute *de gradibus non cumulandis*, 'being now much in esteem for his knowledge [in physic]'. The questions he debated *in vesperiis* and *in comitiis* for the degrees show him to have been interested in the wider philosophical implications of medicine as well as in questions of diagnosis and treatment.[1] These occasions invited some display, perhaps, but Gulston's confidence and informedness must have made any readings he performed with Merton men an interesting experience. After taking his degrees he left Oxford for good; not for him the provincial life of Barnes or Bust. He went on to become Fellow of the College of Physicians of London, and died in 1632, leaving to Merton his very extensive medical library.[2] The contents of this library (like that of John Collins which came to St. John's College, Cambridge) deserve fuller analysis elsewhere; here it is perhaps relevant to remark that a high proportion of the books were published, especially in Basle and in Venice, in the 1550s and 1560s, and may have belonged *en bloc* to some previous owner, while most of the remainder were published before 1600, especially in the 1590s. It would be valuable to be able to establish whether or not many of these books were in Gulston's possession during his tenure of the lectureship.

His successor, William Simonson, was a good college man, repeatedly Vice-Warden and Dean. He held the lectureship for eleven years, scrupulously and regularly renewed, but he took no medical degree, and has left no evidence of medical interests. If he performed the duties of the lectureship, it may well have been in a fairly routine or perfunctory way.

The situation may have improved under his successor, Richard Hawley, who seems to have spent his five years as Linacre lecturer reading medicine, to himself at least, and perhaps to others, for in June 1627 he obtained a Leyden M.D.,[3] returning to Oxford to

---

[1] Clark, *Register*, i. 192.   [2] Merton College Library, card-index of donors.
[3] R. W. Innes Smith, *English-Speaking Students of Medicine at the University of Leyden*, Edinburgh, 1932, p. 110.

incorporate as M.D. there in July. The Leyden records do not reveal
how long he spent there; if it was any length of time, then he was
an absentee during part of his tenure of the lectureship; on the other
hand he may have done most of his medical reading in Oxford,
paying Leyden a brief visit only. That University was in the habit
of granting medical degrees to itinerants, once it had satisfied itself
of their competence. In later years, after he had ceased to be Linacre
lecturer, Hawley stayed on in Oxford as a practising physician.

After Hawley's came the brief tenure of Peter Turner, son of a
physician whose M.D. was from Heidelberg, grandson of the inter-
nationally celebrated botanist and physician William Turner. Peter
Turner, 'a most exact Latinist and Grecian, . . . well skill'd in the
Hebrew and Arabic, . . . a thorough-paced mathematician, . . . excel-
lently well-read in the fathers and the councils, a most curious critic,
a politician, statesman and what not',[1] was a close friend of Sir
Henry Savile, and had held the Gresham Chair of Geometry since
1620. He retained this when he became Linacre lecturer, but relinquished the Linacre lectureship when in 1631 he was made Savilian
Professor of Geometry. His M.D., in 1636, was by royal creation
during the visit of Charles I to Oxford, and was partly in recognition
of the fact that he had been one of the principal architects of the new
Laudian statutes. A perfectionist, he tinkered endlessly with his
writings, and published nothing. He was ejected from Merton by
the Parliamentary Visitors in 1648 and deprived of his Savilian Chair
which went to John Wallis; he died in 1651. Whether or not he had
lectured regularly on Galen between 1628 and 1631 remains obscure;
but his learning and distinction, even at that early date, were considerable.

The same was true of his successor John Bainbridge, who held the
junior lectureship from 1631 to 1636, and the senior one from 1636
to his death in 1643. Bainbridge was a Cambridge M.D. with several
years of medical practice and schoolmastering behind him when
Savile brought him to Oxford in 1619 as first Savilian Professor of
Astronomy. He 'was entred a master-commoner of Merton college,
was incorporated doctor of physic as he had stood at Cambridge,
lived in the said college for some years (the society of which confr'd
on him the senior reader's place of Lynacre's lecture in 1636 . . .)'.[2]
Again, it is not possible to establish for certain whether or not he
regularly lectured; however, his lectures as astronomy professor are

[1] Wood, *Athenae Oxonienses*, iii. 306.   [2] Ibid. iii. 67.

equally hard to discern, but certainly occurred. He was busy learning Arabic at this time, in order to read the Arab astronomers, but
he had been actively interested in medicine as recently as 1622–8,
as letters between him and Hannibal Baskerville, a hypochondriacal
friend, reveal.[1] Bainbridge was evidently a practised and patient
physician. Like Hawley, he had travelled abroad, and for a time he
was enrolled among the English students at Padua.

St. John's, 1560–1647

Those Linacre lecturers of the years 1524–60 who had not died
young had all gone on to become learned men, but more often
divines than physicians. The situation improved between 1560 and
1580, during the tenure of *William Baronsdale*, or *Barnsdale* (1560–8),
Thomas Randall, or *Randolph* (1568–76), and *William Lakyn* (1576–80).

Baronsdale held the lectureship for two consecutive four-year
terms, taking his M.D. at the end, in 1568. He later became a prominent Fellow of the College of Physicians of London, and eventually
its President. Randall too became a Fellow of the College, having
taken his M.D. in 1577 just after his second four-year term as
Linacre lecturer. St. John's College library possesses a copy of
Alexander Trallianus, *De singularum corporis partium vitijs*, in Alban
Thorer's version of 1533 (Basle), with his autograph. Lakyn held
the post for one four-year term, and took his M.D. at the end of this
time. He had earlier obtained his licence to practise.

Almost certainly these three 'read' Galen more or less as Linacre
intended, although it is unlikely to have been daily. The opportunity
to combine the duties of the office, liberally interpreted, with one's
own private reading in preparation for the M.D. was surely too good
to be missed. St. John's was, in these years, on the evidence of the
College registers, maintaining fairly strict academic discipline and
ensuring that its members fulfilled scrupulously their various public
obligations. Under the Masterships of Nicholas Shepheard (1569–
74) and John Still (1574–7), the celebrated Hebraicist Broughton
and the Greek scholar Andrew Downes were elected to fellowships;
Still brought a second Greek scholar, one Bois, to the college 'to be
a future ornament . . . especially in the Greek tongue, then so rarely
known that for part of Mr. Bois' time there were only two in college
that understood it, Mr. Downs and himself'.[2]

---

[1] Oxford, Bodleian Library, Rawlinson MSS., letters, 41, fols. 4–20.
[2] Baker, *History of the College of St. John*, i. 171.

This was an active time in the history of Cambridge medicine too. The 1570 Statutes (which set out in full all the conditions attaching to the Linacre lectureships) had laid down that medical degrees could be obtained, if sufficient evidence of learning was given, without a prior M.A.; this had the effect of making it possible for students to complete the medical course in eleven years from matriculation, or only six if they stopped at the B.M. In practice, many of those who proceeded to medical degrees in later years had not taken advantage of this, and were already M.A. when they started studying medicine; but some were not. The provision facilitated, although it did not in itself cause, a steep rise in the number of medical graduates of the University of Cambridge between 1570 and 1600. This was accompanied, between 1570 and 1580 at least, by the second phase of the boom in the issuing of licences to practise to non-graduates. The Regius professorship of *Thomas Lorkyn* (1564–91) coincided with an active period for medical studies in several colleges. Thomas Moufet, William Harvey, William Gilbert, and John Dee all studied medicine in Cambridge during these years. Lorkyn himself much enlarged the University's medical library with a handsome bequest of 270 books.

Between 1586 and 1595 William Whitaker was Master of St. John's, 'one of the greatest men the college ever had'. Under him 'all indirect courses, especially of bribery . . . were utterly discouraged. . . . This made the college flourish in learning and swarm in numbers.' His own learning 'was diffusive and spread itself over the whole society, where by his example, instruction and encouragement he raised such an emulation amongst his fellows as to make others learned as well as himself; to that degree, that the society in his time was looked upon as something more than a private college.'[1]

It is the more surprising, therefore, that none of the Linacre lecturers between 1580 and 1600 was specifically a medical man. Two of them indeed were relatively undistinguished: *Robert Booth* (1580–8) disappears during his tenure to a rectory in Essex; *Thomas Cooke* (1596–1600) had incorporated at Oxford in 1594, returned to Cambridge and become Proctor in 1595, and thereupon is heard of no more. If he is to be identified with the Thomas Cooke who died at Padua some years later, then this may be a clue to some medical interest on his part; but the matter, and the man, remain obscure.

The other two, however, were by any criterion men of distinction

[1] Baker, *History of the College of St. John*, i. 180, 183, 184.

in the academic world. *Thomas Playfere* (1588–92), later Lady Margaret Professor of Divinity, had held before he became Linacre lecturer almost every other College office—*praelector topicus*, Rhetoric Examiner, Preacher, Hebrew Praelector, Senior Fellow, and Senior Dean. He took his B.D. in 1590 and his D.D. in 1596. In 1594 he had even had time to become a member of the Inner Temple. In 1595 he was 'of greatest fame [of all the Fellows] for learning',[1] but just failed to be elected Master. It is perhaps too much to expect that he could have lectured regularly on Galen during these years. But on grounds of sheer scholarship he was competent to do so, and he did at least possess a copy of the 1538 Basle Greek edition of Galen's works, which survives in St. John's to this day.

Henry Briggs (1592–6) held the Linacre lectureship for four years, before becoming Gresham Professor of Geometry in 1596, and moving to London. In 1619 he moved again, this time to Oxford, to the Savilian Chair of Geometry, and, like Bainbridge, to membership of the common room at Merton. Briggs was undoubtedly a distinguished mathematician; just how far his medical learning went seems impossible to determine on the evidence available.

It is perhaps significant that in the expansion in the number of Cambridge medical graduates between 1560 and 1600, the peak was reached in the University in general after 1580, while the smaller peak in St. John's had been reached and passed between 1560 and 1580, during the lectureships of the three medical men Baronsdale, Randall, and Lakyn: the sag corresponding with the tenure of Booth, Playfere, Briggs, and Cooke. It would be a difficult matter to work out whether this was cause and effect, and indeed, quite which was cause and which effect; but at the least, the coincidence serves once more to show how very fragile a thing a 'medical tradition' in a college was; when the numbers involved were so small, the death or departure of one or two men could mean the extinction of such a 'tradition'.

After 1600 the pattern shifts again. *John Collins* (1600–4) was a most interesting figure, and a genuine medical scholar. Later Regius Professor of Physic (1626–34), Fellow of the College of Physicians of London, anatomy lecturer and practitioner in London and Cambridge, he was at the time of his election as Linacre lecturer still a young man, in the early days of his study of medicine. In March 1606 the College granted him permission 'to travaile (3 years)

[1] Ibid. i. 190.

beyond the seas for his increase in learning, and withall [we] have
given him his grace to be Doctour in Physicke'.[1] He took his degree,
in fact, on his return from Italy in 1608. When he died in 1631 he
left to his apprentice 'several books, such as Gerard's *Herbal*, Vigo's
Surgery and the *Pharmacopoiea Londinensis*' as well as 'all his brewing
vessels'.[2] To St. John's he left his very extensive and wide-ranging
medical library of several hundred books, together with £100 to buy
more. This handsome bequest forms the largest single collection of
medical books in the St. John's library, and must have made it for
the next thirty or forty years one of the best-equipped medical
libraries in Cambridge. The titles include most of the more important medical publications of the previous 100 years, and the collection as a whole deserves a more lengthy analysis.

After Collins came *Robert Allott* (1604–20, and again 1624–35), a
figure who might almost have stepped out of the list of senior
Linacre lecturers elected by Merton. Although he was only about
twenty-nine when he was first elected, Allott continued to hold the
post (with one brief intermission, when it was, oddly perhaps, given
not to a medical fellow but to *Robert Mason*, whose own interests lay
entirely in law, and who was afterwards an associate of the Duke
of Buckingham) for a total of twenty-seven years. During this
time Allott was a well-known medical practitioner in Cambridge.
Whether or not he lectured regularly, there seems to be no means
of knowing; either he was, in effect, an outside tutor to three
generations of medical students, or he was little more than a lay
figure in their affairs. Medical studies in Cambridge were, in terms
of graduates produced, running at a fairly high rate during these
years. John Collins as Regius Professor was admonished in 1628 to
perform an annual anatomy, a duty his predecessor had neglected,
and anatomies were held in March 1628, and in 1631. But the precise nature of Allott's role at St. John's is difficult to discern.

The Linacre lectureship ran into bad days with his three successors. *John Hay* (1635–42) was a Scot, intruded into the College by
Royal mandate in 1634; M.A. of Edinburgh in 1630, and *minister
verbi*, there is no evidence that he had medical interests or qualifications. *John Cleveland* (1642–4) is celebrated as a poet, but not as a
physician; ejected by the Parliamentary Visitors in 1645, he joined
the Royalist army at Oxford, and never, it seems, reappeared in

[1] Baker, *History of the College of St. John*, i. 457.
[2] Rolleston, *The Cambridge Medical School*, p. 146.

Cambridge. *John Bird* (1644–7) is an even more obscure figure, intruded into St. John's by the Earl of Manchester; he may have been the Oxford graduate of this name who took his B.A. from Merton in 1620.

Merton, 1637–1704

Merton too was having its troubles in the 1640s. When Bainbridge was promoted to the senior lectureship in 1636, the name of *Valentine Broadbent*, M.D. of Magdalen and another Oxford practitioner, was put forward. But Broadbent died in March 1637, before he had been elected. The next lecturer was *Nicolas Howson* (1637–40), of whose brief tenure nothing is recorded. He took no medical degree, and was ejected by the Parliamentary Visitors in 1648.

There is some confusion about the identity of the next junior lecturer. According to the Merton College Register for September 1640, it was the *vicecustos Magister Greaves*, that is *John Greaves* the astronomer, who was nominated by Archbishop Laud, acting in his capacity as Visitor. But by August 1643 the 'inferior' lecturer is named as *Doctor Greaves e coll. Omn. Animarum*, that is *Edward Greaves*, his brother. It is possible that John had been letting his brother, who was a medical man, do the lecturing and giving him the stipend, or that some other informal but irregular arrangement was being made, and that the position was recognized, if not regularized, in the register entry of August 1643. In any case the situation was changed in November of that year, when Edward Greaves was elected according to the proper procedure to the senior lectureship, in succession to Bainbridge. Whether or not he lectured regularly, Edward Greaves was intrinsically a promising candidate for the post. M.D. since 1641, he 'practised with good success in these parts'. The words in which Anthony Wood reports his election, 'elected by the Mertonians the superior lecturer of physic in their college, to read the lecture of that faculty in their public refectory',[1] may perhaps indicate that even in Wood's day, let alone in the 1640s, the college expected the lectures to be performed, and performed, what is more, with a certain amount of formality, publicly, in the College hall.

The next junior lecturer was *John Sambach* or *Sambarch*, M.D. since 1641; he held the post for four years, 1643–7. A local practitioner, married to the daughter of the first Printer to the University,

[1] Wood, *Athenae Oxonienses*, iii. 1256.

Joseph Barnes, he has left no trace of his activities as lecturer in the records.

In 1647, 'the King's cause having declined', Edward Greaves left Oxford, being succeeded in the senior lectureship by *Daniel Whistler* (1647–53). Whistler, later a controversial President of the College of Physicians, was certainly one of the ablest men ever to hold one of the Linacre lectureships, but almost certainly also its first real absentee. He had been 'admitted probationer fellow of Merton college in January 1639, where going through the severe exercises then kept up'[1] he had proceeded in arts four years later, having already paid a brief visit to Leyden in 1642; he continued his study of medicine, partly in Oxford, partly abroad, took a Leyden M.D. in 1645, and returned to Oxford and incorporated M.D. there in May 1647. His election to the Linacre lectureship came in August, and was renewed in August 1650 for a further three years. As is well known, Whistler had presented for his doctoral dissertation at Leyden an admirably concise and exact clinical description of rickets, or the 'English disease', which anticipated by five years the longer treatment of the matter published by Francis Glisson, at that time Regius Professor of Physic at Cambridge, but most of his time an absentee. Whistler in Oxford, like Glisson in Cambridge, would have been most valuable to medical studies in the University had he resided. But as Wood points out, 'he read not, because he was practising his faculty in London'.[2] Indeed, the election had come at a busy moment in Whistler's career—it was succeeded almost immediately by his candidature for the College of Physicians, and by his election to the Gresham Chair of Geometry (the fourth Merton man in succession to hold this). He continued to hold his Merton fellowship, although he was absent from Oxford. This was perhaps already a sign of the times. Even so, the fact that Wood remarks upon Whistler's having 'read not' may paradoxically give us some grain of reassurance: at least the phenomenon was worth remarking upon.

Meanwhile the junior lectureship was held by *Richard Lydall* (1647–52), another good college man, later to marry and settle in Oxford as a physician. He succeeded to the senior post in 1653, and held it for a further nine or ten years, until his marriage. He took his M.D. only very late in this period, in 1656, and has left no medical publications, or evidence of any particular learning or

[1] Wood, *Athenae Oxonienses*, iv. 133.   [2] Ibid.

talents. He did, however, become Warden of Merton in 1692, much to the disgust of Anthony Wood who regarded Lydall as depressingly similar to the previous Warden, Thomas Clayton, M.D., Regius Professor of Physic, a third-rate medical man with a grasping wife and too many daughters. Lydall had a wife and daughters too, and as for his intellectual abilities, Wood regarded them with contempt: 'He has been a packhorse in the practical and old Galenian way of physick, knows nothing else, buys no books, nor understands what learning is, or the world.'[1] However, as Linacre lecturer in the 1640s, perhaps this 'Galenical packhorse' (to whom Wood may well have been unfair) had had his uses; at least he survived throughout the exclusions and intrusions of Civil War and Interregnum. And the Lydalls were not a negligible academic family in Oxford; Richard had a brother John, Fellow of Trinity, whose surviving correspondence with John Aubrey, dating from 1648 to 1653, shows him to have been a close friend and associate of Ralph Bathurst, William Harvey, Nathaniel Highmore, John Willis, William Petty, and others in Oxford at that time; the letters discuss questions in anatomy, navigation, horticulture, and astronomy, and refer to chemical and other experiments in natural philosophy.[2] Richard Lydall would have to have been a very dull dog not to have been affected at all by everything that was going on in Oxford in these matters in the very years he was Linacre lecturer, and it seems likely that evidence may yet be found of his involvement in these affairs.

Edmund Dickinson succeeded Richard Lydall in the junior lectureship in 1653, and was scrupulously renewed in it by the College at three-year intervals until 1661. He appears as senior lecturer in 1664, but the precise date of his change of status is not clear from the register. Dickinson, yet another practitioner in the locality, took his M.D. in 1656. During his tenure 'he spent much labour and money in the art of chymistry, kept an operator, and gave out to his acquaintance that he would publish a book thereof, but as yet there is nothing of that nature made extant by him'.[3]

[1] Brodrick, *Memorials of Merton College*, p. 123.
[2] Bodleian Library, Aubrey MSS. 12, fols. 292–319.
[3] Wood, *Athenae Oxonienses*, iv. 477. Dickinson, like Briggs, Bainbridge, the Greaves brothers, and Whistler, was one of those Linacre lecturers who were already during their tenure of the post closely associated with the leading natural philosophers and men of science of their day, and were themselves notable contributors to scientific literature or controversy. Apart from his interest in chemistry during his Oxford days, Dickinson was working on an

After Dickinson came *Richard Trevor* or *Travers* (1662/3–9, senior lecturer 1669–74), M.D. of the University of Padua since 1658, incorporated M.D. Oxford, 1661; about his tenure of the lectureship, no information has come to light. He was followed by a succession of undistinguished men, *Robert Whitehall* (1669–77), *Edward Jones* (1677–8), *Thomas Alvey* (1679–85), *Stephen Welsted* (1685–9), *Charles King* (1689–90), and *Martin Hartopp* (1691–2). Their relative lack of intellectual distinction or of medical or experimental turn of mind is the more to be regretted, in the history of Merton medicine and of Oxford natural philosophy, because they were present in Oxford during two decades when elsewhere in the University these studies were, if not flourishing, at least providing some incidents of interest.

Whitehall, another of the *bêtes-noires* of Wood, had been intruded by the Parliamentary Visitors in 1650. He created a mild stir by his capacity for composing satirical and mocking verse; then removed himself to Ireland under the aegis of Henry Cromwell; and on his return in 1657 had, as Wood incredulously reports, 'actually been created bachelor of physic' by a letter of Richard Cromwell, 'since which time he made divers sallies into the practice of physic, but

investigation into the antiquity of alchemy, and had already published the first of several works in which he explored the implications for philosophy and theology of recent study of the problems of chronology. He practised in Oxford from his rooms in Merton for several years, and then from a house in the High Street, moving to London in about 1664. During this time and later he was a close associate of Robert Boyle. Through the good offices of Arlington he was introduced to King Charles II, who took such a fancy to Dickinson's chemical experiments that he installed him for a time in a small laboratory connected by a staircase to his own private apartments at Whitehall. Dickinson also acted as the King's physician. After 1688 he retired and worked out an elaborate philosophical system, founded not on hypotheses, or experiments, but on principles observed by him to exist in Biblical chronology, or 'Mosaic history'. This work, published in 1702 as *Physica vetus et vera, sive Tractatus de naturali veritate hexameri mosaici*, looks less odd and isolated now than it did before recent disclosures about Isaac Newton's unpublished work on alchemy, philosophical systems, and Biblical chronology, which was occupying much of the great mathematician's private attention in the same few years.

The details available about Dickinson's life and preoccupations reveal him to have been both characteristic and remarkable among the natural philosophers of his day; but there is nothing with which we can piece together a picture of his activities (if any) as Linacre lecturer. The usual silence of the Merton records on the point is especially tantalizing in his case, as in that of Briggs, Bainbridge, and Edward Greaves.

thereby obtained but little reputation'. Whitehall was Linacre lecturer for eight years, presumably during this period, and a resident Fellow of Merton; when he died in 1685 he was buried in the chapel, 'having for several years before hang'd on that house as an useless member'.[1]

Edward Jones took his M.B. in 1662, and his M.D. in 1669, but was then an absentee, retaining his fellowship (and with it, briefly, the lectureship) while dividing his time between his practice in London, and Wimborne in Dorset.

Already the heyday of the lectureships in Oxford is over; we are moving into the eighteenth-century pattern of their decline. However, Thomas Alvey was not a negligible figure in the medical world, however little he did for Merton medicine. M.B. in 1669, M.D. in 1671, Fellow of the College of Physicians of London in 1676, Harveian Orator in 1684, he published in 1680 a conservative but scholarly book on the unexceptionable traditional medical topic of urines.[2] But as Linacre lecturer he can have been of little use since he was absent from Oxford for most of the time.

Stephen Welsted, too, was an absentee. After taking his M.B. in 1685 he was in 1686 given permission by the college to retain his fellowship while being out of residence for three years, the very years he held the lectureship. Martin Hartopp, M.B. 1689, a Cambridge graduate originally, was later to be a physician in Leicester. He travelled in Italy and in 1693 contributed to the *Philosophical Transactions of the Royal Society* a description of an earthquake at Naples.[2] But he had at least the decency to resign the lectureship before his departure. Charles King, son of a physician, took his M.B. at the end of his brief tenure of the junior lectureship in 1689, and went on to become M.D. in 1692, during his longer, and, as far as we know, undistinguished tenure of the senior one, which did not end until his death in 1715.

The last senior Linacre lecturers who belong to this period are *Charles Willoughby* (1674-7), *William Coward* (1685-9), and *Edmund*

---

[1] Wood, *Athenae Oxonienses*, iv. 177–8.

[2] *Dissertatiuncula epistolaris, unde pateat urinae materiam potius e sero sanguinis quam e sero (quod succo alibili in nervis superest) ad renes transmitti*, London, 1680.

[3] *Philosophical Transactions*, No. 202 (July–August 1693), pp. 813–56; Bodleian Library, Lister MSS. 4, fol. 46, is a medical letter from Hartopp to Lister, Jan. 1689/90, in which Hartopp asks advice about some treatment 'for I never could admire those long Gallymophories of Physick our modern Oxford Practice dictates'.

Marten (1689–1704). Willoughby had been one of a batch of ten fellows intruded in 1649–50 under the mandate of the Parliamentary Visitors; they included at least one other medical man, John Arnold, M.D. of Leyden, who later practised in York. Willoughby himself travelled in Italy in the 1660s, taking a Paduan M.D. in 1663, and returning to incorporate at Oxford in 1664. He presented Merton with a handsome *Herbarius siccus* compiled by himself in Italy. This is still in the College's possession, and shows him to have been at the least a careful pupil of some competent botanist, or a careful reader of the botanical classics; the specimens are well mounted and seem to be accurately named. The details of Willoughby's later life are fairly obscure; he practised medicine for a time in Dublin (he was a native of Cork), but it is not clear whether or not he was an absentee during his time as Linacre lecturer.

William Coward took his M.B. just before his election and his M.D. during his tenure. He almost certainly resided. He left Oxford in 1689, although retaining his fellowship, and practised in Northampton and then in London. He became celebrated, even notorious, at the turn of the century, when he became involved in controversy with Locke, and attracted the derision of Swift for his views on the separate existence of the soul. He was suspected of atheism, called to answer for his views at the bar of the House of Commons, and had his book burned by the common hangman. Nothing daunted, he went on to publish in 1706 a book which ridicules the Cartesian notion that the soul may reside in the pineal gland. He possessed one of the most combative and independent intellects of all the Linacre lecturers, and if he did make himself available to Oxford medical students in the 1680s, they must surely have profited from the experience. He was the author, too, of two books on chemical subjects, and a table of medicinal remedies.[1]

---

[1] His works include (apart from the well-known philosophical works *The Just Scrutiny: or a Serious Enquiry into the Modern Notions of the Soul*, and *The Grand Essay*), *De fermento volatili nutritis conjectura rationalis*, London, 1695; *Alcali Vindicatum . . .*, London, 1698; *Remediorum medicinalium tabula*, London, 1704; and *Ophthalmoiatria*, London, 1706, which would suggest that William Munk's dismissive comment (*Roll of the Royal College of Physicians*, 3 vols., London, 1878, i. 513) that Coward was 'more devoted to literary and metaphysical pursuits than to medicine', may be wide of the mark. Indeed, discussion of the role of natural and vital spirits (and the question of what exactly they were) seems to have lain behind some of his philosophical treatment of the difficulties in the idea of an immaterial soul. Coward, like Dickin-

Edmund Marten, M.D. in 1689, is perhaps unlucky in having left no evidence in the College records about his activities while he was Linacre lecturer, but upon his later wardenship Hearne made this damning judgement: 'by a lazy Epicurean Life, and an utter neglect of all Discipline, [he] has very much prejudiced that noble and ancient Seminary'.[1]

St. John's, 1647–1709

After 1647 at Cambridge the position improved. *Wadeson, Stoyte, Paman, Brackenbury*, and *Stillingfleet*, who held the lectureship between 1647 and 1695, all took their M.D. during their tenure, and in some cases at least it is clear that this was more than a mere assumption of status.

Robert Wadeson (1647–51) took his M.D. immediately upon election, perhaps for the sake of decency; but he had been a licentiate of the College of Physicians of London since 1645, and was to be a candidate for their fellowship in 1647. The War interrupted his career. He incorporated at Oxford in 1648, but died in 1654. For the last two years of his lectureship he may have been an absentee from Cambridge, and in any case University and College teaching seems to have been seriously disrupted during these years.

Edward Stoyte (1651–4) took his M.D. in 1651, and for many years lived and practised in Cambridge, where he was also a J.P.

Henry Paman (1654–62, 1670–4, 1678–91) was altogether a more interesting man—or at least has left evidence of his talents and his intellectual interests where Wadeson and Stoyte have not. M.D. in 1658, he obtained permission from the College in November 1662 to keep his fellowship while travelling abroad.[2] He resigned the lectureship. On his return in 1670 he resumed it, and practised and taught in Cambridge until 1677, when, on the translation of his friend Sancroft to Canterbury, he moved to London, and lived in the Archbishop's household in Lambeth Palace. He then became, in rapid succession, F.R.S. and Gresham Professor of Physic. At Gresham 'he attended his province, and read his lectures in person'.[3]

son, deserves further scrutiny in the light of recent work on the strange borderland of theology and natural philosophy in these years. But again, as Linacre lecturer, his lineaments are shadowy.

[1] Brodrick, *Memorials of Merton College*, p. 170.
[2] Baker, *History of the College of St. John*, i. 327.
[3] J. Ward, *Lives of the Professors of Gresham College*, London, 1740, p. 280.

It seems likely, therefore, that he had in his earlier and less elevated days read his Linacre lectures at Cambridge 'in person'; the fact that the College took the trouble to appoint a substitute in his stead during his time abroad from 1662 suggests that they were at this date still regarding the lectureship as a duty and not merely as a sinecure. However, they renewed Paman's tenure for a third time between 1678 and 1691, when, as we have seen, he had moved on to London. For this period at least the lectureship had an incumbent who, although distinguished, was an absentee. Paman was a friend and correspondent of Sydenham, and left the College about forty books, which bear witness more clearly to his cultivated tastes than to his medical learning.[1]

Pierce Brackenbury (1662–70, 1674–8) filled in twice for Paman; he took out his licence to practise medicine in 1662, his M.D. in 1665, and remained a Fellow of the College until his death in 1692; he has left little trace in its records.

Edward Stillingfleet (1691–5), son of the more famous bishop of the same name, took his M.D. in 1692 and was already, thanks perhaps to his father's interest on his behalf, F.R.S. (1688) and Gresham Professor of Physic (1689). But in 1692 he forfeited his Cambridge fellowship, and, more disastrously, his father's favour by his 'marriage with a young gentlewoman'. He practised for a time as a physician at Lynn in Norfolk, until a near-by rectory was procured for him, which he soon exchanged for another. John Ward, author of the *Lives of the Gresham Professors*, thinks that Stillingfleet's truncated career was a pity: 'He wanted not abilities, either of parts or learning' but had spoiled his chances by his ill-timed and ill-regarded match.[2] It may well have been a pity for the Linacre lectureship, too, for had Stillingfleet proved an assiduous teacher (at a time when Cambridge medicine in some of the colleges was not yet moribund) St. John's might have seen the slipping pattern of Paman's last years reversed. But perhaps this is to expect too much, and to hope for an outcome which would have been, if not impossible, very much against the contemporary social grain. As early as

[1] He seems to have been especially interested in history and topography. The books include Froissart's *Histoire et chronique*, Paris, 1579, Inigo Jones, *Stonehenge*, London, 1655, Evelyn's *Numismata*, London, 1697, Edward Browne's *Travels in Europe*, London, 1685, and Dugdale's *Ancient Usage of Bearing Arms*, London, 1682, as well as the works of Isaac Barrow and Jeremy Taylor.
[2] Ward, op. cit., p. 283.

1659 John Edwards of St. John's had remarked 'I might observe how our *Religious Mammonists* grasp at *any thing* where Gain is to be had. They fetch even Physic and Surgery under their Jurisdiction.'[1] The next two Linacre lecturers, while not exactly 'religious Mammonists', cannot be absolved from grasping at gain. To *Thomas Gardiner* (1695–c. 1703), and to *Matthew Prior* (1703–9), poet and diplomatist, the Linacre lectureship seems to have represented an honour, and a small stipend, no more. Certainly Prior was an absentee, and though he was a cultivated man, he was no scholarly physician.

The Decline and Eventual Transformation of the Lectureships, from about 1700

In the course of the eighteenth century there was in the history of the lectureships an undeniable and irreversible decline. The terms of the original endowments and the scale of the stipends came gradually even in the earlier period to have less and less relevance to medical education and to academic status. By 1700 on both counts the lectureships must have seemed to be little more than survivals from a remote part of each college's past, offices more honorific than onerous, something to award as a mark of respect to a medical man in the college, or in the university at large, or even merely as something any Fellow of the college might rely upon as a minor contribution to his income.

There is a certain contrast between the way the lectureships were treated at Merton and at St. John's in this later period. In the contrast we see some of the differences not only between two colleges, but between the two universities, and the fate of medical education in each.

Little pretence was made at Merton after 1703 that the lectureship was anything but a perquisite for one of the Fellows, or for someone else they cared to choose. *John Lydall* (1704–11), son of the late Warden and earlier Linacre lecturer Richard Lydall, had never been a Fellow of Merton, although he had been an undergraduate there, and he did not take his M.B. until 1710; he died in 1711. He had displaced *Thomas Byrom*, who was a Fellow, and who had taken his M.B. in 1698 and his M.D. in 1704, but who apparently held the lectureship for only a few months. Lydall was succeeded in 1711 by

[1] H. Bradshaw, *Cambridge Antiquarian Communications*, iii, 1864–76, 124; quoted by Rolleston, *The Cambridge Medical School*, p. 15.

John Martin, or *Marten* (1711–15 junior, 1715–38 senior), who took his M.B. in 1715 and his M.D. in the following year, and who remained a Fellow of the College until his death. No evidence has come to light about his learning, nor is it known whether or not he practised medicine; references to him in the Merton College register are so rare as to suggest that he may well have been absent from Oxford, at least on and off, for many years.

Gilbert Trowe (1715–38 junior, 1738–56 senior) took his M.B. in 1717, his M.D. in 1723, and became Sherardian Professor of Botany in 1724. He relinquished this last office in 1734, but retained a Linacre lectureship until his death in 1756. He has left little trace upon the history of botanical teaching in Oxford, upon medical history, or upon the records of his College. The Warden and Fellows went through the process of renewing his junior lectureship every three years until 1738, but the senior lectureship was renewed formally only once, in 1741; for the remaining twelve years he simply kept it.

His promotion to the senior position in 1738 found the College unable to fill the junior one with a medical man from amongst their own ranks and, apparently, unwilling to look elsewhere. There was a gap of three years, filled temporarily between 1741 and 1744 by the Warden *Robert Wyntle*, who was indeed a physician, who had taken his M.B. and M.D. in 1726, and who had been, in 1715, one of the first Radcliffe travelling fellows. Wyntle had probably been responsible for advising, perhaps for offering some tuition to Merton men interested in medical study in the 1730s. There seems to be no record of his having taught during his tenure of the lectureship.

Wyntle was succeeded by *Walter Ruding* who held the junior post for two separate terms of three years, and the senior one for a long run of no less than twenty-two. He was a numismatist and antiquary, and compiled annals of the College from its registers and letters. He seems to have had no particular medical qualifications or expertise. In the interval between his two terms as junior Linacre lecturer (1747–53), the holder was *Holland Cooksey*, who remains obscure, and who occupied the post, in any case, for only three of these six years; between 1751 and 1753 it seems to have been vacant.

In 1756 *Joseph Kilner* was elected junior lecturer; his tenure was renewed at triennial intervals until 1767. Like Ruding, he was a good college man, intermittently resident Fellow, and antiquarian. He wrote one book, *The account of Pythagoras's school in Cambridge as in Mr. Grose's antiquities of England and Wales*, n.p., 1790, but seems to have played no part—or has left no evidence of having played any part—in specifically medical tuition at Merton. *William Goodenough* (1767–70), junior lecturer for one three-year term, possessed copies of Cooper's *Anatomy* (1696) and of the 1766 collected edition of the works of William Harvey, both of which are still in Merton's library, but is otherwise obscure.

In 1770 *Samuel Kilner* was elected to the junior lectureship; he held it without formal renewal until his death fifty-five years later, together with the senior one, which came to him in 1789. He did nothing, as far as can be ascertained, for the stipend, over this entire period. This was really the nadir of the endowment's fate. The nineteenth-century holders, including *John Oglander* and *Edward Capel* (a military man, but at least with an interest in medicine), were almost all absentee. In 1857, under the ordinances of the Royal Commission on the University, the Linacre lectureships disappeared, and were replaced by a chair in physiology, to be called the Linacre chair, and to be attached to Merton College.

At St. John's the story was not quite the same. The medical tradition of Merton had flickered and virtually died in the course of the eighteenth century. In St. John's too, it grew dim, and as the numbers of undergraduates at the College and at Cambridge altogether shrank, there was a danger that medicine, always studied by relatively few, would cease altogether to be read or taught. But this never quite happened; indeed, it has recently been argued that Cambridge medicine right up to 1760 was in a healthier state, in a few protected corners of a few colleges, than the traditional judgement, or the University records alone, would suggest.[1] One certainly cannot establish, where the Linacre lecturers appointed by St. John's between 1710 and 1908 were active in medical teaching, that they

---

[1] A. W. Rook, 'Medicine at Cambridge, 1660–1760', pp. 107–22. He demonstrates convincingly that St. John's was, in terms of the number of medical graduates it produced, one of the leading—if not the leading—medical colleges in Cambridge at that time. However, numbers fell off seriously soon after 1700, and it was between 1700 and 1760 that colleges found more and more difficulty in enforcing residence for the Fellows; by the middle of the century they seem to have more or less given up the attempt. G. Rolfe, who held the Chair of Anatomy from 1708, seems to have been a perpetual absentee, as was Thomas Martyn, Professor of Botany from 1762 to 1825. On the other hand, John Martyn, Regius Professor from 1733 to 1761, did lecture, at least at first; he also translated some of the works of Boerhaave.

were so active precisely because they regarded it as their duty as Linacre lecturer. One must concur with the view that in this period the lectureships as such cannot be shown to have contributed effectively to medical education in Cambridge. It is, however, the case that the active medical figures, even in the doldrums of the mid to late eighteenth century, included one or two men who happened, among other offices, to hold that of Linacre lecturer.

Edmund Waller (1710–14, son of a physician, himself a St. John's man from the palmier days of the 1680s, practising in Newport Pagnell), took his M.D. in 1712 and remained a Fellow until his death in 1745; his tenure looks like the earlier pattern of the fairly recent M.A., still in residence, holding the lectureship while reading for his own medical degree.

Richard Wilkes (1716–20) has left no record of M.D., or even or M.B., but practised later in Wolverhampton, and was the author of several medical books.[1] When he was elected, however, he had not yet taken his M.A., and unless he was an autodidact with an unconventional early career, he can hardly have been much help as an adviser to young men at much the same stage in their medical studies as he was himself.

George Edward Wilmot (1720–4) took his M.D. in 1725, and relinquished his fellowship. He went on to become Fellow of the Royal College of Physicians (1726), F.R.S. (1730), Harveian Orator (1735), Physician-general to the Army (1740), and physician to the Crown. He was made a baronet in 1759.

Lancelot Newton (1724–32), a Fellow of eight years' standing at the time of his election, later went on not to a medical degree, but to the LL.D., in 1728.

Henry Goddard (1732–4) was young when he was elected, having taken his M.A. earlier in the same year. He did proceed to the M.D. in the end, but not until 1753. He had ceased to be a Fellow in 1735, and had gone to practise in Yorkshire, being succeeded by *William Heberden* (1734–8).

Of all the Linacre lecturers at Cambridge in the eighteenth century, Heberden was certainly the one who did most (although not, essentially, because he was Linacre lecturer) for medical education

---

[1] *A Treatise on Dropsy*, London, 1730, new edn., 1777, and *A Letter to the Gentlemen, Farmers, and Graziers of the County of Staffordshire on the Treatment of the Distemper now Prevalent among Horned cattle and its Prevention and Cure*, London, 1743.

in the University at large. He lectured regularly—in itself an unusual thing to do—between about 1734 and 1748, for the last ten years in the Anatomy School. His lectures covered a wide variety of medical topics, including *materia medica*. He left to St. John's a very fine display cabinet, which he had perhaps used as much for demonstration purposes as for actual dispensing, and which contained in numerous drawers and small cupboards carefully labelled examples of the entire conventional *materia medica* of the day. Notes taken at one of his lectures by Erasmus Darwin survive in St. John's, and deserve further scrutiny elsewhere. The substance of another of his lectures, or rather lecture courses, was published by Heberden in 1745 under the title Ἀντιθηριακά: *an Essay on Mithridatium and Theriaca*. At least one of Heberden's Cambridge pupils, Robert Glynn Clobery, copied his master's example in making a practice of offering regular lectures in Cambridge in the second half of the century.[1] It may well be the case that St. John's, by affording Heberden the Linacre lectureship in the years immediately before he took his M.D., had at least given him the opportunity to start on so auspicious a course. But the opportunity itself had not proved enough in earlier cases, nor was Heberden's example to affect his successors in the post. He was unusual amongst them, although thirty or forty years earlier he would not have been a unique figure in Cambridge medicine generally. It was only recently (a change since the time of Vigani, James Keil, and Stephen Hales) that even privately organized lectures and demonstrations for medical students had become rare; even between 1690 and 1730, however, the situation described in 1759 by Richard Davies, M.D., already obtained:

The Arts subservient to Medicine have no appointments to encourage teachers in them. Anatomy, botany, chemistry, and pharmacy have been but occasionally taught when some person of superior talents has sprung up, and has honoured the University by his first display of them there before his passage into the world.[2]

As in the case of the Linacre lectureships, the endowments existed, but had not proved incentive enough to keep the able men in the university world. Nor had that world proved willing to exact from the incumbents a regular performance of their duties, whether

[1] Rolleston, op. cit., pp. 18–19.
[2] R. Davies, *The General State of Education in the Universities with a particular view to the Philosophical and Medical Education, set forth in a letter to Dr. Hales, being Introductory to Essays on the Blood*, Bath, 1759; Rolleston, op. cit., pp. 14–15.

literally or liberally interpreted. Too often, medical education had had to rely on the 'person of superior talents', like Heberden, 'before his passage into the world', and upon the prevailing ethos in a college at a given time.

Heberden moved on in 1748, but he had already been succeeded in the Linacre readership by *Thomas Clerke* (1738–45). Clerke was a brand-new M.A. who took no medical degrees later, but decided instead to seek membership of the Inner Temple.

His successor was *Samuel Hutchinson* (1745–53), another quite junior appointment. He stood, unsuccessfully, for the Chair of Anatomy in 1746, and died in 1753.

Thomas Gisborne (1753–7) may have been rather more use to St. John's men who consulted him about their medical studies (if such there were), since he was at least intent upon becoming a medical practitioner himself. In 1757 he became physician to St. George's Hospital, taking his M.D. in 1758, becoming Fellow of the Royal College of Physicians in 1759, and delivering the Gulstonian lectures at the Royal College in 1760.

Although Thomas Gisborne kept his St. John's fellowship until his death in 1806, he had ceased to be Linacre lecturer as early as 1757, when, as we have seen, he left Cambridge; this is an indication, perhaps, that at St. John's the post was still regarded as something a young man held for a few years only, when he was preparing for his own M.D.

His successor *John Cam* (1757–63) fits fairly well into this pattern too; he held the lectureship for six years, until he moved away from Cambridge, relinquishing his fellowship at the same time (perhaps because he married). He never bothered to take any medical degree, but he became a practitioner in his home town of Hereford, where his father had been a surgeon.

George Ashby (1763–7) was an older Fellow of the College, having taken his M.A. as early as 1748, and indeed having been a Bachelor of Divinity since 1756. He was a man of wide-ranging scholarly interests, an antiquary, bibliographer, topographer, and local historian as well as a divine, rather similar in his tastes to John Kilner and Walter Ruding at Merton. He was in some matters a radical, an advocate of university reform who argued, for example, in favour of college Fellows being allowed to keep their fellowships after marriage. Certainly the fact that they were not allowed to do so had helped perpetuate a situation where it was difficult to keep more than a handful of scholars in Oxford and Cambridge beyond their early thirties, obliged as they were, if they wished to marry, to seek preferment or a secular livelihood elsewhere.

Ashby was followed, for a matter of at the most two years, by *Walter Ludlam* (1767–9), son of Richard Ludlam, M.D., earlier of St. John's. Walter Ludlam was already in 1767 a man of 50, Bachelor of Divinity since 1749, and unsuccessful contender for the Lucasian chair of mathematics in 1760. His medical learning, if it existed, is not in evidence, and it seems unlikely that he was ever actively involved in the teaching of medicine at St. John's. But he was an astronomer, and well informed about a variety of problems in physics, and interested in technical inventions and in all kinds of machinery. He published several books, and was a regular contributor to the *Philosophical Transactions* in the 1760s. In 1767–8, while he was Linacre lecturer, Ludlam was certainly in Cambridge, and was busy making astronomical observations, as we know from an account of them, together with a description of some astronomical instruments, which he later published.[1]

In 1769 began the long tenure of the Linacre lectureship by *Isaac Pennington*. He retained it until his death in 1817, combining it from 1775 with a faculty fellowship in medicine, from 1773 until 1793 with the chair of chemistry, from 1785 with a post as physician to Addenbrooke's Hospital, and from 1793 with the Regius chair of physic. There is no sign that he gave any regular course of lectures during this long period, although he fulfilled the vestigial duty of the Regius professor which was to deliver a 'determination' or short formal speech in Latin at the end of the Physic Act, when a Doctor of Medicine was admitted. Commentators have been virtually unanimous in lamenting the institutional languor which was characteristic of Cambridge medicine in the second half of the eighteenth century, and Pennington has received a share of the blame. One must concur. And yet, he lived an intensely busy life as a Cambridge physician and University dignitary, his world was one in which medical questions, practical and intellectual, if not necessarily pedagogic, were actively discussed, while the very large library of medical (and other) books he bequeathed to St. John's suggests that he

[1] His *Rudiments of Mathematics*, London, 1785, was for many years a standard Cambridge textbook. In 1765 he had been one of the 'three gentlemen skilled in mechanics' who had reported to the Board of Longitude on the merits of John Harrison's chronometer.

went to considerable lengths to keep his own medical learning up
to date. The bequest includes an especially impressive collection of
medical works published in Edinburgh, mostly between 1780 and
1800, and a formidable *ensemble* of English medical books, not only
from the London presses, but from Bath, Liverpool, the two universities, and elsewhere; the emphasis is on clinical descriptions of particular diseases, many of them in short monograph form, and again,
nearly all have publication dates of between 1770 and 1815. These
two collections must be almost unique of their kind, outside Edinburgh at least; their contents, their origin, and the way they came
into Pennington's hands are all problems worth proper investigation
elsewhere (were they perhaps complimentary copies sent to the
Regius Professor, or did Pennington himself collect the library
together?). In any case, their presence in St. John's in the early
nineteenth century must have made it one of the best-equipped
medical libraries in the country. Perhaps one should pause before
dismissing Pennington as a malign, or at best a negative power, in
the history of Cambridge medicine; the matter needs further inquiry.

During the nineteenth century, there were seven more Linacre
lecturers, chosen with good judgement by the College (not necessarily from among their own members), for almost all of them later
turned out to be prominent figures in the Cambridge, or the London, medical world.

John Haviland (1817–22 and 1824–47) is well known as the
reinvigorator *par excellence* of Cambridge medicine and physiology,
advocate of the organized provision by the faculty of a whole system
of regular lecture courses, anatomical demonstrations, clinical
tuition, and examinations; a man who would surely have been after
Linacre's own heart (or perhaps even more that of John Caius).

Sir Thomas Watson (1822–4) enjoyed a highly successful later
career as Fellow and President of the Royal College of Physicians
and Physician-in-Ordinary to Queen Victoria; he was author of *The
Principles and Practice of Physic* (1843), which remained a standard
textbook for two generations or more.

Henry Thompson (1847–51) was a noted clinical innovator at the
Middlesex Hospital. These four men, and their successors *George
Paget*, *John Buckley Bradbury*, and *Sir Donald Macalister*, are given
further mention below.[1]

---

[1] See below, Margaret Pelling, 'The Refoundation of the Linacre Lectureships in the Nineteenth Century', p. 288.

In 1908 the lectureship was made an annual appointment; the College decided to invite each year 'a man of mark in the medical profession' to give a single public lecture, in Cambridge, on some topic of specialized or of general medical interest. That has continued to be their practice to this day.

How then, should one conclude? The Linacre lectureships surely did, for a long period in their history, make some contribution to medical education. They did, at the very least, provide a small additional stipend for young members of Merton and St. John's who wished to go on with their medical studies, and who had been allowed a fellowship already for this purpose. They did, perhaps, help to secure the presence for a little longer in the universities of medically learned men (or serious beginners in medical learning), who might otherwise have earlier moved elsewhere. They did, perhaps, keep some local practitioners in touch with the university, and one supposes (although it cannot be demonstrated) with would-be and actual students of medicine. Conversely, the presence of men with university associations among the practitioners may have made it easier for a young man actively seeking some experience of seeing patients at the bedside, or of visiting with a physician an apothecary's dispensary, to obtain such experience. But the Linacre lectureships, as such, cannot alas claim any specific credit here. Medical studies in both universities were far from being as exiguous, or as conservative, as some critics have supposed. New evidence is continually coming to light of the presence, intermittently, in colleges or in private households, of individuals, coteries, groups of friends and correspondents, even professional teachers, some of them foreigners like Stahl and Vigani, who offered to the interested the opportunity of discussing and learning about not only basic 'consensus' physic, but also many of the medical and philosophical controversies of the day. The opportunities for clinical tuition in both Oxford and Cambridge were a little better than its virtual absence from the formal syllabus would suggest, but scanty enough. On the other hand, for medical book-learning, there was probably more than a student could digest in the libraries of Merton and St. John's—and for this individual Linacre lecturers should take some share of the thanks.

Linacre's endowments had not succeeded entirely as he would have wished. The colleges and the universities in general continued, in spite of their benefactors, to depend until the nineteenth century on young college tutors and on the odd 'person of superior talents' before his 'passage into the world'. The entire system of examinations and qualifications had to be overhauled before the problem was solved; and, even then, clinical tuition had to be sought in larger hospitals in London. If the Linacre lecturers, or some of them, contributed individually to medical teaching in their day, one has nevertheless to concur in the judgement that the lectureships as such (after the early episode of the founding of Regius chairs) failed to influence the course of medical education. That the Linacre lecturers included few men of distinction has been shown to be patently false; there were nonentities, or men whom the accidents of the survival of evidence have made appear as such; and there were men of mediocre talents among them; but the able, the learned, and the subsequently successful are not few; it is medical scientists of the first, or even the second rank who are lacking.

Whether or not the 'happy inheritor(s) of the bequest' received their 'money gladly and made no pretence of work' has proved to be a difficult question to answer. The silence of the college records on the point lends itself, at different epochs, to subtly different, and never wholly demonstrable, conclusions; all one can say is that it seems unlikely that all the lecturers 'made no pretence of work'. Both colleges had periods when they produced a spate of medical graduates, with whose welfare someone must have been concerned. But the work was almost certainly never the daily reading upon the works of Galen which Linacre himself had so much desired.

Addendum to p. 247:

It may be evidence that the style 'Linacre lecturer' was, on one occasion at least, adduced as proof of respectability in the medical world, that *John Bird* (1644–7), who left no trace of his Cambridge activities, nevertheless styled himself in 1657, in a letter written from Sion College, and printed in James Cooke's edition in English of the *Select Observations on English Bodies; or, Cures both Empericall and Historicall, . . . First, written in Latine by Mr. John Hall Physician, living at Stratford upon Avon. . .* , 'pridem in Academia Cantabrigiensi Medicinae Prelector Linacerianus'. He recommends to the reader the remedies here published on the ground that they are not taken 'from other men upon Trust' but are based upon Hall's own clinical experience, and upon 'Observations' which 'are the Touch-stone for the trying of what ever is not good, and what Current in Physik'.

I am grateful to Charles Webster for drawing my attention to this letter.

The Refoundation of the Linacre Lectureships in the Nineteenth Century

MARGARET PELLING*

THE PRESENT VOLUME, WHICH DEALS PRIMARILY with events in which Linacre directly participated, is not the appropriate place for an extensive essay on a nineteenth-century subject. Nevertheless it is important to note that Linacre has exercised a continuing influence, not primarily by virtue of his published works, but because of an acquired mythological stature. This reputation has proved remarkably durable. Medical men and others even in the modern period have identified themselves with Linacre with the result that the name of the Tudor reformer has been commemorated in various ways in modern reforms, in particular by the lectureships and College at Oxford, and to a lesser extent, the lectureship at Cambridge. Linacre and his bequests are not directly relevant to these later developments, but the innovators have often believed that their foundations were established in accordance with the ideals of Linacre.[1]

It should perhaps be stressed that, notwithstanding the appearance in 1835 and 1881 of biographies of Linacre, his period was to nineteenth-century medical men quite remote. They took, for fairly specific reasons, a much greater interest in Sydenham and in Harvey, although their view of conditions in, and the achievements of, the seventeenth century was in general idealized rather than informed.

---

* Research Assistant, Wellcome Unit for the History of Medicine, Oxford University.

[1] It will be assumed throughout that the reader is already acquainted with the situations described elsewhere in this volume by Dr. Fletcher and Dr. Lewis.

Similarly, they did not, on the whole, have an accurate knowledge of the conditions prevailing at the universities at much earlier periods.

The broader context to which the reader is now referred is that of the Victorian movement for university reform, and the campaign for systematic instruction in scientific subjects both as an essential element in general education, and as a preparation for various professions. The two latter questions are, as we shall see, in many ways distinct from each other, and from the question of medical reform, which is also involved.

Neither scientific nor medical schools could be said to have existed in Oxford during the first half of the nineteenth century, in spite of the strenuous efforts of a few individuals. The impetus created by William Buckland, Charles Daubeny, James Adey Ogle, and others had died out by 1830, owing, it has been suggested, to the counter-attraction exerted by newer institutions. Oxford produced an average of only two graduates a year in medicine between 1828 and 1848; there was no examination in the (optional) School of Natural Sciences until 1853. The reform movement, which was well developed within and outside the universities before the Commissions of 1850, had so far been otherwise occupied.[1] Various changes in the examination statutes had been enacted, but without real benefit to the subjects under discussion. Linacre's was merely one of the least noticeable examples of endowments in scientific subjects which served no useful purpose except to supplement stipends. The professorships and readerships in existence before 1850 had been founded from time to time over 300 years by various persons and institutions outside the University and were usually, by the later time, inadequately endowed.[2]

The government investigations of the 1850s represent the most concerted attempt on the part of the State to redirect the activities of the universities since the Interregnum. By 1850 the lack of scien-

---

[1] On this and other aspects of change in Oxford during the nineteenth century, see W. R. Ward, *Victorian Oxford*, London, 1965. Ward makes very little mention of either science or medicine. See also J. Sparrow, *Mark Pattison and the Idea of a University*, Cambridge, 1967, and G. V. Cox, *Recollections of Oxford*, London, 1870.

[2] For a (not wholly accurate) list, see *Oxford University Commission: Report of the Commissioners Appointed to Inquire into the State, Discipline, Studies and Revenues of the University and Colleges of Oxford*, Parliamentary Papers, 1852, xxii. 119–20.

tific instruction in existing institutions, and the absence of institutions specifically designed to teach and support science, had become for many an issue of national importance. The comparison was of course chiefly with the methods and achievements of the German scientific establishment. The Commissions announced by Lord John Russell in 1850 therefore investigated this as well as other issues relating to the suppression of privilege and abuses. It was felt that Oxford could with a little adjustment provide a home for those best fitted to make a career of scientific research; a compromise solution would thereby be reached in which 'a Professorship would . . . become a recognised Profession'.[1]

The importance of Henry Acland[2] in the wider context of reform should not be overestimated. Nevertheless, the particular recommendations of the Commissioners with respect to the School of Physical Science were based on proposals first broached by him at a meeting of the British Association in Oxford in 1847.[3] Acland had taken his degree at Oxford, and returned to the University as Dr. Lee's Reader in Anatomy (an appointment belonging not to the University but to his old college, Christ Church) in 1844. His views were determined largely by his own experience, and his career in medicine had itself been launched on the advice of Sir Benjamin Brodie (1783–1862), who also aroused his interest in the subject of medical reform.[4]

Acland believed that the fundamental principles of natural science should be part of the liberal education of every Oxford student; he did not think it was proper for Oxford to provide students with strictly professional qualifications. Nor was Oxford the place to establish an independent medical school, in spite of medicine's claim to being considered one of the learned professions. Instead, medical students should undertake the preliminary part of their education in as broad a manner as possible, under the civilizing influence of the University, before proceeding to the rigours of clinical training

[1] Ibid., p. 122.

[2] Sir Henry Wentworth (Dyke) Acland (1815–1900), Regius Professor of Medicine at Oxford, 1858–94. F.R.S. 1847; F.R.C.P. 1850; President of the General Medical Council, 1874–87. See J. B. Atlay, *Sir Henry Wentworth Acland, Bart. . . . A Memoir*, London, 1903. For a variety of contemporary accounts, see A. G. Gibson, *The Radcliffe Infirmary*, Oxford, 1926.

[3] H. W. Acland, *Remarks on the Extension of Education at the University of Oxford*, Oxford, 1848.

[4] Idem, *Oxford and Modern Medicine*, Oxford, 1890, pp. 12–13, 21.

in the metropolis. The University should relinquish its licensing powers, and concentrate on establishing 'complete *practical* teaching' in every department of 'Natural Science', first for the general education of all classes and secondly for the medical students working for 'every grade of the profession'.[1] Science in Oxford was to be 'founded within the walls' of a single institution, the Museum,[2] which would imitate in philosophical principle the Hunterian Museum in London, then under the supervision of Acland's friend, Richard Owen. For a time the energies of promoters of science at Oxford became almost exclusively absorbed in lobbying for such a museum.[3]

Acland's view of science was in no way utilitarian; although he stressed the importance of practical work, he was concerned to demonstrate to students such broad philosophical and moral principles as the unity of nature. Acland persisted in these views, and they largely determined the form of medical teaching in Oxford into the twentieth century.

The Commissioners 'appointed to inquire into the State, Discipline, Studies and Revenues of the University and Colleges of Oxford' reported in 1852. As part of its schemes for 'establishing an active Professoriate' (in combination, it was hoped, with a reformed tutorial system), the Commission recommended not only that existing endowments be rationalized, but that some colleges should suspend a number of their fellowships in order to provide stipends for 'Professor-Fellows'. The Linacre lectureships are not mentioned, either in the body of the Report or in the brief testimony submitted to the Commissioners by Merton College.[4] Acland himself had thought first not of Merton but of All Souls, 'the College of Linacre and Sydenham'.[5] In the Report, Magdalen and Corpus were first called upon to aid in the endowment of professorships, because of

[1] P.P., 1852, xxii. 131–2; Acland, *Oxford and Modern Medicine*, pp. 21–2.

[2] Acland's use of the term 'museum' stressed its older meaning, then almost obsolete, of a building devoted less to the preservation and exhibition of objects than to the 'pursuit of learning'.

[3] On the museum question see Atlay, *Memoir*, pp. 197–226; H. W. Acland and J. Ruskin, *The Oxford Museum*, 1st edn., London, 1859; 3rd full edition, with additions, London, 1893.

[4] It is doubtful whether the existence of Linacre's endowment was known outside Merton before March 1855. See below.

[5] P.P., 1852, xxii. 625. Acland was considering here the support of medical students. Elsewhere he 'could not say' what available funds there might be for the support of professors (ibid., p. 623).

their wealth and because of 'the intention of the Founders that some revenue be so applied'. The Commissioners then nominated Merton and All Souls, and possibly New College and the Queen's College, on the grounds that their revenues, even after some appropriation, 'would be more than sufficient for the greatest number of Undergraduates which they are ever likely to accommodate'. Moreover, the principle in question had been established at the first two of these colleges by the Visitors in the time of Henry VIII and of Edward VI.[1]

A minority of the Fellows at Merton and in particular the Warden, Robert Bullock Marsham,[2] had wished at the outset to refuse all information to the Commissioners,[3] but a more co-operative spirit prevailed and by 1853 (after the publication of the Report) this had been quite palatably institutionalized as an internal committee[4] set

[1] Ibid., pp. 207–8.

[2] Robert Bullock Marsham (1785–1880), nephew of 1st Earl of Romney. B.A. (Christ Church), 1807; Fellow of Merton, 1811; dean, 1824; Warden, 1826–80; barrister-at-law (Lincoln's Inn), 1817; D.C.L. 1826. Because of his regard for the Irish Church and his protectionism Marsham was put forward as a candidate for parliament against Cardwell and Gladstone in 1847, and he failed as the Heads of Colleges' candidate against the last-named in 1852 (receiving only 25 of 55 Merton votes). Ward describes him as 'a man of moderate talents and small influence' and ascribes his candidature to his being one of the few Heads not in holy orders (Ward, *Victorian Oxford*, pp. 172 and 143, and *passim*). The standard history of his College has almost nothing to say about him, in spite of the length of his tenure as Warden (B. W. Henderson, *Merton College*, University of Oxford College Histories, London, 1899). Marsham contended, in his own words, for 'law and ancient usage': see his *A Letter Relating to the Oxford University Bill, Addressed to the Right Honourable the Earl of Derby, Chancellor of the University of Oxford*, Oxford, 1854, in which it is maintained that the proposed increase in the professoriate, as well as the Bill and the Royal Commission itself, was not only novel and unconstitutional but unnecessary.

[3] Oxford, Merton College. Merton College Register, 1850, meeting of 14 December. I am grateful for permission to quote from the College's records.

[4] This committee consisted of the Warden and Messrs. Randolph, Eaton, Wilkins, and Walton. An earlier committee, specifically set up to compose a reply to the Commissioners' letter of questions, comprised Messrs. Cockerell and Farrer (who had both opposed the Warden) and Randolph and Eaton. The Warden declined to act on this committee (ibid., 1853, meeting of 12 April; 1850, meeting of 14 December). The administrative work of reform was carried out principally by Randolph and Eaton. Although clearly opinion in the College was divided, it is necessary in view of what follows to reverse the favourable tendency of Henderson's account of Merton during the period of reform (Henderson, *Merton College*, pp. 167–9).

up to consider suggestions for altering, 'where expedient', the 'present system of the College'. In response to the Commissioners' specific recommendations, it was resolved, in part, that

If it shall appear that the University is unable to provide, from its own resources, the means of endowing a sufficient number of Professorships . . . this College would, on its part, be disposed to entertain favourably proposals for supplying the deficiency by proportionate contributions from the several Colleges according to their means and circumstances . . .

Inasmuch as the College has not at present, nor is likely for sometime, to have any surplus funds applicable to the foregoing purposes, it should be enabled to raise them by a corresponding diminution in the number of fellows.[1]

Clearly, the College would rather limit the number of Fellows than reduce its corporate income, and thereby the income of each Fellow.

The Executive Commissioners[2] appointed under the Oxford University Act of 1854 began meeting in August of that year. Negotiations between the College, the Commissioners, and the Visitor of the College (the Archbishop of Canterbury) on all matters of reform continued throughout 1853–7.[3] In reply to the Commission's first routine inquiries the College drew up an amended set of resolutions, one of which was that the forming of any definite plan with respect to supporting an increased professoriate should be deferred until matters of principle had been decided upon between the Commission and the University; that a suitable scheme should 'if possible' be agreed to, and afterwards submitted to the colleges for their co-operation, 'if needed'.[4] At the same time the College announced

[1] Merton College Register, 1853, meetings of 17 May and 27 October. Cf. 'Correspondence respecting the proposed measures of improvement in the Universities and Colleges of Oxford and Cambridge', P.P., 1854, l. 226.

[2] These were the Earl of Ellesmere, Lord Harrowby, the Bishop of Ripon (C. T. Longley), the Dean of Wells (G. H. S. Johnson), Sir John Coleridge, Sir John Awdry, and Mr. Cornewall Lewis. Lewis was replaced in late 1855 by Edward Twisleton. The secretaries were Goldwin Smith, and S. W. Wayte, Fellow and tutor at Trinity College. See Ward, *Victorian Oxford*, pp. 206–7.

[3] See especially the resolution concerning the admission of 'medici', Merton College Register, 1854, meetings of 8 June and 31 October.

[4] Ibid., meetings of 4 December and 6 December. A form of these resolutions was first decided upon on 17 May 1853, after the College had heard the report of the 'internal' committee, and included those already quoted. Subsequent amendments were partly the result of decisions taken by the Archbishop of Canterbury as to the College's powers of amending its statutes.

its own plan for the improvement of its 'educational department' by the appointment of four praelectors or tutors. There being, as already stated, 'no available surplus income', it was proposed that this scheme (estimated to cost £624 a year) should be financed by the 'temporary suspension' of a limited number of fellowships.[1] The College persisted in opposing this plan to that of the Commissioners throughout the negotiations of 1855–6.

It may be noted that the resistance of a minority in Merton, and even of its Warden, to the proposals of the Universities Commissions was not so much absolute as informed by a determination that the College's resources should remain in the College's hands and be applied to the benefit of the College rather than of the University at large. The way in which Merton was forced to support the Linacre professor has a peculiar attraction, but it is in other ways a typical example of the clash of interests within Oxford.[2]

The existence of a trust under which estates at Newington and Doctors' Commons were charged annually with 'two stipends of £12 and £6 payable to two lecturers in medicine for the benefit of the University' was revealed as it were inadvertently by the Warden in his reply to the Commissioners' second routine request, for information as to the income and properties of the colleges.[3] Marsham further stated that the trust (unnamed) had not been fulfilled for many years, although attempts had been made to render it available; that the College still desired to achieve this, and contemplated the possibility of a scheme's being devised for the purpose in connection with the professoriate.[4] In June 1855 Marsham and Randolph[5] met the Commissioners to discuss 'the financial state and prospects' of Merton College. Although the 'Linacre trust' was

---

[1] Ibid., meeting of 6 December.

[2] For the immediate context, see Ward, *Victorian Oxford*, chapter 9: 'The Triumph of Reform and the Executive Commissioners'.

[3] The question which elicited this information read: 'To what trusts in favour of others than members of your Foundation is any part of your property subject?' (Merton College Register, 1854, meeting of 11 December).

[4] Ibid.; Public Record Office (P.R.O.), MSS. of Oxford University (Executive) Commission. H.O. 73.42: Merton College. Warden to Commission, received 3 March 1855.

[5] J. J. Randolph, b. 1817. B.A. (Christ Church), 1838; Fellow of Merton, 1840; tutor and dean, 1841; bursar, 1842; sub-warden, 1846; barrister-at-law (Lincoln's Inn), 1844. Randolph was evidently acquainted with both Goldwin Smith and Wayte, and the Commission's communication was with him rather

evidently not the main subject of discussion at this meeting,[1] it is clearly at this point that the Commissioners' knowledge of the endowment began to be a source of embarrassment to the College. Goldwin Smith warned Randolph after the conference that the Commissioners would wish 'to know the substance of the deeds relating to the foundation of the Linacre Lectureships',[2] and on I August the subject of the 'Lineacre [*sic*] Trust' was for the first time specifically raised at a meeting of the Warden and Fellows.[3]

  Not recorded in the minutes of this or any other meeting is the part played by Edmund Hobhouse, then a Fellow of Merton.[4] Hobhouse was in personal communication with the Commissioners, and a close friend of at least one of them (Sir John Coleridge) and possibly another (S. W. Wayte).[5] On the day after the meeting of I August Hobhouse wrote returning two letters on the subject of the Linacre trust which he had caused to be read at the meeting; and

than with the Warden, especially on confidential matters (H.O. 73.38, G. Smith to Warden, 10 December 1856). Given Marsham's attitude this is scarcely surprising, but there is also evidence that Randolph was actively sympathetic to the Commissioners' designs.

 [1] I have found no detailed account of events at this meeting, but see H.O. 73.42: Merton College. Warden to Ellesmere, 6 July 1855; and next note. Formal records of negotiations between Merton and the Commission are fewer and more nominal than in the case of other colleges because of the degree of personal acquaintance between some of the parties involved.

 [2] H.O. 73.38, Letter Book for March 1855–March 1857. G. Smith to Randolph, 28 June 1855.

 [3] Merton College Register, 1855, meeting of I August.

 [4] Edmund Hobhouse (1817–1904). B.A. (Balliol), 1838; B.D. 1851; D.D. 1858. Stood for Merton fellowship at wish of his father, Henry (of Hadspen House; Under-Secretary of State for Home Department); elected 1841. Bishop of Nelson, New Zealand, 1858–65. Hobhouse intervened in various College matters, being anxious to make College life 'a more efficient instrument of religion and learning'. He had also some interest in science, having attended Oxford lectures on natural science while studying theology at Durham, 1838–40, as well as professorial lectures on chemistry, anatomy, and mineralogy during 'a general course of study' at Oxford, 1840–1. See *Dictionary of National Biography*; memoir by his son, Walter Hobhouse, in his *Sermons and Addresses*, London, 1905. Hobhouse was also a patient of Acland, although this may be of no significance here.

 [5] See records of Hobhouse's attempts to convert St. Alban Hall and St. Edmund Hall to the use of poor clergymen's sons intending to enter the ministry: Oxford, Bodleian Library, MS. Top. Oxon. d. 35. Both Wayte and Coleridge contributed to Hobhouse's schemes. See also Ward, *Victorian Oxford*, pp. 204–6.

reporting that it had been agreed it was 'very desirable to initiate a Proposition from the College side of the Question' and that he could 'venture to promise . . . that a Proposition will issue from a half-yearly meeting at the end of October'.[1] Hobhouse's promise was made good even before this, at a meeting of 28 September in which the College agreed to offer to disgorge annually the sum of £400 towards defraying the salaries of 'such Medical Lecturers or professors' as the Commissioners might select, on condition that the College be allowed to suppress two Fellowships for the purpose. This decision was taken 'having regard as well to the circumstances of the Lineacre [*sic*] Trust endowment as to the expediency of increasing the endowments of the Professoriate in the University'. As before, the College requested power to suppress the same number of fellowships in order that the proceeds might be applied to 'educational improvements' within the College itself.[2]

By this time the Commissioners, and a majority of Fellows, evidently felt that the College's behaviour with respect to the Linacre trust placed it under a moral obligation to co-operate with the Commission. Others, however, were more concerned to know whether or not the College had sufficiently fulfilled its legal obligations in the case. On 29 September Randolph presented the College's latest proposals at a meeting of the Commission held in Oxford, after which it was conveyed to the College through its representative that the Commissioners 'did not feel justified in accepting the view at present taken by the College of the Linacre Trust' as a basis of the arrangement respecting its contribution to the professoriate, and that, since on this depended all other arrangements, it was 'useless' at present to discuss any scheme for the endowment of College lecturers (that is, the 'praelectors or tutors', who would serve only the College, not the University). The college's offer of £400 per annum was therefore declined. In reply to a further query, Goldwin Smith told Randolph that he understood the Commission to dissent from both the legal and the moral view of its obligations with respect to the Linacre foundation taken by the College, but that he would obtain an opinion from Mr. Justice

---

[1] H.O. 73.42: Merton College. Hobhouse to [member of Commission], 2 August 1855.

[2] Merton College Register, 1855, meeting of 28 September. The suppression of fellowships was itself a controversial matter elsewhere; see Ward, *Victorian Oxford*, pp. 162, 192–3.

Coleridge.[1] Coleridge's reply forestalled an attempt by the College
to display the original documents—a copy of the Will, a Deed Poll,
and two Indentures[2]—to the Commissioners as self-evident reasons
for its position.[3] The Commissioners, Coleridge said, were anxious
to assist and guide the College as far as possible, but felt they could
properly suggest nothing until an opinion had been obtained upon
'a case fully stated' as to the position of the College with regard to
the Linacre property.[4] Accordingly, at the end of October, the College put a case and the documents before its own legal adviser.[5]

The moral if not the legal case against the College must have
depended to a large extent on the increase in value of Linacre's
property over a considerable period, since the College maintained
on various occasions and in particular in the case presented to Rolt
that the stipulated sums, £6 and £12, had been paid without
intermission up to 1840.[6] Since 1840 the College had 'retained the
stipends in its own hands' and nothing had been done beyond the
payment of certain fees on behalf of students attending University
lectures.[7] Presumably the income per annum in excess of £18 had
for a very long time been made part of the corporate assets and
consequently the income of the College.[8] It is difficult to assess how

[1] H.O. 73.38, G. Smith to Randolph, 1 October 1855; idem to idem,
3 October 1855.
[2] See above, John M. Fletcher, 'Linacre's Lands and Lectureships', pp.
107–97.   [3] Merton College Register, 1855, meeting of 4 October.
[4] H.O. 73.38, G. Smith to Randolph, 5 October 1855.
[5] Rolt, Q.C. Merton College Register, 1855, meeting of 25 October.
[6] See especially Randolph's reply to a specific query of the Commissioners:
H.O. 73.41, Register of Letters Received, letter of 5 April 1856, received
7 April; H.O. 73.42: Merton College, 'Copy . . . Case for the opinion of
Mr Rolt, Q.C. . . .'. See also below, p. 276 n. 1.
[7] H.O. 73.42: Merton College, Case for Rolt.
[8] I have not been able to discover that the income from Linacre's estates
was ever entered separately at this time. Newington (which presumably
included the manors of Traces and Frognall) and Doctors' Commons merely
appear in the main rent-roll. There is no evidence that even after the Commission's investigations the income from these sources was ever specifically
applied to the support of the Linacre professor. In 1881 benefactions dating
from before 1827 which had previously been subject to special trusts were
made part of the 'general corporate property' of the College, but no mention
of Linacre's endowment was made on this occasion ('Universities of Oxford
and Cambridge Act, 1877 (Oxford). Twenty-six Statutes made by the
University of Oxford Commissioners . . . for the . . . Colleges in that University', P.P., 1882, li. 130, 132 (434, 436)).

much this excess might have been, especially as the College obviously felt obliged to account only for the amount of the stipends.
Merton claimed to have no documents to show the value of the
benefaction in 1524 or in 1549, but submitted that others of 1540,
and of 1559 and later, gave a value (annual income) of £24 clear.[1]
In the case given to Rolt and eventually to the Crown Law Officers,
no statement about the current value of the properties (let alone any
indication of what the excess had amounted to over several centuries) was given other than that it was 'now considerably greater'
than in the sixteenth century.[2] Elsewhere the Warden described the
endowment as having 'turned out profitable' for the College.[3] It can
perhaps be assumed that the Commissioners, who were generally
tactful in their dealings with the colleges,[4] would not have pressed
Merton so hard had they not been able to determine that the profits
enjoyed by the College were indeed considerable.

Evidence of the College's good intentions towards the trust was
somewhat meagre, although it is unfair to blame Marsham and his
contemporaries for the deficiencies of previous centuries or for the
difficulty experienced in establishing science teaching in the early
nineteenth. Appointments to the lectureships had been made up
until 1840, although admittedly no lectures had been read for many
years previous to that date.[5] The College also claimed to have made
'attempts by negotiation with the medical authorities of the university to render the lectureships available . . . but in consequence of

---

[1] H.O. 73.42: Merton College, Case for Rolt. 1524 is the year of Linacre's
death; 1549, that in which Tunstal transferred Linacre's property to Merton.
1540 is the date of the abortive agreement with Brasenose; 1559, that of the
first appointment of a lecturer at Merton. See above, Fletcher, op. cit., p. 146.

[2] H.O. 73.42: Merton College, Case for Rolt. I owe to Mr. John Burgass
of Merton College the information that 'No. 4 Knight Rider Street' (the
Doctors' Commons estate) was sold by Merton in 1862 for £2,528. The
original statement made to the Commissioners by the Warden gave the
current 'estimated value' of the Newington and London estates respectively
as £613 and £580. (Ibid., Warden to Commission, received 3 March 1855.)

[3] Ibid., Warden to Wayte, 3 July 1856.

[4] Ward, *Victorian Oxford*, p. 209.

[5] H.O. 73.42: Merton College, Case for Rolt. The 'Senior Linacre' and
'Junior Linacre' appointments recorded each year for the period 1822–39
involved six Fellows, one of whom (Capel) held the senior 'lectureship'
1822–9, 1831–2, 1834–8; another, Whish, held one or the other of the appointments for 14 years consecutively. From 1840 both positions are recorded as
vacant. Merton College Register, 1822–42.

the insufficiency of the stipends, without effect'.[1] The existence of
the trust had been disclosed, to the Executive Commissioners if not
during the more public proceedings of 1850–2, and the Warden had,
as already noted, made some statement of good intent, more or less
nullified by his and the College's later behaviour. As the College
itself implied, the strength of its position rested not on moral but
on legal grounds, and, in some quarters, on its willingness to put
forward its own schemes for reform. A certain flexibility was given
to the situation by the circumstance that the terms of Tunstal's
agreement with Merton had apparently never been embodied in the
College's Statutes.[2]

It cannot be said of the College that a majority within it desired
to make no change in the administration of Linacre's endowment.
Rolt was informed that Merton wished to 'augment the stipends to
secure the delivery of competent lectures and to connect them per-
manently with the Medical Professorships of the University'. This

[1] H.O. 73.42: Merton College, Case for Rolt. During the period of
'Academical reform' (Goldwin Smith), before the Tractarian movement,
Merton had revised its financial affairs at some length and also set up a
committee of five including the Warden, Cockerell, and J. R. Hope (allegedly
the moving spirit at this time), to make up from the documents a complete
set of 'College laws' as well as to report on 'the objects of the Foundation'.
This investigation resulted primarily in resolutions aimed at increasing the
number and commitment of clerical Fellows (Merton College Register, 1837,
meeting of 30 March; 1838, meeting of 20 April; 1839, meeting of 5 April;
Henderson, *Merton College*, pp. 167–8). These resolutions failed of their effect
but more radical suggestions (e.g. that of Compton, that Fellows should
engage in the professions of law and medicine) failed more completely
(Merton College Register, 1846, meetings of 3 June and 14 November). On
23 April 1840, in the course of similar business, it was resolved 'that measures
be taken . . . to ascertain in what manner *the annual sums appointed for Linacres
lectureship* [*sic*] may be applied with most advantage, and that in the meantime no appointment be made to these offices'. The Principal of the Post-
masters (Bigge) was asked to prepare a report on the subject. (Ibid., 1840,
meeting of 23 April. My italics; see below.) There is no record in the Register
either of Bigge's report or of any approach made to the University.

[2] The College makes this assertion in the case put to Rolt, and it is borne
out by the absence of any reference to Linacre in the statutes referred to by
Commissions in the 1850s (which were not provided by Merton, but put
together from published and MS. sources outside the College). *Statutes of the
Colleges of Oxford; with Royal Patents of Foundation, Injunctions of Visitors, and
Catalogues of Documents . . . Preserved in the Public Record Office. Merton College.*
Printed by desire of Her Majesty's Commissioners, Oxford/London, 1853.
See also above, Fletcher, op. cit., pp. 143–6.

statement could, however, be interpreted to mean something very much less than had already been offered by the College. The point of law to be determined by Rolt is defined more overtly:

> Whether, after determining the amount payable in respect of the lectureships, it will be a sufficient execution of the Trust if such amount be paid in augmentation of the salaries of the medical professors on condition that lectures be read, not on the original books but according to present needs.[1]

One might at this point credit the College with at least a scrupulous regard for Linacre's expressed wishes, except that a few lectures would not at all have met current needs, and lecturing alone was perhaps the least of the expenses involved in medical education.

Rolt's brief opinion, given at the end of the year, was cast entirely in terms of the College's observance of the letter of the law. The construction of the original documents was, he thought, 'doubtful', but the College 'could not be obliged by any court to go beyond' the stipends of £6 and £12. The plan suggested was, in his view, a 'sufficient execution'; it represented indeed a deviation sufficient to render necessary the previous sanction of the Court in Chancery, but 'for practical purposes' the College could 'rely that should the matter be ever hereafter questioned the past application of the Income according to the proposed scheme will be sanctioned and confirmed by the Court'.[2] In sum, Rolt's opinion could be interpreted as implying that the College might fulfil all its legal obligations with respect to Linacre's endowment merely by contributing £6 and £12 respectively to the annual incomes of the medical professorships already in existence in the University; and it seems certain that the Warden at least had never contemplated anything else, even at the time of his disclosure of the existence of Linacre's trust. Doubtless the College could have expected other arrangements brought about by the Commission to render this procedure more effective than it had been judged in 1840.

On receipt of Rolt's favourable opinion, the College sent off the case, the opinion itself, and copies of the original documents to the Commission. The reaction of the Commissioners can only be inferred from their immediately (as they were increasingly having to

[1] H.O. 73.42: Merton College, Case for Rolt.
[2] Ibid. The 'proposed scheme' was of course the plan suggested by the College in the case put to Rolt, not that proposed to the Commissioners in September and involving an annual expenditure of £400.

do) seeking a legal opinion of their own, from the Crown Law
Officers. This second opinion was unequivocal and its terms may
have surprised the Commissioners themselves. Referring principally
to the conditions under which Linacre intended his estates to be
conveyed to the Mercers' Company, the Law Officers stated that
the *only* purpose of the bequest was the support of professorships,
and that 'the *whole* of the income derived from *all* the lands conveyed
to Merton College was applicable and ought to be devoted to the
endowment and maintenance of the Professors and Schools of Medicine in the University of Oxford'.[1] Not content with this, the
Officers went on to declare that 'the application which has hitherto
been made of the rents of the Estates appears to have been a breach
of trust on the part of Merton College, to whom great blame is
attributable for their neglect of this important Charity'. The opinion
concluded with a course of action to be taken against the College
by the Attorney-General to ensure the 'due application of the
whole of the rents and profits of the devised estates'.[2]

Apparently no such drastic action was necessary. The opinion of
the Law Officers was forwarded to the College in March 1856, and
on 31 May the Commissioners informed Merton that

having regard to the obligation of the College in respect of the Linacre
Trust, and also to their own duties in regard to rendering portions
of the Property or Income of the Colleges available to purposes for the
benefit of the University at large . . . the Commissioners are of opinion
that £800 a year will not be too large a sum to be contributed to the
Professoriate by Merton College.

It was to be left to the College whether the contribution should be
made by annexing certain professorships to the College or, as
proposed by the College itself in the first instance, by its paying
over the sum of £800 a year to the University for application to the
purposes of the professoriate.[3] Randolph, or the College through
Randolph (although there had been no College meeting), made some
reply to this communication and the Commissioners, after recon-
sidering the subject, made in response the more specific proposal
that 'there shall be in Merton College a Professor of Physiology, to

[1] H.O. 73.42: Merton College, 'Case in the Matter of Merton College re
Linacre's Estate. For the Opinion of the Attorney and Solicitor General . . .'.
My italics.
[2] Ibid.
[3] H.O. 73.38: Wayte to Warden, 31 May 1856.

be called the Linacre Professor, with a salary of £800 a year'. The nature and title of the professorship, now defined for the first time, were both evidently the suggestion of the Commissioners. Doubtless they took advice on this matter, possibly from Acland who had met the Commissioners in February at his own request, to discuss matters raised by the Commission in the questionnaire sent out to existing Oxford professors in December of the previous year.[1] Wayte's letter to Randolph stated in explanation merely that a professorship of physiology was 'generally considered necessary', and that the subject seemed sufficiently cognate with those specifically mentioned by Linacre as the object of his foundation. Wayte added, perhaps rather largely, that the University already had foundations for medicine and anatomy.[2] On 24 June the College met and agreed to both the Commission's proposals, only resolving 'that such Linacre Professor be not a Fellow of the College', and that the endowment should be raised as the College had first suggested, that is by the suppression of fellowships, rather than by a subtraction from the corporate income of the College.[3] The Commissioners wrote immediately to express their satisfaction and to empower the suppression not only of the four fellowships required to endow the Linacre Professor but of two more, for the College's purposes of 'augmenting the Scholarships and instituting new [College] Lectureships'.[4]

The Warden continued, though without visible effect, to show his resistance to these events. His personal view, submitted in a lengthy letter to Wayte early in July, was that the bequest, having been offered first to the Mercers and then to Brasenose, was in no respect connected with Merton and that the College must have accepted it merely as a speculation. It might even have represented a loss to Merton, since the stipends would have had to be paid no matter what the income from Linacre's estates. In the Warden's opinion, Linacre had made no deposition of the residue; and the 'ablest counsel', consulted at the suggestion of the Commissioners themselves, had merely confirmed the College's view that its liability did not extend beyond the two annuities. Marsham was

[1] H.O. 73.41: Acland to Wayte, received 9 February 1856; H.O. 73.40: Minute Book, p. 88.

[2] H.O. 73.38: Wayte to Randolph, 12 June 1856.

[3] Merton College Register, 1856, meeting of 24 June; H.O. 73.42: Merton College, Randolph to Wayte, 25 June 1856. But see below, p. 280.

[4] H.O. 73.38: Wayte to Warden, 27 June 1856.

here able to cite the example of St. John's College, Cambridge, which had also never increased the amount of the lecturers' stipends above that specified by Linacre himself. Given the conflict of legal opinion, the Warden concluded, the College ought not to be charged to the extent or in the manner proposed without the decree of the Court in Chancery. Even if that Court decided against the College, only Chancery was truly able to license such a deviation from the intentions of both Linacre and Walter de Merton as was represented by the proposed Professorship of Physiology. A lectureship held on the conditions of a fellowship was in all respects a more proper institution than a life professorship, and the College was of course as capable of making a good appointment as any board of electors. Marsham added that if, for some reason, professors were thought the most desirable of all aids to education, then they should be financed out of the profits of the University Press.[1]

Further negotiation between the College and the Commission, largely on financial questions, was still necessary and the ordinance setting up the Linacre professorship had to be sealed separately and as late as April 1857. However, the delay was owing less to the resistance of the Warden or even to the College's objection to the proposed gradual restoration of its suppressed fellowships, than to the Commission's communications with the University authorities as to the relation in which the Linacre professorship was to stand to the other professorships of cognate subjects.[2] For example, the Commissioners were suggesting in October 1856 to the Hebdomadal Council that the foundation of a professorship of physiology at

---

[1] H.O. 73.42: Merton College. Warden to Wayte, 3 July 1856. The Warden did not receive a (formal) reply until October, when Goldwin Smith wrote that the Commissioners regretted Marsham could not approve their measures but that they still felt it desirable to adhere to the arrangement as accepted by a majority of the College (H.O. 73.38: G. Smith to Warden, 13 October 1856).

For another attempt from a different quarter on the recently disclosed profits of the Press, see Atlay, *Memoir*, pp. 202–3, 206 n.

[2] H.O. 73.38, G. Smith to Warden, 5 December 1856; 20 February 1857; and pp. 277 ff. See also H.O. 73.44: Part I: University, and ibid., Part II End: University. The College's objection to restoration was ostensibly that the income fixed for the reconstituted fellowships, £250 a year, would not attract worthwhile candidates. Its real objection was probably to the diminution in all incomes of fellowships which would be caused by restoration (see also above, p. 270).

Merton would enable Council to propose to the University the consolidation of existing medical professorships of small value, with a view to the adequate endowment of a professorship of medicine.[1] The establishment of Merton's professorship should be seen as part of a context in which the Commission, after protracted consultation and negotiation, prepared a plan for the extension of the professoriate involving contributions to it of £600 a year and over in the case of six colleges, and of the income of one fellowship in the case of five more.[2] The part of this plan which concerned Merton succeeded, because, one could say, of Merton's abuse of the Linacre endowment; other parts did not.[3] It should, however, be emphasized that Merton would have been asked to contribute to the support of the professoriate regardless of the existence of Linacre's trust.

The ordinance published in June 1857 provided that, in the case of Merton,

the emoluments of certain Fellowships within Merton College, being the third, fifth, seventh and ninth, which should fall vacant after the approval of the said Ordinance . . . shall, to an amount not exceeding 800 l. *per annum*, be applied to the maintenance within the said University of a Professorship of Physiology, . . . to be called the Linacre Professorship of Physiology.[4]

Election to the professorship was vested in the Visitor and the Warden of Merton, the Presidents of the Royal Colleges of Physicians and of Surgeons, and the President of the Royal Society. The University was to define the professor's duties by statute; the professor was not to engage in the practice of medicine or surgery.[5] Later, the University to some degree accepted responsibility for

[1] H.O. 73.38, G. Smith to Vice-Chancellor, 13 October 1856.

[2] This plan was first presented as a whole to the colleges in July, and to Hebdomadal Council in October 1856 (ibid., pp. 277 ff.). For Council's reply, see H.O. 73.44: Part I: University, Vice-Chancellor to Commission, 11 November 1856. Council's reaction to the Linacre professorship proposal in particular was that it would be 'advantageous' to the University.

[3] For some verdicts on the work of the Executive Commission, see Ward, *Victorian Oxford*, p. 209; Atlay, *Memoir*, pp. 250–1.

[4] 'Oxford University: Ordinances framed by the Oxford University Commissioners, under 17 and 18 Vict. c. 81, in relation to New . . . and Merton Colleges, respectively', P.P., 1857, Sess. 2, xxxii. 138 (292).

[5] That the professor should not practise was a recommendation of Hebdomadal Council as well as the request of the College (H.O. 73.44: Part II: University, Vice-Chancellor to Commission, 20 March 1857; H.O. 73.41: Warden to Commission, 2 April 1857).

the teaching of anatomy[1] (not necessarily human anatomy) by the transfer of the Tomlins Readership in Anatomy (1624) and the Aldrichian Professorship of Anatomy (1803), from the Regius to the Linacre professorship, which then became known as the 'Linacre Professorship of Anatomy and Physiology'. The intention was that the lesser endowments should provide the salary of an assistant to the Linacre professor.[2]

The first Linacre professor, George Rolleston,[3] had taken a first in Greats in 1850 and then been diverted into medicine by the offer of a fellowship founded in 1846 for the 'furtherance of study in law and physic'. After an absence he returned to Oxford, was appointed a physician at the Radcliffe Infirmary, and Dr. Lee's Reader on the election of Acland to the Regius professorship in 1858. Rolleston's appointment as Linacre professor (1860) coincided with the opening of the University Museum, and he at once became responsible for all the biological teaching within it as well as for the collections which were finding a home there. Rolleston had practised as a physician but he was temperamentally much better suited to research, and he immediately became engaged in 'Biological work of the widest kind' (Acland). The results of this work appeared as *The Forms of Animal Life* (1870). To the large areas assigned to him by statute—physiology, human and comparative anatomy—Rolleston added another, the then comparatively new science of anthropology, in which he was personally much interested. 'Biology' in its less wide sense, he once explained, was equivalent to the older and previously more common word, 'physiology'; but in its wider sense, it included animal and vegetable physiology, and anatomy, ethnology, anthropology, scientific zoology, and taxonomic botany.[4]

Rolleston was obviously, on philosophical grounds, an enemy to

---

[1] See H. M. Sinclair and A. H. T. Robb-Smith, *A Short History of Anatomical Teaching in Oxford*, Oxford, 1950.

[2] H.O. 73.44: Part II: University, Vice-Chancellor to Commission, 1 April 1857. The intention was carried out in that in 1860 Charles Robertson, already an associate of Rolleston, was appointed 'Aldrichian Demonstrator of Anatomy' and keeper of the physiological collection in the Museum (Sinclair and Robb-Smith, op. cit., p. 60 and App. I).

[3] George Rolleston (1829–81). M.B. 1854; M.D. 1857; F.R.C.P. 1859. See George Rolleston, *Scientific Papers and Addresses*, ed. W. Turner with a biographical sketch by E. B. Tylor, 2 vols., Oxford, 1884.

[4] G. Rolleston, *Address to the Biological Section of the British Association. Liverpool, September 14th, 1870*, London, 1870, p. 7.

specialization in science, and Acland was later to deplore the removal of his influence in this respect. However, he had been accused of over-diversification well before his death in 1881, and with more and more justification, since the sciences in which he was most interested were growing rapidly. He had himself advised the sub-division of his professorship[1] and this was also recommended by Lord Salisbury's Commission in 1877. A friend and pupil, H. Nottidge Moseley,[2] who had travelled as a naturalist with the *Challenger* expedition (1872–6), accordingly became Linacre Professor of Human and Comparative Anatomy; E. B. Tylor,[3] author of *Researches into the Early History of Mankind and the Development of Civilisation*, 1865, and *Primitive Culture: Researches into the Development of Mythology, Philosophy, Religion, Art and Custom*, 1871, and a keeper in the University Museum since 1883, was made Reader in Anthropology in 1884; and in 1883, after a delay, John Burdon Sanderson[4] came from University College, London, to become the first Waynflete Professor of Physiology, a post supported by Magdalen College.[5] It is clear that, for the most part, the successive incumbents of posts in science subjects in Oxford were drawn from a small group interconnected either through the pupil–teacher relationship or because the younger man was already in some other, often informally established, post in the University.

[1] Printed letter from George Rolleston to the Vice-Chancellor of Oxford University, dated 7 May 1873 and beginning 'Dear Mr. Vice-Chancellor . . .' (no other title, date, or place; unpaginated). There is a copy of this open letter in 'Oxford Science, 1858–1893', a bound volume of offprints, leaflets, etc. in the Library of the Museum of the History of Science, Oxford.

[2] Henry Nottidge Moseley (1844–91). Gained a 1st class in Natural Sciences School under Rolleston, 1861; on a Radcliffe Travelling Fellowship (1869) to Vienna and Leipzig; F.R.S. 1879. See an obituary by his friend E. Ray Lankester in *Nature*, 26 November 1891, pp. 79–80.

[3] Sir Edward Burnett Tylor (1832–1917), first Professor of Anthropology at Oxford, 1896. See A. Lang in *Anthropological Essays Presented to Edward Burnett Tylor*, Oxford, 1907.

[4] Sir John Scott Burdon Sanderson (1828–1905). Studied in Paris under Bernard; M.D. Edinburgh, 1851; F.R.C.P. 1878; Professor of Practical Physiology and Histology at University College, London, 1871; Jodrell Professor of Physiology, 1874; Regius Professor of Medicine at Oxford, 1895–1903. See Lady John Scott Burdon Sanderson, J. S. Haldane, and E. S. Haldane, *Sir John Burdon Sanderson, a memoir . . . with a selection from his papers and addresses*, Oxford, 1911.

[5] The Waynflete professorships were first projected in 1855. See above, pp. 268–9.

It should not be imagined that the initiative enforced by the Act of 1854 was sufficient to establish a flourishing Natural Science School in Oxford, or that the developments which did take place were entirely satisfactory. One obvious barrier to progress was the independent status of the University. By contrast with Germany, the English universities were private institutions, which received little State aid. Furthermore, as was implicit in the work of the Commissions of the 1850s, Oxford University as an institution had very few resources and was therefore at the mercy of the rich and largely independent colleges. Statutory changes were made only to be stultified in operation by the lack of continuous provision for the scientific instruction of students within the colleges. The colleges, again, were most unwilling to devote fellowships or other revenue to the support of research workers in scientific and other subjects, and this was a major obstacle as late as 1895.[1] It was, as Burdon Sanderson in particular discovered, one thing to be appointed a professor, and another to be given the financial support necessary for accommodation, equipment, and the appointment of junior staff. Gladstone's Commission of 1872–4 was a tardy admission of the importance of financial factors.

Another problem experienced by Acland and Rolleston was the growing opposition of many of the medical profession to the development of what Acland called 'a purely scientific school of biology' at Oxford. The highest pitch of the controversy over the so-called 'lost medical school' coincided with the consideration of the Medical Act Amendment Bill by the General Medical Council, of which Acland was then (1878) President and Rolleston a long-standing member.[2] The Council, a much criticized body, was at this time being condemned as unrepresentative by vocal members of the profession who demanded direct independent representation or at least that the Council should include representatives of the provincial medical schools. Not much interest had been taken in Oxford affairs in the 1850s, before the passing of the first Medical Act which set up the Council; but by the late 1870s it appeared to some medical men that the medical school which they had always seen as at least potentially

[1] See, e.g., E. Ray Lankester, Preface to *Linacre Reports*, ii, 1895; F. Max Müller, *My Autobiography: A Fragment*, London, 1901, pp. 260–1.
[2] On medical reform in general, see J. Simon, *Public Health Reports*, ed. E. Seaton, 2 vols., London, 1887; and the unsatisfactory W. H. McMenemey, *The Life and Times of Sir Charles Hastings*, London, 1959.

present at Oxford had been stolen from them, and its revenues per-
verted, by the Regius Professor of Medicine and the Linacre Professor of Anatomy and Physiology. Part of their resentment may
have been caused by the knowledge that, without allies in the
universities (whose medical schools were, to them, most justly seen
as provincial medical schools), there was no possibility of breaking
the power of the only other licensing bodies, the London corporations. More generally, the situation at Oxford aroused the fear,
always dormant in the minds of physicians, that medical research
and teaching would fall into the hands not of specialized medical
scientists but of specialists outside the profession.

A lively and often rather discreditable debate ensued, which is
best documented in the pages of the *British Medical Journal*. The
Journal, being the organ of the society which had grown out of the
Provincial Medical and Chirurgical Society, took an active part in
the affair. In spite of the personal nature of the attacks made upon
him, Acland made no attempt to reply to his critics until many years
later. In 1890, he expressed the hope that Dr. Burdon Sanderson
would 'resist the pressure put upon him to restrict his wide purposes and deep scientific insight into the principles of life, within
the supposed limits of study proper for a provincial Medical School',
and then went on to reflect that

some of us, perhaps, overvalued the total effect on human nature of
material investigation and natural knowledge . . . Reaction is beginning. I trust it will not go too far. We are taking, moreover, a utilitarian path. In our zeal for technical and practical progress, under the
pressure of insular over-population, we are praising our Science chiefly
for its material advantages, not for its truth and its discipline.[1]

In the meantime, both Rolleston and Acland were defended by their
pupils, and others expressed their belief in the benefits of 'domesti-
cating . . . professional study in a place of general culture'[2] or in the
leavening effect of the more mature Oxford student upon his wilder
London counterpart. As when the question was first raised (in a few
minds) in the 1850s, much surprisingly inconclusive discussion
centred on the possibility or otherwise of using a comparatively
small local hospital like the Radcliffe Infirmary as a teaching hospital. Analogies with German practice were, as on all similar occasions,
employed. At the end of the controversy, it was apparent that a

[1] Acland, *Oxford and Modern Medicine*, pp. 32, 40.
[2] Acland quoting Goldwin Smith, ibid., pp. 25–6.

body of informed opinion favoured an expansion of medical studies at Oxford, some requiring the establishment of a complete medical school, and others merely the greater development of anatomy and physiology.

No great changes followed this controversy; rather, there was a gradual accumulation of men at Oxford with particular interests in medical science, and an eventual resumption of the relations between the medical faculty and the Infirmary.[1] Burdon Sanderson is often given credit for refounding the Oxford Medical School,[2] but Sanderson's own intention was merely to make pathology (with a unique bias towards practical work) the special study at Oxford, and he took no interest in the clinical side of teaching. With respect to the teaching of anatomy, the Linacre professor was first given, at Sanderson's instigation, the assistance of a Lecturer in Human Anatomy, who was to teach the medical students; then, following the succession to the Linacre chair of E. Ray Lankester[3] in 1891, the title of the professorship was altered to exclude any reference to human anatomy. Lankester, as the Linacre Professor of Comparative Anatomy, reserved for himself only 'the treatment of man's structure as part of the general science of morphology'.[4]

Moseley's term of active service as Linacre professor had been short; Lankester made more of an impression. While still Jodrell Professor of Zoology at University College, London, but also tutor and Fellow at Exeter College, Oxford, he had taken part in the 'lost medical school' controversy, stressing the indivisibility of theory and practice[5] and the necessity therefore of close ties between

---

[1] Acland held the Lichfield Clinical Professorship as well as the Regius. See Atlay, *Memoir*, pp. 241–4. Gibson finds that 'clinical teaching was in abeyance' for most of the latter half of the century, and states that the connection between the medical school and the Infirmary was at its loosest about 1880. Gibson, *The Radcliffe Infirmary*, pp. 267, 261.

[2] See, e.g., *Dict. Nat. Biog.*; K. J. Franklin, 'A Short Sketch of the History of the Oxford Medical School', *Annals of Science*, i, 1936, 431–46.

[3] Sir Edwin Ray Lankester (1847–1929). Gained 1st class in Natural Science School, 1868, with H. N. Moseley and under Rolleston; Radcliffe Travelling Fellowship, 1870. Studied in Vienna, Leipzig, Naples. Jodrell Professor of Zoology at University College, London, 1874; F.R.S. 1875. Director of the natural history departments and keeper of zoology in British Museum, 1898. See *Dict. Nat. Biog.*

[4] E. Ray Lankester, 'Human and Comparative Anatomy at Oxford', *Nature*, 26 October 1893, p. 617.

[5] Lankester cites Billroth in this connection: *British Medical Journal*, 1878

the medical faculty and the Infirmary. He was, however, thinking less of the functioning of an independent medical school than of the needs of resident research workers. As may be seen in a review by him of the work of Metchnikoff, 'a biologist revolutionising medicine' by comparative work on invertebrates, Lankester thought that the education of physicians, physiologists, and medical scientists generally was far too narrow. Zoology, comparative anatomy, and embryology were ignored.[1] Many medical men did not of course agree with Acland, Rolleston, or Lankester about the extent of scientific knowledge and experience desirable in a medical training.

The manner in which Lankester urged the claims of pure science and of research as a profession, and criticized the indifference and parsimony of the University, made him notorious. 'For the purpose of affording evidence to members of the University not conversant with the literature of Comparative Anatomy, that the laboratories and collections under his charge [were] being made the means of producing new knowledge', Lankester published a short series of *Linacre Reports*[2] which comprised accounts of original contributions made by his students (most of them previously published in the *Quarterly Journal of Microscopical Science*, of which he was then editor).[3] The *Oxford Magazine* thought this 'striking *Apologia pro scientia sua*' not calculated to remove the prejudice in favour of 'the proper study of mankind' of 'students of historical and other sciences'.[4]

Lankester resigned the Linacre chair in 1899. In the present century, his post matured into the Linacre Professorship of Zoology in the Faculty of Biological and Agricultural Sciences, having become a professorship of zoology and comparative anatomy in 1915, and changing its title to the present form in 1961.

(i), p. 245. For a letter by Billroth to 'an English *confrère*' in reply to 'inquiries respecting the advisability of extending the Medical Faculty in Oxford', see ibid., pp. 271–2.

[1] *Nature*, 31 March 1892, pp. 505–6.
[2] The 'medallion portrait' of Linacre used on the cover of the Reports was obtained for Lankester by J. F. Payne, who like his friend had been a pupil of Rolleston, and who was from 1899 Harveian Librarian at the Royal College of Physicians. See Margaret Pelling, 'Published References to Thomas Linacre', below, p. 346; Preface to *Linacre Reports*, i, 1894.
[3] Ibid.
[4] *Oxford Magazine*, xii, no. 14, 1894, 216.

The history of the establishment of modern science and medicine at Cambridge has obvious similarities but is of equal interest.[1] Very generally, it may be said that the natural sciences were more slowly, and medicine more readily, established there. As to differences in method, the Cambridge don Leslie Stephen wrote (anonymously) in 1865 that the Oxford reformer was apt to be 'a democrat in kid gloves', admiring metaphysics and general principles, and inclining to the 'coxcombry of politics'. Of his own university Stephen said, 'We introduce reforms when we want them and make no fuss about them.'[2]

Unfortunately, there is not even the most tenuous connection between Linacre and changes at Cambridge. The income from Linacre's estate was perceptible until quite recently, but was used throughout the nineteenth century straightforwardly to augment the incomes of medical fellows of St. John's College or (on two occasions) the incomes of members of the medical faculty. Only seven persons are concerned: Sir Isaac Pennington, who held the 'Linacre Readership' from 1767 to 1817; John Haviland, Regius Professor of Medicine from 1817 to 1851 (1817–22, and again 1826–47); the well-known London physician Thomas Watson (1822–6); Henry Thompson (1847–51); George Paget, Regius Professor 1872–92 and one of the (three) progenitors of the modern medical school at Cambridge (1851–72); John Buckle Bradbury (1872–94); and (Sir) Donald MacAlister (1894–1907).[3] J. F. Payne, writing in 1881 in a biography of Linacre, refers to the 'Linacre Reader of Pathology', no doubt because the then recipient, J. B. Bradbury, was giving lectures in pathology and medical anatomy at that time. Payne found this application of Linacre's endowment not discreditable, since 'the present Linacre Reader of Pathology fills with credit a chair most inadequately endowed, and has revived at Cambridge the public teachings of a study perfectly congruous with, though different from that which was intended by the founder'. He added that it was 'impossible to doubt that Linacre looked forward to

[1] Much less has been written on the subject of reform in Cambridge, but see here H. D. Rolleston, *The Cambridge Medical School: A Biographical History*, Cambridge, 1932, and A. Rook (ed.), *Cambridge and its Contribution to Medicine*, London, 1971.

[2] [L. Stephen], *Sketches from Cambridge, By a Don*, London, 1865, p. 138.

[3] All these details may be found in the chapter on the 'Linacre Lectureship in Physic' in Rolleston, *The Cambridge Medical School*. See also above, R. G. Lewis, 'The Linacre Lectureships subsequent to their Foundation', pp. 261–2.

founding what should essentially be a school of medicine in each University'.[1]

No relation could be expected to subsist between Linacre's original design and the needs of the nineteenth century other than the generic one suggested here by Payne. It would of course be absurd to charge the Victorians with misappropriation because the Linacre professor at Oxford is no longer a member of the medical school. One may note, however, that Linacre intended his lectures to be given for the benefit not of particular colleges but of the University as a whole and that some capital was made of this by nineteenth-century reformers.[2]

In 1865, St. John's College sold outright the property which they had (it seems imprudently) exchanged for that originally settled on them by Linacre.[3] According to H. D. Rolleston, the College records do not show how the sum realized was invested; but in 1908 a new arrangement was instituted, on the same general plan as the Rede Lectureship (a Cambridge foundation, also dating from 1524), whereby a single 'Linacre Lecture' was to be given annually by a 'man of mark', usually a distinguished member of the medical profession. The honorarium was fixed at 10 guineas.[4] These lectures have frequently been of a literary or reflective character, but have also been made the vehicle for original communications. Appropriately, the first and one of the most distinguished contributions in this series was William Osler's lecture on Thomas Linacre, which perfectly represents the persistence of the humanist ideal in twentieth-century medicine.[5]

[1] Payne, Introduction to *Galeni Pergamensis de temperamentis et de inaequali intemperie libri tres Thoma Linacro Anglo interprete*, Facsimile edn., Cambridge, 1881, pp. 32–3. For a contribution by Payne to the 'lost medical school' controversy, see *British Medical Journal*, 1878 (i), pp. 138–40.

[2] See above, pp. 271 ff. This was so in general in that the reformers of the earlier period, like their opponents, cited precedent whenever possible. Cf. the case of the better-known lectureships founded by Waynflete and Fox (e.g., P.P., 1852, xxii. 325, 207–8; and above, pp. 268–9).

[3] Payne, *Galeni . . . de temperamentis*, p. 32; Rolleston, *The Cambridge Medical School*, p. 7.

[4] Rolleston, p. 219.

[5] *Thomas Linacre*, Cambridge, 1908. For a complete list of the lectures to 1931, see Rolleston, *The Cambridge Medical School*, pp. 219–20. For some others, see Pelling, below, pp. 338, 348–52.

Thomas Linacre: A Bibliographical Survey of his Works

GILES BARBER*

I. *Linacre's Personal Publishing History*

ALTHOUGH LINACRE MAY HAVE SPENT SOME TIME with Aldus Manutius, the Venetian printer, at the end of his stay in Italy and may have been so concerned in the latter's work that in the preface to the 1497 *editio princeps* of Aristotle Aldus wrote of him as 'Thomas Anglicus homo et Graece et Latine peritissimus', he does not seem to have published anything before his return to England in 1499. Of several projects in hand that year, including translations of the commentary of Simplicius on Aristotle's *Physics* and that of Alexander of Aphrodisias on the *Meteorologica*,[1] he seems first to have completed that of the *Sphaera* of Proclus. Linacre dedicated this work to Arthur Prince of Wales (who was to die in 1502), since, as he puts it, of all his present lucubrations this was the text most likely to help the Prince with his literary and other studies. An undated manuscript copy of the work written in a fine italic hand with initials in the English style survives in the library of Trinity College, Cambridge.[2]

Linacre must, however, also have sent his translation to Aldus for printing, and it was included by the latter at the end of the volume of collected astronomical texts which was completed in October

---

* Fellow of Linacre College, Oxford. Librarian, The Taylor Institution, Oxford University.

[1] P. O. Kristeller, *Catalogus translationum et commentariorum*, Washington, 1960, i. 100.

[2] M. R. James, *The Western Manuscripts in the Library of Trinity College, Cambridge*, Cambridge, 1901, ii. 347 (MS. 936).

1499. Before the Greek and Latin texts Aldus printed not only Linacre's dedication but also his own letter to Alberto Pio present-ing Linacre's work to their friend, and a similar letter from William Grocyn to himself. The whole work is therefore closely connected with Linacre's Italian period and friends.

Since the fifteenth century the Greek text Σφαῖρα has generally been ascribed to Proclus (A.D. 410–85), the chief representative of the later Neoplatonists and commonly surnamed Diadochus by reference to his being the 'successor' of Plato. However, it has been suggested by P. Tannery that the text was really an extract, made by a Byzantine monk, from the work of the earlier Stoic philosopher, Geminus of Rhodes.[1]

A. Proclus, *De sphaera* 1499.

General title: Iulii Firmici Astronomicorum libri octo integri, & emen| dati, ex Scythicis oris ad nos nuper allati. | Marci Manilii astronomicorum libri quinque. | Arati Phaenomena Germanico Caesare interprete cum com-| mentariis & imaginibus. | Arati eiusdem phaenomenon fragmentum Marco T.C. interprete. Arati eiusdem Phaenomenon Russo Festo Auienio paraphraste. | | Arati eiusdem Phaenomena graece | Theonis commentaria copiosissima in Arati Phaeno-| mena graece. | Procli Diadochi Sphaera graece| Procli eiusdem Sphaera, Thoma Linacro Britanno interprete. |

A first colophon at the end of the Firmicus text is dated June 1499 but the second, on sig. T8, reads: Venetiis cura, & diligentia Aldi Ro. Mense octob. | M.ID. Cui concessum est ab Ill.S.V. ne hos | quoq; libros alii cuiquam impune for-| mis excudere liceat. |

Collation: Folio. *⁶a–g¹⁰, h¹², 2a–2h¹⁰, 2i–2k⁸, A–D¹⁰, E¹², F⁶, G–M¹⁰, N⁶, [2] N–S¹⁰, T⁸.

The Greek text of Proclus occupies S6 verso to S9 verso and the title to Linacre's translation on T1 reads: PROCLI DIADOCHI SPHAERA, ASTRONOMI | AM DISCERE INCIPIENTIBVS VTILISSIMA. | THOMA LINACRO BRITANNO INTER-| PRETE, AD ARCTVRVM, CORNV-| BIAE, VALLIAEQVE ILLVSTRIS|SIMVM PRINCIPEM| *******|*****|***|*|. On T1 verso and T2 are Aldus's and Grocyn's letters and on T2 verso

[1] *Catalogue général des livres imprimés de la Bibliothèque nationale*, Paris, 1937, cxliii, col. 174.

Linacre's dedication to the Prince of Wales. The text occupies T3 to T6 verso, with the index on T7.

Linacre's edition of Proclus was an immense success and was reprinted almost at once in Wittenberg, Reggio Emilia, Leipzig, and Paris. The first English edition appeared in 1522, two years before Linacre's death. It is noticeable that of all his works the Proclus was the most consistently popular, some thirty editions appearing in the sixteenth century at an almost regular rhythm of three or four each decade.

The other translations which, according to Aldus, Linacre had in hand never reached print and it seems likely that in the next ten years he was too busy for such pursuits. Indeed, the whole history of his next book is shrouded in mystery and even the date of its publication is uncertain.

B. Linacre, *Progymnasmata grammatices vulgaria* [1511?]. Edition of *c.* 1515 described.

> Title-page: (Black letter) ¶ Linacri progymnasmata | Grammatices vulgaria |
> Collation: 12⁰, A⁶, b–f⁶, g⁴. Unpaginated.
> Contents: A1 title; A1ᵛ poems by Linacre, T. More, W. Lily; A2 text; g² ¶ Erroris quorūdam in hoc opusculo Recognitio; g3ᵛ blank; g⁴ ¶ Empryntyd in Londoñ on ye sowth syde of | paulys by Johñ Rastell with ye priuylege | of our most suuerayn lord kyng Henry | the. VIII. grauntyd to the compyler | therof that noo man in thys hys | realme sell none but such as the same cōpyler makyth pryn- | tyd for ye space of ii. yeere. | ; g4ᵛ John Rastell's mark.
> References: *STC* 15635. The only copy recorded is that in the British Museum (G.7569) which was the Heber-Grenville copy.

The traditional tale concerning this book is that when John Colet founded St. Paul's School in 1509 an elementary grammar was required for the pupils, and that Linacre wrote the *Progymnasmata* with this in view. Colet, however, apparently rejected the work as being too advanced for his pupils. The best evidence of this incident is a letter written by Erasmus to Colet on 13 September 1511 in which he writes:

> De Linacro cave ne cui temere credas; nam ego certis argumentis habeo compertum illum observantissimo in te esse animo, et de reiecta

grammatica non magnopere laborare: quanquam id est hominum ingenium, ut suis quisque scriptis, ceu parentes filiis, impensius faveat. Quod si quid etiam ea res hominem movet, tua dexteritatis erit dissimulare neque refricare eam cicatricem, vultuque et consuetudinis alacritate magis quam excusatione, praecipue per alios facta, revocare; hoc pacto, si quid illi dolet, id tempore sensim evanescet. Sed nae ego egregie impudens, qui haec tibi, hoc est sus Minervae.[1]

The valuable insight which this letter supplies helps to date the disagreement, but it is not made clear whether the rejected grammar was already printed at that date. The evidence of the three prefatory poems in the book is equally difficult to interpret.

> Linacri ad praeceptores [p̄rie] et pueros
> Primum haec quae patria libuit conscribere lingua
> Haud quamquam inuitus perlegito Angle puer
> Nec tibi concisus videar si forte quibusdam
> Ista legis missis que potui adstruere
> Sic placitum est de te primum cepisse periclum
> Ad normam explesse: an semi repleta queas
> At tu preceptor qui multa nouata notabis
> Quorum nec ratio hic sat sua constiterit:
> Inde laboraris nolim. mox illa dabuntur
> Quis tibi perlectis: fiet in hisce satis
> Ergo vel ista cubans ambas securus in aures
> Interea pueros qualiacunque doce.

> Thome mori in progymnasmata linacri
> Qui leget hec sensim docti precepta linacri
> Dicere (si teneat que legit inde) volet
> Post tot grammatices immensa volumina paruus
> Non tamen incassum prodiit iste liber
> Exiguus liber est. Sed gemme more nitentis
> Exiguo magnum corpore fert precium.

> Guliel. Lilij in progymnasmata Grammatic.
> Linacri a plagiario vindicata.
> Pagina que falso latuit sub nomine nuper
> Que fuit ex multo commaculata luto
> Nunc tandem authoris perscribens nomina veri
> Linacri dulces pura recepit aquas.

These poems evidently provide points of value. Firstly it is

[1] D. Erasmus, *Opus epistolarum Des. Erasmi Roterodami*, ed. P. S. Allen, 12 vols., Oxford, 1906–58, i. 467.

interesting that both Linacre and More should, rather apologetically, stress the brevity of the work and that the former should excuse himself to the schoolmaster with the promise of a more extended work to be published shortly. More important, however, is William Lily's poem where we learn that Linacre must be defended from the accusation of plagiarism since, as it appears, the text of this work had already been published earlier but under some form of false name and with many errors.[1] These remarks are clearly both invaluable and tantalizing, as with so many similar contemporary references. We do not know what book is referred to, nor whether it bore someone else's name or a pseudonym. It is, however, evident that there was a form of the *Progymnasmata* earlier than the surviving text and it seems reasonable to suggest that such a work, probably produced before September 1511, was the 'reiecta grammatica' to which Erasmus refers. Evidently something went disastrously wrong with the book and it may be that Colet had rejected it arbitrarily either in ignorance of the fact that it was by Linacre or because he too considered it 'multo commaculata luto'.

Whatever the explanation of the mystery of the first edition, the problem of dating the *Progymnasmata* as we know it from the only surviving copy remains. The powerful triumvirate of Linacre, More, and Lily, all coming together to preface this small work, combined with the apologetic tone of the poems and the forecast of a fuller work to come (possibly the *Rudimenta grammatices* of Linacre's last years), suggest that there was something rather vindicatory about this edition. Linacre, still much interested in grammar, may after a few years have wished to rectify the slur on his reputation (whatever it was) of the earlier edition. By his use of the perfect tense Lily suggests that the first edition had appeared some years back, while Linacre's comment looks forward to his work of 1523. Lily being High Master of St. Paul's, Colet's foundation, one might wonder whether the book would be republished during the latter's lifetime. Colet died on 15 September 1519, but since it would seem that it was Linacre who was the injured party and that Colet was prepared to humour him (as we know from a brief reply to Erasmus' letter quoted above),[2] it would seem that little can be pinned on this.

---

[1] These may well have included some perpetuated here, for the examples of the third, fourth, and fifth declensions given in the *Progymnasmata* appear, correctly, in all editions of the later *Rudimenta* as those of the fourth, fifth, and third declensions respectively. [2] Allen, ii. 479.

A further contribution which, although it is in many ways as imprecise, is nevertheless of value, comes from looking at what is known of the printer, John Rastell. The varied and interesting career of this printer, decorator, adventurer, and lawyer has attracted some attention.[1] Rastell was born about 1475, was educated at the Middle Temple, married Thomas More's sister Elizabeth some time before 1504 and moved shortly afterwards to Coventry. Returning to London, he printed More's translation of *The lyfe of Johan Picus, Erle of Myrandula*, possibly in 1510. He served in the French war of 1512–14 and visited France again some time in 1515 or 1516. In March 1517 he sailed on a voyage to Newfoundland but the crew mutinied and the ship put in at Waterford. Rastell remained in Ireland until some time in the summer of 1519 and in September of that year started paying rent for his next shop, at Paul's gate in Cheapside. None of his early productions is dated but those with the St. Paul's address, like the *Progymnasmata*, are generally attributed to the years 1512–19. If we assume that the book was printed a few years after the row of 1511, and when Rastell was in London, it must have been done either in the period late 1514 to March 1517 or in the summer of 1519. Comparison of the state of the printer's device used here (a), in *STC* 9599 [1514?] (b), and in *STC* 9517.7 [dated 1519] (c), suggests this order of publication (a, b, c). The revised *STC* dates the *Progymnasmata* we are concerned with here, (a), as [1512] but, in the light of the prefatory poems, this date seems a little early, and it is suggested that *c.* 1515 is preferable. Thus it is clear that, although no copy survives, Linacre's first original composition was some form of the *Progymnasmata* dating before September 1511, and it is on this dating that the record of the only surviving copy of the later edition has been placed here in the sequence of Linacre's works.

With his next publication Linacre entered on his translations of Galen which were to prove remarkably popular in the next three decades.

---

[1] See, amongst others, A. W. Reed, *Early Tudor Drama*, London, 1926, pp. 1–28; H. J. Graham, 'The Rastells and the Printed English Law Book of the Renaissance', *Law Library Journal*, xlvii, 1954, 5–25; and A. H. King, 'The Significance of John Rastell in Early Music Printing', *The Library*, 5th ser. xxvi, 1971, 197–214. I am also greatly indebted to Miss K. Pantzer, at the Houghton Library and in charge of *STC* revision, for advice on this and other entries.

c. Galen, *De sanitate tuenda libri sex* 1517.

   Title-page: CVM PRIVILEGIO | AD QVADRIEN | NIVM. |
   [Within woodcut frame with portraits of Galen and Linacre and
   a shield bearing the arms of Paris University at the top, and
   knotwork below the central circular wreath] Galeni de sanitate
   tu= | enda Libri sex | Thoma | Lina | cro Anglo Interprete. |
   ∴ ∴ | ∴ | [Below frame] Habetur venale sub pellicano in vico
   Iacobeo. | (See Frontispiece.)
   Collation: Folio; a–i⁶, K–M⁶, N⁸.
   Contents: a1 title-page, a2 dedication to Henry VIII (Lond. XVI.
   Cal. Quintiles. 1517), a3 Linacrus ad lectorem, a4 text, N6 Im-
   pressum Parisiis per honestum virum Guilielmum Rubeum
   Typographum. Anno nostre reparationis. M.D.xvij. undecimo
   calendas Septembris, N6ᵛ errata; N7ᵛ blank.

Some copies (Adams G103) have in the colophon the error
'Impressnm' and the last page numbered 72, others (Adams G104)
have both errors corrected. The book was printed in Paris by
Guillaume Le Rouge (Rubeus), a well-known printer who had
worked at Troyes in 1491 and 1492, and it was probably one of his
last productions. It appears that there had been a suggestion that
it was to be printed by Bade, for Erasmus wrote to Guillaume Budé
on 21 February 1517: 'Thomae Linacri lucubrationes ex officina
Badiana propediem exituras dici non potest quam gaudeam. Nihil
ab eo viro expecto non absolutissimum omnibus numeris. Deum
immortalem, quod saeculum video brevi futurum! utinam contingat
reiuuenescere!'[1]

In his long dedication of the translation to Henry VIII Linacre,
describing himself as 'medicus suus', relates how the king's splen-
dour and glory attract gifts, 'alius generosus equos, alius insignes
canes, alius aurum argentum', and stresses how his gift shows that
he works for the king even when he is not in his presence. The
dedication copy does not seem to have survived although that which
bears a manuscript extra dedication (sig. a1ᵛ) to Wolsey (British
Museum, C 19 e. 15) bears an old Royal Library shelfmark, no. 1115.
This copy is on vellum, is rubricated and decorated throughout,
and the title-page is richly illuminated in gold, silver, red, and blue,
with the royal arms at the foot. Finally after the colophon the mark
of the printer Le Rouge is, appropriately enough, in red.

[1] Allen, ii. 479.

The binding of Wolsey's copy, of concentric rows of arabesque tools and fleurs-de-lis, gilt and decorated in blue, is attributable to the same French workshop employed for the dedication copies of Linacre's next book. A rather plainer copy in the library of the Royal College of Physicians bears a more natural-sounding manuscript dedication to Richard Fox, Bishop of Winchester, 'antistes humaniss. et gravissime'.

In his dedication of the *De sanitate tuenda* Linacre writes 'Delegi igitur potissimum ex iis quae nuper verti' and it is therefore not surprising that since he apparently had a number of them ready he published virtually one translation a year for the rest of his life.

D. Galen, *Methodus medendi*, 1519

Title-page: Cum priuilegio Regio Ad quadriennium. | [Within a frame of woodcut borders decorated with angels and monsters and bearing bottom centre the name DIDIER | MAHEV.] GALENI | METHODVS MEDENDI, VEL | DE MORBIS CVRANDIS. | THOMA LINA- | CRO ANGLO INTER-PRETE. | LIBER QVATVORDECIM. | In fine apposuimus quae ipse | Linacer recognouit in | opere De sanitate | : tuenda. : | ∴ | M.D.XIX. |

Collation: Folio; +⁸, 2+⁸, A–M⁸, N¹, X⁸, y–z⁸, 2A⁶.

Contents: +i title-page, +iᵛ Iani Lascaris (ten-line poem, begins Omnigenos Paean), +ii G. Budaee Thoma Lupset Anglo s.d., +v Index, 2+8 (Dedication to King Henry VIII), A1 text, 2A4 Desiderius Maheu studiosis S.D. (corrigenda), 2A5ᵛ Ad lectorem. Pauca haec Lector studiose quae in opere de sanitate tuenda per incuriam sūt omissa (corrigenda to *De sanitate tuenda*), 2A6 end of corrigenda and colophon, Lvtetiae, Sumptu Godefridi | Hittorpi Spectata fi | de Mercatoris apud | Desiderium Ma | Heu. Mense iu | nio anno | M.D.XIX. | ∴ | .

Some copies bear on 2A6ᵛ: EME FRVERE ET | VALEBIS PAN | CRATI | CE |. The text is very roughly printed, and was probably put in to bear the blank page and should not have been inked. It would seem that some jovial compositor was commenting 'Profit from me and you will be as healthy as an athlete.'

The dedication copy presented to Henry VIII and another with an extra dedication to Wolsey, both printed on vellum and sumptuously illuminated and bound, formed part of the old Royal Library (nos. 1201 and 531 respectively) and are now in the British Museum

(C 19 e. 17 and 16). Although the covers of the King's copy were remounted, possibly in the eighteenth century, the binding is in good condition and is a most impressive piece, bearing the Royal Arms and in large letters the motto DIEU ET MON DROYT (see Plate IV). Both volumes have attracted attention as bindings alone and are now ascribed, like the presentation copy to Wolsey of the 1517 *De sanitate tuenda*, to the French 'Louis XII–François I' bindery.[1] The bindings now grouped together and attributed to this workshop are fine examples of the traditional French style with rolls and small tools used in predominantly vertical patterns. In these early days of gold tooling the new technique is often combined with blind-stamped work. The bindery clearly did much royal work and was earlier thought to have been at Blois, where Louis XII usually held court, but it is now considered to have been in Paris and may have been that of the publisher Simon Vostre, who died in 1521.

The title-page of the book is colourfully illuminated in gold, blue, red, and green while the dedication is sumptuously treated with the King's name in gold on red and Linacre's in gold on blue. In the text the same manuscript hand has marked all the printed errata and also made some other corrections.

It is tempting to think that the publication of Linacre's next translation from Galen may have been prompted by political considerations. The *De temperamentis et de inaequali intemperie* were printed not in France like the other Galen translations but by John Siberch's new and short-lived press at Cambridge. The work was dedicated to the Pope, Leo X, and the letter of dedication is dated September 1521. Leo X, born Giovanni de' Medici, had in his youth had lessons with Angelo Poliziano which Linacre was allowed to share, as the translator naturally recalls. However, more immediately it should be noted that in this last year of his life (1521) Leo X had formally excommunicated Luther in January, had been sent Henry VIII's *Assertio septem sacramentorum* in May, and was to confer on the King the title of Defender of the Faith in October of the same year. It is also known that as early as March 1521 Linacre had made some request to the Pope and that this had been

---

[1] See J. Guignard, 'L'Atelier des reliures Louis XII (Blois ou Paris?) et l'atelier de Simon Vostre' in *Studia bibliographica in honorem Herman de la Fontaine Verwey*, Amsterdam, 1968, pp. 202–39 (all three Linacre bindings are illustrated on plates IV and V), and H. M. Nixon, *Sixteenth-Century Gold-Tooled Bookbindings in the Pierpont Morgan Library*, New York, 1971, pp. 9–12.

granted.[1] What is not known, however, is what the favour was and one might suppose that he had merely asked for permission to dedicate the book to the Pope. Whether or not there was any concealed diplomatic purpose behind Linacre's action, it is interesting to note the preoccupations of Linacre's circle at the time. A final link with the royal circle which is worth recording is that the vellum copy of the *De temperamentis* now in the Bodleian (Arch. A e. 71) and probably originally presented to Cuthbert Tunstal, Bishop of London, is in a presentation binding using the same panel-stamps with which the London stationer John Reynes decorated the eleven surviving presentation copies of Henry VIII's book.[2]

E. Galen, *De temperamentis et de inaequali intemperie* 1521.

Title-page: [within a border, McKerrow and Ferguson 10] CALENI [*sic*] PERGAMEN= | SIS DE TEMPERA= | MENTIS, ET DE IN= | AEQVALI INTEMPE | RIE LIBRI TRES | THOMA LINACRO | ANGLO INTER= | PRETE∴ | ⸮⸮? | Opus non medicis modo sed et | philosophis oppido ℥ | necessariū | nunc primum prodit in lucem | CVM GRATIA | & Priuilegio. | ,',', | ·⸵· |

Collation: 4°. π⁴, 2⁴, A–P⁴, Q⁶(−Q5,6), R⁴, S⁶.

Contents: πI title-page; πIᵛ dedication to Pope Leo X, dated London Nonis Septembris; π2ᵛ contents; AI text of *De temperamentis*; RI text of *De inaequali intemperie*; S5 errata; S6 colophon (Impressum apud praeclaram Cantabrigiam per | Ioannem Siberch. Anno.M.D.XXI. |); S6ᵛ printer's device.

Two issues of this work have been identified; in the first, which lacks the translation of *De inaequali intemperie*, signature Q has six leaves with the colophon 'Impressum apud praeclaram Cantabrigiam per Io | annem Siberch. Añ.M.D.XXI' and a woodcut of the Adoration of the Shepherds on Q5 verso, and a device and date on Q6 verso; in the second issue (to which belong the two extant vellum copies) Q5, 6 have been cancelled, the end of the text has been reprinted on RI and the book continues as described.[3] The vellum copies also lack the text initial on AI.

[1] S.P.D., Henry VIII, 3, pt. I, nos. 1204, 1275.

[2] J. B. Oldham, *Blind Panels of English Binders*, Cambridge, 1958, panels HE 21 and 22.

[3] O. Treptow, *John Siberch, Johann Lair von Siegburg*, translated by T. Jones, Cambridge, 1970, p. 55.

It is thought that one of the two other books with Greek which Siberch published earlier in 1521 was the first printing of Greek in England, but it has also been claimed that Linacre's translation was the first English book with a copper-engraved title-page.

Although Siberch left Cambridge the following year Linacre did not return to having his books printed on the Continent but turned, for the rest of his life, to the famous London printer, Richard Pynson. The latter was a Norman by birth and appears to have learnt his trade in Rouen. He established himself in London between 1486 and 1490 and remained there until his death in 1530. He became King's Printer in 1508, in which year he used the first roman type to be seen in England, but if he included among his books the *Canterbury Tales* and much popular reading matter in English, his main interest lay in legal publishing of which he had a virtual monopoly. As the printer of Henry VIII's *Assertio* it was perhaps natural that Linacre should turn to him although the other great London printer, Wynkyn de Worde, specialized in what was to be Linacre's field, grammar books, and was the printer of Colet, Erasmus, and Lily.

Two out of Linacre's next three publications are undated and while it is likely that they are all close together in time, the exact sequence seems difficult to establish. Linacre had been rewarded with livings from early on in his career but it was apparently only in 1521 that he became an ordained priest, perhaps on his appointment as Rector of Wigan. In March 1522 he became a canon of St. Stephen's, Westminster, but resigned the office in November of the same year, possibly selling it (as was done), or possibly on account of ill health. Some time in 1523 he was appointed tutor to the future Queen Mary I, then seven years of age. In his dedication of Galen's *De naturalibus facultatibus*, dated 25 May 1523, Linacre offers Archbishop Warham the early fruits of the leisure he has now been allowed, possibly a reference to the ecclesiastical preferment he had received. He refers too not only to his ill health but also to certain important business, and one wonders whether this might not be the preparation of the *Rudimenta grammatices* for the Princess. The date of his appointment is not known but would seem, from a reference to him by his fellow tutor, Vives, to have been before October 1523. It is possible therefore that the *Rudimenta*, the shape of which was hinted at in Linacre's prefatory poem to the

Progymnasmata, preceded the *De naturalibus facultatibus.* The *De pulsuum usu* is dedicated to Wolsey and was probably a New Year's gift to the other primate, then at the height of his power. Following Linacre's remarks to Warham, offering him the first fruits of his leisure, it is now suggested that the dedication to Wolsey is later in date and therefore probably refers to New Year's Day 1524, the work itself dating from the last months of the previous year.

The *Rudimenta grammatices* is another work of which there survives only one imperfect copy of what is probably the first edition and, indeed, but one copy of the only other contemporary edition in English. The *Short Title Catalogue* has for long listed under number 15636, and as [n.d.], the edition described on the title-page as 'castigata denuo' (British Museum C21b37(1)), and under number 15637, and also as [n.d.], the other unique British Museum copy (C21b37(2)), which was also printed by Pynson. This ordering of the two copies would imply the existence of an earlier edition, presumably of 1523, of which no copy has survived. It is, however, now suggested that the second of these surviving editions, *STC* 15637, is in fact this missing first edition. Firstly, it is printed on vellum, which would argue some more special purpose or audience and be more likely to precede the paper 'castigata denuo' edition. Secondly it collates, rather unusually, [a]–e, A–E (signature a is wanting). Signature e4 verso ends that part of the text on declensions and then adds: In aedibus Pynsonianis cum Priuilegio, before continuing in noticeably disproportionate large capitals with William Lily's poem to Princess Mary which ends at the bottom of the page. The following page, signature A1, starts with the proper section heading 'Generally of Construction . . .'. It seems clear therefore that for some reason unknown the *Rudimenta* was printed in two parts, first signatures a to e and then A to E. The first text finishing half-way down e4 verso, a short colophon was printed and the remaining half-page filled out with the poem, the heading of which was printed in large capitals to fill out space. In the paper 'castigata denuo' edition the signatures run regularly A–M⁴ and the declension text, finishing on G2, is mysteriously, and pointlessly, followed by Lily's poem (the colophon was, however, omitted). The priority of the vellum copy edition would thus seem to be established.[1]

[1] Miss K. Pantzer dates *STC* 15636, the 'castigata denuo' paper edition, as [1525] and points out that the Paris 1533 edition appears to follow it. She

F. Linacre, *Rudimenta grammatices* [1523?].

Title-page (of later edition): [Within a border McKerrow and Ferguson 7] ☙ RUDI= | MENTA GRAMMA= | tices Thomae Linacri di= | ligenter castigata denuo. | ∴ |
Collation: 4°. [a]–e⁴, A–E⁴. Only recorded copy wants sig. a.
Contents: (sig. a wanting), b1 text (begins: singular, is, the gen. eius . . .), e4ᵛ colophon (In aedibus Pynson. cum priuilegio.), W. Lily, poem to Princess Mary (begins: Inclyta progenies Angliae . . .), A1 text (begins: GENERALLY OF CON= | STRVCTION. For the ioynyng . . .), E4ᵛ colophon: Impress. Londini In aedibus Pynsonianis. Cum priuilegio a rege indulto. The later edition also contains on M4 Ricardi Hirtii, in Rudimenta grammatices, Thomae Linacri, Epigramma (12 lines) and the colophon: IMPRESS. Londini in aedibus Pynsonianis. Cum priuilegio a rege indulto, and on M4ᵛ the printer's mark.

This is further substantiated by minor textual differences between the two, the vellum edition being closer to the *Progymnasmata* early text and the 'castigata denuo' edition being apparently slightly rewritten in a fuller manner. Thus both early texts have: 'The verb is declined with modes, tenses, persons, and numbers. Modes be V. the indicative . . .' which in the other becomes 'A verb is a part of speech declined with . . . and betokeneth to be to do . . .'. George Buchanan's famous Latin translation, which appeared first in 1533, was probably based on the vellum text. Professor McFarlane has pointed out that Buchanan's version was probably on the syllabus of the colleges where he taught and that its success suggests that it was used in other establishments too.[1] The translation may have been inspired by Estienne's edition of the *De emendata* in 1527, or perhaps Gentian Hervet, a former pupil of Linacre's and at one time a teacher at the Collège de Guyenne, played some part.

dates *STC* 15637 as [*c.* 1525], adding 'probably earlier than 15636'. The hesitation about dating it earlier still arises from its typography since the 70 mm textura W⁵ᶜ used with the 80 mm roman is otherwise only known from *STC* 3361 which, from its connection with Wyer, must be a very late Pynson production.

[1] I. D. McFarlane, 'George Buchanan and French Humanism' in *Humanism in France* (Manchester, 1970), ed. A. H. T. Levi, p. 313.

G. Galen, *De naturalibus facultatibus* 1523.

Title-page: GALENI | PERGAMENI | DE NATVRALIBVS | FACVLTATIBVS | LIBRI TRES, | THO. LINA= | CRO AN= | GLO | INTERPRETE. |

Collation: 4°. A–Z⁴, &⁴; ff. 1–96.

Contents: A1 title-page, A1ᵛ dedication to William Warham, Archbishop of Canterbury (undated), A2 text, &3 colophon (Impress. Londini in aedibus Ricardi Pynsoni | regij Impressoris. Anno uerbi incarnati millesimo quingentesimo uigesi= | mo tertio. Octauo Calen. | Iun. Cum priuile= | gio a rege in= | dulto. | ·,· |), &3ᵛ and 4 blank, &4ᵛ printer's device.

H. Galen, *de pulsuum usu* [1523/4].

Title-page: [within a border, McKerrow and Ferguson 7] GALENI PERGAME= | ni de pulsuū usu Tho. | Linacro Anglo | interpre | te. |

Collation: 4°. π⁴, A–C⁴, D².

Contents: π1 title-page, π1ᵛ dedication to Cardinal Wolsey (undated), π2 Elenchus sequentis operis, A1 text, C4ᵛ colophon (LONDINI in aedibus pinsonianis, cum priuilegio a rege indulto), D1 Index errorum, D2ᵛ blank.

As we know from the dedication of the *De naturalibus facultatibus*, Linacre had been ill for some months before he died on 20 October 1524, leaving his major original work, the *De emendata structura Latini sermonis*, ready for the press. The book bears no dedication and no outstanding presentation copies are known. A brief and unsigned prefatory word merely warns the reader of the printer's lack of experience in printing Greek.

I. Linacre, *De emendata structura* 1524.

Title-page: [within a woodcut border, McKerrow and Ferguson 8] THOMAE | LINACRI BRITAN= | NI DE EMENDATA | STRVCTVRA LA= | TINI SERMO= | NIS LIBRI | SEX. | ♜ |

Collation: 4°. π², A–2D⁴, 2E⁶, A–S⁴, 2T⁶; ff. *1–2, 1, 2–113, 114,* I–LXXVIII.

Contents: π1 title-page; π1ᵛ preface to the reader, errata etc. π2ᵛ regestrum operis; A1 text; 2T6ᵛ colophon (Londini apud Richardum Pynsonum mense Decembri. M.D.XXIIII. Cum priuilegio regio).

The woodcut border used on the title-page, showing Mucius Scaevola and Lars Porsenna, is copied from a design by Hans Holbein and bears his initials (see Plate V).

About the same time Pynson also printed the last of Linacre's translations of Galen. The anonymous preface-writer lists the previous ones (not in chronological order) and adds: 'Multa item alia a se versa reliquit, quae, quod ante obitum non erant aedita, verendum est ne in manus studiosorum nunquam exeant. Grammaticam vero absolutissimam paulo ante mortem calcographis excudendam commiserat.' No more Galen texts appeared, however.

J. Galen, *De symptomatum differentiis* 1524.

Title-page: [within a border, McKerrow and Ferguson 7] GALENI| PERGAMENI DE| symptomatum differen=| tijs liber unus.| EIVSDEM DE SYM=| ptomatum causis libri tres| Thoma Linacro Britan=| no interprete.| ∵|
Collation: 4°. A–Y⁴, Z⁶.
Contents: A1 title-page; A2 preface (Studioso lectori . . .); A3 errata; B1 text of *De symptomatum differentiis*; F1ᵛ text of *De symptomatum causis*; Z5ᵛ colophon (Impress. Londini in aedibus Pynsonianis. An. Christi. 1524: cum priuilegio a rege indulto); Z6ᵛ printer's mark.

The last of Linacre's translations to appear in print did so together with a revised version of the *De naturalibus facultatibus*. In his preface the editor, Johann Winther, calls Linacre 'deum immortalem quo viro' and goes on to say that these texts had not yet appeared in either France or Germany but that 'Petrus Bellus ducis Vendoviensis physicus, nuper ex Anglia primus, quo cum oratoribus Christianissimi Gallorum regis profectus est, una secum eos faustis avibus advexit'. However, the text had had to be much corrected. Further information about this interesting intermediary appears unfortunately to be lacking.

K. Paulus Aeginetae, *De diebus criticis* 1528.

Title-page: GALENI PER=| GAMENI DE NATVRALI=| bus facultatibus libri tres.| De pulsuum vsu liber vnus.| Item & quaedam Pauli Æginetae,| de diebus criticis.| Thoma Linacro Anglo interprete.| [printer's mark]| PARISIIS| Apud Simonem Colinaeum| 1528|

Collation: 16°. a–m⁸, n⁴.

Contents: A1 title-page; A1ᵛ preface (Guinterus Ioannes Andernacus, lectori S., undated); a2 index; a8 Linacre's dedication of 1523; b1 text of *De naturalibus facultatibus*; 15 text of *De pulsuum usu*; m8ᵛ EX PAVLO AE= | GINETA DE CRISI, ET CRITI' | cis siue decretorijs diebus, eorūmque si= | gnis, Tho. Linacro Anglo interprete. | ; n4 colophon (Hos quatuor Galeni perutiles libellos nunquam prius in Gallia visos & stylo elimatione a Guinterio Ioanne Andernaco perpolitos, excusit Simon Colinaeus: Anno salutis humanae millesimo quingentesimo vicesime octauo, mese vero Decembri).

It will be seen that the twenty-five to thirty years covering Linacre's original publications was a remarkably interesting and important period in the development of European humanism. Linacre's publishers included Manutius in Italy, Gourmont, Le Rouge, Maheu, and Colines (with Bade, Estienne, and Wechel within the next five years) in France, and Rastell, Siberch, and Pynson in England. A few separate editions of Linacre translations appeared in Italy in the early decades of the century but these soon died out, possibly overtaken by the Giunta edition of Galen which incorporated them, and only one of Linacre's grammatical works was ever published there. It is also noticeable that the English editions of his works all come in the last years of his life or very shortly after. German interest, however, if never very high, was remarkably constant, reaching a slight peak in the 1530s, 1540s, and 1550s. The vast majority of the editions both of Linacre's own works and of his translations appeared of course in France where, after a slow start, Robert Estienne and Christian Wechel together with the Lyonnese printers were very active, particularly in the 1530s and 1540s. Indeed, it is remarkable how Linacre's own works fell abruptly out of fashion everywhere from roughly 1560 onwards while the Galens, although sharing the same peak period, straggle on to the end of the century. Proportionately, Proclus was by far the most constant seller.

In number of editions Linacre's own *De emendata* has a handsome lead as the most popular of his works with the Proclus just leading Buchanan's version of the *Rudimenta*, of which the English text had strangely little success. Although Linacre's own work was undoubtedly famous his fame was evidently considerably enhanced by Buchanan's translation.

Linacre's publications are also very representative of his times for another reason, some being large and well-produced folios while others are small octavos or duodecimos of which hardly a copy survives and which show every sign of hasty production. Linacre, the doctor, familiar and friend of kings, popes, archbishops, and cardinals as well as of scholars, was in a position to dedicate his works to the mighty and to call on the finest binders of his day to decorate his presentation copies. Other books, and noticeably his own works, were more humbly produced for scholars and friends. The schoolbook for Princess Mary is a more homely production of the latter kind, a small book for a young girl, in presentation as in the style of writing and choice of examples, unimposing, friendly, and intimate. How far Linacre was responsible for these details is unknown since, except for his friendship with Manutius, little remains of his relations with his printers or publishers. He may have chosen Rastell because of the latter's connections with More, and it is conceivable that he met Siberch when Wolsey visited Cambridge in 1520, but in other cases he was evidently prepared to let friends abroad see his work through the press. It is also noticeable that he does not appear to have had a hand in any of the numerous re-editions of his works but to have been more interested in producing new ones. Whatever the flood of later editions tells us of contemporary taste, the impression left by Linacre's personal publishing history is not that of the old grammarian, 'a Grecian, a latinist, a mathematician, a philosopher', referred to by Erasmus in his *In Praise of Folly*, 'who after three-score years' experience in the world, had spent the last twenty of them only in drudging to conquer the criticisms of grammar, and made it the chief part of his prayers, that his life might be so long spared till he had learned how rightly to distinguish betwixt the eight parts of speech'; we retain more an impression of a practical, exact, and human scholar.

2. *Checklist of Editions of Works Written or Translated by Thomas Linacre*

The aim of this chronological checklist is to record all editions of Linacre's works and translations for which a location, or at the least a detailed description, is available. The holdings of the British Museum (BM), the Bibliothèque Nationale, Paris (BN), and the Bodleian Library (Bod.) are recorded together with the locations of other outstanding or unique copies. For the separately published translations of Galen the list is largely based on the work of R. J. Durling. Besides the standard bibliographical references the following abbreviations have been used:

Buisson [F. Buisson], *Répertoire des ouvrages pédagogiques du XVIe siècle (Bibliothèques de Paris et des départements)*, Paris, 1886; reprinted Nieuwkoop, 1962. I am indebted to Professor I. D. McFarlane for reference to this work which gives French locations.

Durling R. J. Durling, 'A Chronological Census of Renaissance Editions and Translations of Galen', *Journal of the Warburg and Courtauld Institutes*, xxiv, 1961, 230–305. Locations of numerous copies are given.

Hoffmann S. F. G. Hoffmann, *Bibliographisches Lexicon der gesammten Literatur der Griechen*, 2. Ausgabe, Leipzig, 1839.

Osler Sir William Osler, *Bibliotheca Osleriana*, reprinted with addenda etc., Montreal, 1969.

M. A. Shaaber, *Check-list of works of British authors printed abroad, in languages other than English* (New York, Bibliographical Society of America, 1975), was also used but appeared too late for references to be added to each entry.

Checklist

1499 Proclus, De sphaera (Gk. & Lat.). *In* Firmicius (J.), *Astronomicorum libri octo*, Venice, Aldus Manutius, fol. Hain＊14559, Renouard, *Aldes* 1499.3, Osler 7492, Proctor 5570, *BMC* v. 560, Klebs 405. See part 1, description A.
BM, BN, Bod.

1502 Proclus, De sphaera.
Wittenberg, [H. Sertorius & N. Marschalk], 4°.
The second book printed in Wittenberg where the university was founded the same year. Marschalk was an ardent scholar and probably in touch with Aldus Manutius. See D. E. Rhodes, 'Two early German editions of Proclus', *Beiträge zur Geschichte des Buches und seiner Funktion in der Gesellschaft, Festschrift für Hans Widmann* (Stuttgart, 1974), pp. 178–82. I am indebted to Dr. D. E. Rhodes of the British Library, London, for assistance with a number of points. Bayerische Staatsbibliothek, Munich

1503   Proclus, De sphaera (Gk. & Lat.). *In* Firmicius (J.), *Astro-nomicorum libri octo*, Reggio Emilia, F. Mazalis, fol. Sander 2783, Norton, p. 86.
        The title-page follows that of the 1499 Venice edition but the BN copy (Rés. g. V. 28), which appears to be complete, lacks the four last texts including the Proclus.
                                                                BN

[1503/4]   Proclus, De sphaera.
           [Leipzig, M. Landsberg] 4°.
           Hain 13387, Proctor 2982, *BMC* iii. 643, Klebs 807. See Rhodes, op. cit.   BM

[1510?]   Proclus, De sphaera.
           Paris, E. Gourmont, 4°.   Bod.

[1511   Linacre, Progymnasmata grammatices vulgaria.]
           Postulated date of the 'reiecta grammatica'.

1511   Proclus, De sphaera.
           Vienna, H. Vietor & J. Singiener, 4°.   BM, Bod.

1512   Proclus, De sphaera.
           Cracow, F. Ungler, 4°.
           No copy located but recorded in detail by Hoffmann, 3, 293.

[*c.* 1515]   Linacre, Progymnasmata grammatices vulgaria.
           London, J. Rastell, 4°.
           STC 15635 (as [1525?] revised to [1512]). See part I, description B.   BM

1515   Proclus, De sphaera.
           Cologne, H. de Nussia, 4°.
           No copy located but recorded by Hoffmann 3, 293.

1517   Galen, De sanitate tuenda.
           Paris, G. Le Rouge, fol.
           Two states, Adams G103 (uncorrected) and G104 (corrected). Osler 372. See part I, description C.
                                        BM, BN, Bod.

1519   Galen, Methodus medendi.
           Paris, D. Maheu for G. Hittorp, fol.
           Osler 366. See part I, description D.   BM

1521   Galen, De temperamentis et de inaequali intemperie.
           Cambridge, J. Siberch, 4°.

STC 11536. Two issues, corrected and uncorrected.
Melanchthon's vellum copy is now in All Souls College,
Oxford. See part 1, description E. BM, Bod.

[1522] Proclus, De sphaera.
London, R. Pynson, 8°.
STC 20398.3. BM

[1523] Linacre, Rudimenta grammatices.
London, R. Pynson, 4°.
STC 15637 (revised date *c.* 1525, probably before 15636).
See part 1, description F. BM

1523 Galen, De naturalibus facultatibus.
London, R. Pynson, 4°.
STC 11533. See part 1, description G. BM

1523 Galen, De temperamentis et de inaequali intemperie.
Paris, S. Colines, fol.
Renouard, *Colines*, pp. 51–2. BN, Bod.

1523 Galen, De sanitate tuenda.
Venice, heirs of A. Bindoni, 4°.
Osler 373. BM, BN

1523 Proclus, De sphaera (Gk. & Lat.). *In* Dionysius Periegetes,
Orbis descriptio (etc.).
Basle, J. Bebel, 8°.
Adams D 645. BM, BN, Bod.

[1523/4] Galen, De pulsuum usu.
London, R. Pynson, 4°.
STC 11534. See part 1, description H. BM, Bod.

1524 Linacre, De emendata structura Latini sermonis.
London, R. Pynson, 4°.
STC 15634. See part 1, description I.
The Nicholas Udall–Herbert–Sebright–Heber–Britwell
copy is now at the Folger Library. See also 1968.
BM, Bod., Linacre College, Oxford

1524 Galen, De symptomatum differentiis, de symptomatum
causis.
London, R. Pynson, 4°.
STC 11535. See part 1, description J. BM

[1525]   Linacre, Rudimenta grammatices . . . diligenter castigata
          denuo.
          London, R. Pynson, 4°.
          STC 15636 (as 1525). See also 1971.   BM

1525   Proclus, De sphaera (L. Vitalis Supplementum).
          [Bologna], C. Achillini, 8°.
          See also *Short Title Catalogue of Books printed in Italy and of
          Books in Italian printed abroad 1501–1600 held in selected North
          American Libraries* (Boston, 1970), ii. 651.
                              Bayerische Staatsbibliothek, Munich

1526   Galen, Methodus medendi.
          Paris, C. Chevallon, 8°.   BM, BN

1526   Galen, De sanitate tuenda (Paulus Aegineta, De uictus
          ratione quolibet anni tempore utili).
          Cologne, E. Cervicornus for G. Hittorp, 8°.
          Osler 374, 442.   BM

1527 [really 1528] Linacre, De emendata structura Latini sermonis.
          Paris, R. Estienne, 4°.
          Adams L 682; Buisson; Osler 5054; Renouard, *Estienne*
          1528.8.
          The colophon is dated 13 Calend. Febr. 1528.   BM, BN

1527   Galen, De temperamentis, De inaequali intemperie.
          [Paris, S. Dubois], 16°.
          STC 11537. Two variant issues; see R. J. Durling, 'Un-
          signed Editions of Galen and Hippocrates: Further Light
          on an Elusive Printer', *The Library*, 5th Ser. xvi (1961),
          55–7.   BM; National Library of Medicine, Bethesda

1527   Galen, Terrapeutica [Methodus medendi].
          Venice, G. B. Pederzano, 4°.
                              All Souls College, Oxford;
                              Royal College of Physicians, London

1528   Galen, [seven items *in*] Opera (ed. J. Rivirius).
          [? Lyons, no printer], 4°.
          Vol. iii contains Linacre's translations of the De tempera-
          mentis, de inaequali intemperie, de naturalibus facultati-
          bus, de pulsuum usu, de tuenda sanitate, de symptomatum
          differentia, methodus curandi. Osler 353.

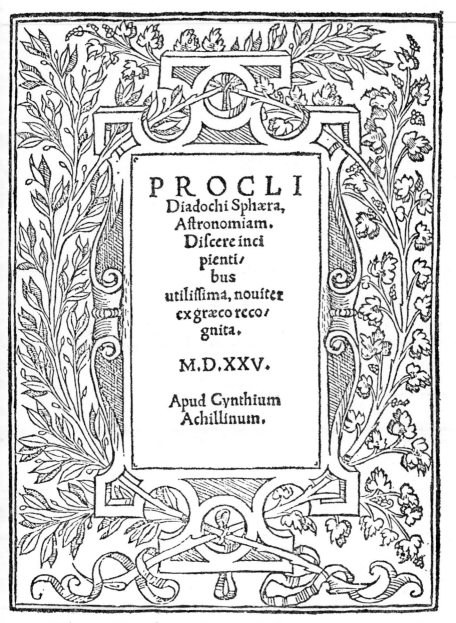

PROCLI
Diadochi Sphæra,
Aſtronomiam.
Diſcere inci
pienti,
bus
utiliſſima, nouiter
ex græco reco,
gnita,

M.D.XXV.

Apud Cynthium
Achillinum.

FIG. I. Title-page of Linacre's translation of pseudo-Proclus, *De Sphaera*, as printed in Bologna 1525. (See p. 310)

1528   Galen, De temperamentis, de inaequali intemperie.
Paris, J. Bade, 4°.
Renouard, *Badius*, p. 460.   BN

1528   Galen, De differentiis symptomatum, de causis sympto-
matum.
Paris, S. Colines, 8°.
Renouard, *Colines*, p. 121.   BM

1528   Galen, De naturalibus facultatibus, de pulsuum usu.
Paulus Aeginetae, de diebus criticis.
Paris, S. Colines, 8°.
Renouard, *Colines*, pp. 121–2. See part 1, description K.
BM

1529   Linacre, Index in sex Thomae Linacri de emendata struc-
tura libros.
Paris, R. Estienne, 4°.
Renouard, *Estienne* 1529.9.   BM, BN, Bod.

1529   Galen, [six items *in*] Opera.
Basle, A. Cratander, fol.
Includes Linacre's versions of De temperamentis, De
inaequali intemperie, Methodus medendi, De sanitate
tuenda, De naturalibus facultatibus, De pulsuum usu.
Bod.

1529   Paulus Aeginetae, De crisi, & diebus decretoriis, eorumque
signis. *In* A. Thylesius, *Libellus de coloribus*.
Paris, C. Wechel, 8°.   BN, Bod.

1529   Paulus Aegineta, De crisi, & diebus decretoriis. *In* J.
Actuarius, *De urinis* [etc.].
Basle, A. Cratander, 8°.   BM

1530   Linacre, De emendata structura Latini sermonis.
Basle, A. Cratander, 4°.
Adams L 683; Buisson; Osler 5055.   BM, BN

1530   Galen, De sanitate tuenda.
Paris, S. Colines, fol.
Renouard, *Colines*, p. 158.   BN, Bod.

1530   Galen, Methodus medendi.
Paris, S. Colines, fol.
Renouard, *Colines*, p. 156. Finely produced with a magnifi-
cent engraved title-page. Mr. Alistair Smith of the

National Gallery, London, has identified the men wearing 'eastern hats' in the left and right panels of the upper engraved border as saints Cosmas and Damian, the patron saints of physicians, as indicated by the initials S.C. and S.D. above. For further discussion of the dress and accoutrements of these saints see M. L. David-Danel, *Iconographie des saints médecins Come et Damien* (Lille, 1958) especially pp. 184–5, 199–200. The letters MMC below the lower panel depicting Christ healing a leper may stand for *Miserere mei Christe*. See Plate VI.

BM, BN, Bod.

1530   Galen, Terrapeutica [Methodus medendi].
Venice, G. Pencio da Lecco, 16°.   BN

1531   Linacre, De emendata structura [Latini sermonis.]
Wittenberg, J. Luft, 8° (? 12°).
Buisson.   Staatsbibliothek, Augsburg;
Bibliothèque municipale, Mende

1532   Linacre, De emendata structura Latini sermonis.
Cologne, J. Soter, 8°.
Buisson.   Bayerische Staatsbibliothek, Munich

1532   Linacre, De emendata structura Latini sermonis.
Paris, C. Wechel, 8°.
Adams L 685; Buisson.   St. John's College, Cambridge

1532   Linacre, De emendata structura Latini sermonis, cum praefatione P. Melanchthonis.
Wittenberg, J. Clug, 8°.
Royal College of Physicians, London

1532   Galen, De pulsuum usu. *In* Opera de pulsibus (translated by H. Croeser and T. Linacre).
Paris, S. Colines, fol.
Renouard, *Colines*, p. 195.
The arms of François I are painted on the title-page of the Bibliothèque nationale copy.   BN

1532 [really 1533] Linacre, De emendata structura Latini sermonis. 2a ed.
Paris, R. Estienne, 4°.
Adams L 684, Renouard, *Estienne* 1533.5. Title-page date 1532 but colophon of 19 Cal. Feb. 1533.   BM, Bod.

1533   Linacre, De emendata structura Latini sermonis.
        Paris, C. Wechel, 8°.
        Buisson.   University Library, Edinburgh

1533   Linacre, Rudimenta grammatices, ex Anglice sermone in
        Latinum versa, interprete Georgio Buchanano.
        Paris, R. Estienne, 4°.
        Adams L 699; Buisson. The first edition of this very
        popular version.   BM, Bod.

1533   Linacre, Rudimenta grammatices (tr. G. Buchanan).
        Paris, C. Wechel, 8°. (See Fig. 3.)
        Adams L 700.   Bod.

1534   Proclus, De sphaera.
        Paris, C. Wechel, 8°.
        Osler 3740.   BM

1535   Proclus, De sphaera (Gk. & Lat.). *In* C. J. Hyginus,
        Fabularum liber.
        Basle, J. Herwagen, fol.   BM, BN, Bod.

1536   Linacre, De emendata structura Latini sermonis.
        Cologne, J. Gymnich, 12°. Universitäts-bibliothek, Basle

1536   Linacre, Rudimenta grammatices (tr. G. Buchanan).
        (*With* J. L. Vives, De ratione studii puerilis.)
        Paris, R. Estienne, 4°.
        Buisson; Renouard, *Estienne* 1536.7.   BN

1536   Proclus, De sphaera (Gk. & Lat., scholiis Zieglerii expli-
        catus). *In* Sphaerae atque astrorum coelestium ratio.
        Basle, J. Walder, 8°.   BM, BN

1537   Linacre, Rudimenta grammatices (tr. G. Buchanan).
        (*With* J. L. Vives, De ratione studii puerilis.)
        Paris, R. Estienne, 8°.
        Adams L 701; Renouard, *Estienne* 1537.6.   BN

1537   Linacre, De emendata structura Latini sermonis. 3a ed.
        Index copiosissimus.
        Paris, R. Estienne, 4°.
        Adams L 686; Buisson; Renouard, *Estienne* 1537.7.   BN

1537   Linacre, Rudimenta grammatices (tr. G. Buchanan).
        (*With* J. L. Vives, De ratione studii puerilis.)
        Paris, C. Wechel, 8°.   National Library of Scotland

1537   Galen, De naturalibus facultatibus.
Paris, C. Wechel, fol.   BM

1537   Galen, De temperamentis, De inaequali intemperie. Cum
isagoge per J. Sylvium.
Paris, C. Wechel, fol.   BM

1537   Galen, (Introductio in pulsus), De pulsuum usu.
Paris, C. Wechel, fol.   BM

1538   Linacre, Rudimenta grammatices (tr. G. Buchanan).
(*With* J. L. Vives, De ratione studii puerilis.)
Paris, R. Estienne, 4°.
Adams L 702; Renouard, *Estienne* 1538.2.
Royal College of Physicians, London

1538   Galen, Terrapeutica [Methodus medendi].
Venice, A. de Tortis, 16°.
Royal College of Physicians, London;
Wellcome Historical Medical Library

1538   Galen, Methodus medendi.
Paris, widow of C. Chevallon, 8°.
Osler 367, 368.   BM, BN

1538   Galen, De temperamentis, De inaequali intemperie.
Basle, T. Platter, 8°.   BN

1538   Galen, De inaequali intemperie. *In* Calani Centurione (P.),
Paraphrasis in librum Galeni de inaequali intemperie.
Lyons, S. Gryphius, 8°.
National Library of Medicine, Bethesda

1538   Galen, De sanitate tuenda.
Paris, widow of C. Chevallon, 8°.
Osler 375   BM, BN, Bod.

1539   Linacre, De emendata structura Latini sermonis.
Lyons, heirs of S. Vincent, 8°.
Adams L 687; Baudrier v. 15; Buisson.   BM, Bod.

1539   Linacre, De emendata structura Latini sermonis.
Basle, N. Brylinger, 12°.   Staatsbibliothek, Augsburg

1539   Linacre, De emendata structura Latini sermonis.
Cologne, J. Gymnich, 8°.   Stadtbibliothek, Nuremberg

RVDIMENTA

GRAMMATICES

THOMÆ LINACRI,
ex *Anglico ſermone in*
Latinum uerſa,
Georgio Buchanano Scoto Interprete.

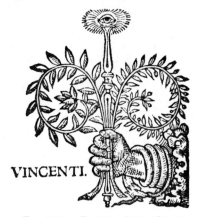

VINCENTI.

LVGDVNI,

Apud Hæredes Simonis Vincentij.

M. D. XXXIX.

FIG. 2. Title-page of George Buchanan's translation of
Linacre, *Rudimenta grammatices*, Lyons, 1539
(See p. 317)

1539 Linacre, Rudimenta grammatices (tr. G. Buchanan). (*With* J. L. Vives, De ratione studii puerilis.) Lyons, heirs of S. Vincent, 8°. (See Fig. 2.) Adams L 703; Baudrier v. 15. A finely printed edition by J. Barbou. BN, Bod.

1539 Linacre, Rudimenta grammatices (tr. G. Buchanan). Basle, N. Brylinger, 12°.

        Hessische Landesbibliothek, Wiesbaden

1539 Galen, De inaequali intemperie (ed. J. Agricola *Ammonius*). Basle, B. Westhemer, 8°. BM, BN

1539 Proclus, De sphaera (Gk. & Lat.). Strasburg, W. Rihel, 8°. BM

1540 Linacre, De emendata structura Latini sermonis. Paris, R. Estienne, 4°. Adams L 688; Buisson; Renouard, *Estienne* 1540.4. BM

1540 Linacre, Rudimenta grammatices (tr. G. Buchanan). Paris, R. Estienne, 4°. Adams L 704; Buisson. BM

1540 Galen, De sanitate tuenda. Paris, C. Wechel, fol. Bod.

1540 Galen, De temperamentis, de inaequali intemperie. Paris, C. Wechel, fol.

     Hunterian Museum, University Library, Glasgow

1541 Linacre, De emendata structura Latini sermonis. Lyons, S. Gryphius, 8°. Buisson. Wadham College, Oxford

1541 Linacre, De emendata structura Latini sermonis. Paris, C. Wechel, 8°. University of Pennsylvania

1541 Linacre, Rudimenta grammatices (tr. G. Buchanan). Paris, R. Estienne, 8°. Wadham College, Oxford

1541 Linacre, Rudimenta grammatices (tr. G. Buchanan). Lyons, S. Gryphius, 8°. Boston Athenaeum

1541 Galen, [five items *in*] Opera. Venice, Junta, fol. Contains De temperamentis, De pulsuum usu, De naturalibus facultatibus, De sanitate tuenda, Methodus medendi. BM, BN

1541   Galen, De naturalibus facultatibus.
        Paris, C. Wechel, fol.   BN

1541   Galen, (Introductio in pulsus ad Teuthram) De pulsuum
        usu.
        Paris, C. Wechel, fol.   BN

1541   Galen, De sanitate tuenda, nunc recens annotationibus a
        Leonharto Fuchsio illustrati [*sic*].
        Tübingen, U. Morhard, 8°.
        Osler 376.   BM, Bod.

1542   Linacre, De emendata structura Latini sermonis. Basle,
        N. Brylinger, 8°.   Yale University (Medical School)

1542   Linacre, Rudimenta grammatices (tr. G. Buchanan).
        Basle, N. Brylinger, 8°.   BM

1542   Linacre, Rudimenta grammatices (tr. G. Buchanan).
        Paris, C. Wechel, 8°.   University of Pennsylvania

1543   Linacre, De emendata structura Latini sermonis.
        Cologne, J. Gymnich, 8°.   Bod.

1543   Linacre, De emendata structura Latini sermonis.
        Paris, M. de Porta, 8°.   BM, BN

1543   Linacre, De emendata structura Latini sermonis.
        Paris, J. Bogard, 8°.
        Buisson.   University Library, Cambridge

1543   Linacre, De emendata structura Latini sermonis.
        Basle, N. Brylinger, 8°.
                         Bayerische Staatsbibliothek, Munich

1543   Linacre, De emendata structura Latini sermonis.
        Magdeburg, M. Lotter, 8°.
                         Universitätsbibliothek, Heidelberg

1543   Linacre, Rudimenta grammatices (tr. G. Buchanan).
        Paris, M. de Porta, 8°. Buisson.   BN

1543   Linacre, Rudimenta grammatices (tr. G. Buchanan).
        Paris, J. Bogard, 8°.
        Buisson.   Bibliothèque municipale, Chaumont

1543   Proclus, De sphaera. Addita sunt Prolegomena J. Schoneri.
        Leipzig, J. Bärwald, 8°.
                         Royal College of Physicians, London

1544   Linacre, De emendata structura Latini sermonis.
Lyons, S. Gryphius, 8°.
Adams L 689; Baudrier viii. 191; Buisson.   BM

1544   Linacre, Rudimenta grammatices (tr. G. Buchanan).
(*With* J. L. Vives, De ratione studii puerilis.)
Lyons, S. Gryphius, 8°.
Baudrier viii. 191; Buisson; Osler 5062.
Musée Calvet, Avignon;
Edinburgh University Library

1544   Proclus, De sphaera.
Paris, P. Gromors, 8°.   BN

1545   Linacre, De emendata structura Latini sermonis (ed. J. Camerarius).
Leipzig, V. Papst, 8°.   Staatsbibliothek, Bamberg

1545   Linacre, Rudimenta grammatices (tr. G. Buchanan).
(*With* J. L. Vives, De ratione studii puerilis.)
Paris, A. Girault, 8°.   BM

1545   Galen, De temperamentis, de inaequali intemperie.
Paris, C. Wechel, fol.   University Library, Aberdeen

1546   Linacre, Rudimenta grammatices (tr. G. Buchanan).
(*With* J. L. Vives, De ratione studii puerilis.)
Paris, R. Estienne, 8°.
Buisson. Renouard, *Estienne* 1546.11, suggests that this book was announced but never published. However, the copy cited below appears to have been J. A. de Thou's and to be that in (A. A. Renouard), *Catalogue de la bibliothèque d'un amateur* (Paris, 1819), ii. 32, since it bears the signature A. A. Renouard 1799.
Royal College of Physicians, London

1546   Linacre, Rudimenta grammatices (tr. G. Buchanan).
Lyons, S. Gryphius, 8°.
Buisson.   Bibliothèque municipale, Aurillac

1546   Linacre, Rudimenta grammatices (tr. G. Buchanan).
Paris, C. Wechel, 8°.
Watkinson Library, Trinity College, Hertford, Conn.

1546   Galen, De naturalibus facultatibus.
Paris, C. Wechel, fol.   Bibliothèque Mazarine, Paris

1546   Galen, Methodus medendi.
            Lyons, G. Roville, 16°.
            Baudrier ix. 127.   BN

1547   Linacre, Rudimenta grammatices (tr. G. Buchanan).
            Paris, R. Estienne, 4°.
            Buisson; Renouard, *Estienne* 1547.5.   BN

1547   Galen, De naturalibus facultatibus.
            Antwerp, J. van der Loe, 8°.   BM

1547   Galen, De sanitate tuenda.
            Lyons, G. Roville, 16°.   BM, BN

1547   Galen, Methodus medendi.
            Lyons, G. Roville, 16°.
            Baudrier ix. 133.   University Library, Manchester

1547   Galen, De temperamentis, De inaequali intemperie. *In*
            Thriverus (H.), *Commentarii in omnes Galeni libros de tem-*
            peramentis.
            Lyons, G. & M. Beringos, 16°.   BM, Bod.
            —— [another issue.]
            Lyons, G. Roville, 16°.
                          National Library of Medicine, Bethesda

1548   Linacre, De emendata structura Latini sermonis.
            Lyons, S. Gryphius, 8°.
            Adams L 690; Baudrier viii. 228.
                          BM, University Library, Cambridge;
                                     Linacre College, Oxford

1548   Linacre, De emendata structura Latini sermonis.
            Leipzig, V. Papst, 8°.
                  Zakład narodowy imienia Ossolińskich, Wrocław

1548   Linacre, Rudimenta grammatices (tr. G. Buchanan).
            Lyons, S. Gryphius, 8°.
            Buisson.   Bibliothèque municipale, Le Havre

1548   Galen, De sanitate tuenda.
            Lyons, G. Roville, 16°.
            Baudrier ix. 141; Osler 377.   BN, Bod.

1548   Paulus Aeginetae, De crisi, & diebus decretoriis. *In*
            Actuarius (J.), *De urinis* [etc.].
            Paris, J. Gazeau, 8°.   BM

1549 Linacre, De emendata structura Latini sermonis.
Cologne, J. Gymnich, 8°.
      Royal College of Physicians, London;
        Worcester College, Oxford

1549 Galen, De sanitate tuenda.
Lyons, G. Roville, 16°.
Baudrier ix. 1953; Osler 378.   BM, Bod.

1549 Galen, De temperamentis, De inaequali intemperie.
Paris, [widow of] J. Gazeau, fol.
       Faculté de Pharmacie, Paris

1549 Galen, De temperamentis, De inaequali intemperie.
Lyons, G. Roville, 16°.
Baudrier ix. 153; Osler 387.
      University Library, Cambridge

1549 Galen, De temperamentis. *In* Quercetanus [Duchesne]
(E.), *Acroamaton in librum Hippocratis de natura hominis
commentarius.*
Basle, J. Oporin, 8°.   BM, BN, Bod.

1549 Galen, (Introductio in pulsus) De pulsuum usu.
Lyons, G. Roville, 16°.
Baudrier ix. 152.   BM, BN, Bod.

1549 Galen, [Eight items *in*] Opera. 4 vols.
Basle, J. Froben, fol.
Contains Linacre's translations of De temperamentis, De
pulsuum usu, De naturalibus facultatibus, De sanitate
tuenda, De differentiis & causis morborum symptoma-
tumque [Bks. 3–6 by Linacre], De inaequali intemperie,
De medendi methodo.   Bod.

1549 Galen, Methodus medendi.
Lyons, G. Roville, 16°.
Baudrier ix. 150.   BN

1549 Proclus, De sphaera (Gr. & Lat.). *In* Hyginus (C. J.),
Fabularum liber.
Basle, J. Herwagen, fol.   BM

1550 Linacre, De emendata structura Latini sermonis.
Paris, R. Estienne, 8°.

Adams L 691; Buisson; Osler 5056; Renouard, *Estienne* 1550.10.
Perhaps the best-known and most widely held edition of this work. The BN copy (Rés. p. X. 71) has a fine, slightly later, binding of olive morocco with onlaid decoration which bears the name of the author, Thomas Linacre, on the upper cover and the date 1551 on the lower.
BM, BN, Bod.

1550   Linacre, Rudimenta grammatices (tr. G. Buchanan). Paris, R. Estienne, 8°.
Adams L 705; Buisson; Osler 5063; Renouard, *Estienne* 1550.9.   BM, Bod.

1550   Galen, De pulsuum usu. Lyons, G. Roville, 16°.
Baudrier ix. 172.   BM, Bod.

1550   Galen, De naturalibus facultatibus. Lyons, G. Roville, 16°.   BM, BN

1550   Galen, Opera [2nd ed. See 1541]. Venice, heirs of L. A. Junta, fol.   BM, BN

1551   Linacre, Rudimenta grammatices (tr. G. Buchanan). Lyons, S. Gryphius, 8°.
Adams L 706.   University Library, Cambridge

1551   Linacre, De emendata structura Latini sermonis. R. Estienne, 12°.
Buisson.   Bibliothèque municipale, Meaux

1551   Linacre, De emendata structura Latini sermonis. Leipzig, V. Papst, 8°.
Bayerische Staatsbibliothek, Munich

1552   Linacre, Rudimenta grammatices (tr. G. Buchanan). (*With* J. L. Vives, De ratione studii puerilis.) Lyons, S. Gryphius, 8°.
Adams L 707; Baudrier viii. 263; Buisson.   BM

1553   Linacre, De emendata structura Latini sermonis. Basle, N. Brylinger, 8°.
Osler 5057.   Exeter College, Oxford

1553   Linacre, De emendata structura Latini sermonis. Magdeburg, M. Lotter, 8°.
Universitätsbibliothek, Düsseldorf

1553   Galen, De inaequali intemperie. *In* Busennius (A.), *In C. Galeni librum de inaequali intemperie commentaria.*
Antwerp, J. Richard [Ryckaert], 8°.   BM, BN, Bod.

1553   Galen, Methodus medendi.
Lyons, G. Roville, 16°.
Baudrier ix. 203; Osler 369.   BM

1553   Proclus, De sphaera.
Paris, M. Le Jeune, 4°.   BM, BN

1553 (really 1554) Proclus, De sphaera (Gk. & Lat.).
Antwerp, J. van der Loe, 8°.   BM

1554   Linacre, Corpus emendatae structurae Latini sermonis libri sex contractum per Ioannem Rutherum.
Basle, J. Oporin, fol.   Trinity College, Dublin

1555   Linacre, De emendata structura Latini sermonis.
Lyons, S. Gryphius, 8°.
Adams L 693; Baudrier viii. 281–2; Buisson.
Clare College, Cambridge

1555   Linacre, De emendata structura Latini sermonis.
Cologne, B. Fabricius, 8°.
Adams L 692.   St. John's College, Cambridge

1555   Linacre, De emendata structura Latini sermonis, recognita a J. Camerario.
Leipzig, V. Papst, 8°.
Osler 5058 records his copy as bound in pigskin and stamped 'P.M. 1555', possibly Philippus Melanchthon's copy.   Royal College of Physicians, London

1556   Linacre, De emendata structura Latini sermonis (ed. J. Camerarius).
Leipzig, V. Papst, 8°.   Staatsbibliothek, Bamberg

1556   Linacre, Rudimenta grammatices (tr. G. Buchanan).
Paris, widow of M. de Porta, 8°.   BM

1556   Galen, Opera [3rd ed. See 1541].
Venice, Junta, fol.   Bod.

1556   Proclus, De sphaera (Gk. & Lat.).
Paris, M. Le Jeune, 4°.
The John Rylands Library copy (in red morocco) bears the arms of J. A. de Thou.   BN

1557   Linacre, De emendata structura Latini sermonis.
Venice, P. Manutius, 8°.
Adams L 694; Osler 5059; Renouard, *Aldes* 1557.14.
BM, BN, Bod.

1557   Linacre, De emendata structura Latini sermonis.
Cologne, P. Horst, 8°.   Stadtbibliothek, Mainz

1558   Linacre, Rudimenta grammatices (tr. G. Buchanan).
Paris, M. Menier, 8°.   Yale University

1558   Galen, De temperamentis, De inaequali intemperie (ed.
J. Sylvius).
Lyons, G. Roville, 16°.   BN

1559   Linacre, De emendata structura Latini sermonis.
Leipzig, heirs of V. Papst, 8°.
Universitätsbibliothek, Göttingen

1559   Linacre, De emendata structura Latini sermonis.
Lyons, heirs of S. Gryphius, 8°.
Adams L 695. Buisson. The British Museum copy has
manuscript notes by I. Casaubon.   BM

1559   Linacre, Rudimenta grammatices (tr. G. Buchanan).
(*With* J. L. Vives, De ratione studii puerilis.)
Lyons, heirs of S. Gryphius, 8°.
Adams L 708; Baudrier viii. 295.   BM

1559   Galen, De sanitate tuenda.
Lyons, G. Roville, 16°.
Baudrier ix. 255.   Bod.

1560   Linacre, De emendata structura Latini sermonis.
Basle, N. Brylinger, 8°.
Buisson; Osler 5060.
Royal College of Physicians, London

1560   Galen, De naturalibus facultatibus (De naturalium facul-
tatum substantia).
Lyons, G. Roville, 16°.
Baudrier ix. 265.   BN

1560   Proclus, De sphaera.
Paris, G. Cavellat, 8°.
Osler 3741.   BN

1561   Galen, De naturalibus facultatibus.
       Lyons, G. Roville, 16°.
       Baudrier ix. 275. A reissue of the 1560 edition.

1561   Proclus, De sphaera (Gk. & Lat.) [with other texts].
       Basle, H. Petri, 8°.   BM, BN

1562   Proclus, De sphaera.
       Paris, G. Cavellat, 8°.
       Recorded by Hoffmann 3.293.

1563   Paulus Aeginetae, De crisi & diebus decretoriis, eorumque
       signis. *In* Actuarius (J.), *De urinis.*
       Basle, heirs of A. Cratander, 8°.
       Recorded by Hoffmann 3.45.

1564   Linacre, De emendata structura Latini sermonis.
       Leipzig, heirs of V. Papst, 8°.   Jesus College, Oxford

1565   Galen, Opera [4th ed. See 1541].
       Venice, heirs of L. A. Junta, fol.   BN, Bod.

1565   Galen, De temperamentis. *In* Lopez Canario (E.), *In libros
       Galeni de temperamentis commentaria.*
       Alcala de Henares, P. Robles, and F. Cormellas, fol.
       Palau^2 viii. 140881.   BM

1566   Linacre, [Rudimenta] grammatices compendiosa per
       quaestiones explicatio, a Gregario Molnar.
       Claudiopoli [= Cluj (Kolozsvár), Romania], G. Heltai,
       8°.   Kegyesrondi Központi Könyvtár, Budapest
       This version, apparently a text with commentary, re-
       printed in 1578, may have been the original form of
       Molnar's *Elementa grammatices Latinae* of which there
       were fifteen editions in the seventeenth century. See P.
       Berg, *George Buchanan and his Influence in Hungary*, Buda-
       pest, 1944, pp. 8–11. I am indebted to Professor I. D.
       McFarlane for this reference.

1569   Linacre, De emendata structura Latini sermonis.
       Leipzig, heirs of V. Papst, 8°.
       Osler 5061.   Stadtbibliothek, Nuremberg

1570   Proclus, De sphaera (Gk. & Lat.). *In* Hyginus (C. J.),
       Fabularum liber.
       Basle (officina Hervagiana), fol.   Bod.

1571   Galen, [seven items *in*] *Epitome Galeni* (operum per A. Lacunam collecta).
Basle, T. Guarinus, fol.   BM

1573   Linacre, De emendata structura Latini sermonis.
Leipzig, heirs of V. Papst, 8°.
Staatsbibliothek, Bamberg

1576   Galen, Opera [5th ed. See 1541].
Venice, heirs of L. A. Junta, fol.   BN

1578   Linacre, [Rudimenta] grammatices compendiosa per quaestiones explicatio, a G. Molnar, recognita, et a plurimis mendis repurgata.
Claudiopoli [= Cluj (Kolozsvár), Romania], G. Heltai, 8°.
See Berg, op. cit., under entry for 1566.

1578   Proclus, De sphaera (Gk. & Lat.). *In* Hyginus (C. J.), *Fabularum liber*.
Paris, J. Parant, 8°.   BM, Bod.
A variant bears Paris, G. Julian. Adams H 1254, 1255.

1579   Proclus, De sphaera (Gk. & Lat.).
Breslau, J. Scharffenberg, 8°.
Universitätsbibliothek, Göttingen

1580   Linacre, De emendata structura Latini sermonis (ed. J. Camerarius).
Leipzig, J. Steinman, 8°.
Adams L 697.   St. John's College, Cambridge

1580   Galen, Methodus medendi.
Lyons, G. Roville, 16°.
National Library of Medicine, Bethesda

1583   Paulus Aeginetae, De crisi, & diebus decretoriis.
Basle, Heirs of A. Cratander, 8°.
University Library, Cambridge

1585   Proclus, De sphaera (Gk. & Lat.).
Basle, S. Henricpetri, 8°.   BM, Bod.

1586   Galen, Opera [6th ed. See 1541].
Venice, heirs of L. A. Junta, fol.   BM, Bod.

1589   Proclus, De sphaera (Gk. & Lat.). *In* [Proclus and others,] *Astronomica veterum scripta isagogica Graeca et Latina.*
[Heidelberg], (H. Commelinus), 8°.

Some copies bear 'In officina Commeliana', others 'In officina Sanctandrea'. BM, Bod.

1591 Linacre, De emendata structura Latini sermonis (ed. J. Camerarius).
Leipzig, M. Lantzenberger, 8°.
Adams L 698; Buisson. BN

1592 Galen, De temperamentis [Bk. 3 only]. *In* Valles (F.), *Commentaria.*
Cologne, F. dei Franceschi & G. B. Ciotti, fol. BN
Reissued in 1593 (BM) and 1594 (BN).

1596 (really 1597) Galen, De temperamentis, De naturalibus facultatibus. *In* Segarra (J.), *Commentarii physiologici.*
Valencia, P. P. Mey, fol.
Palau[1] vi. 482. The title-page is dated 1596 but the work was censored on 2 February 1597. BM

1597 Galen, Methodus medendi [Bks. 1–6 only]. *In* Pacius (F.), *Commentarius in sex priores libros Galeni Methodus medendi.*
Vicenza, G. Greco, fol. St. John's College, Cambridge
A variant bears Vicenza, R. Meietti, 1598 (BN)

1597 Galen, Opera [7th ed. See 1541].
Venice, heirs of L. A. Junta, fol.

1600 [Linacre], Syntaxis figurata, ex secundo et sexto libro Thomae Linacri excerpta.
Frankfurt a. d. Oder, A. Eichorn, 12°.
Stadtbibliothek, Braunschweig

1608 Proclus, De sphaera (Gk. & Lat.). *In* Hyginus (C. J.), *Fabularum liber.*
Lyons, J. Degabiano, 8°. BM, Bod.

1609 Galen, Opera [8th ed. See 1541].
Venice, heirs of L. A. Junta, fol. BM

1609 Galen, Methodus medendi. *In* Pacius (F.). *Commentarius* [etc.] Vicenza, G. Greco, fol. BM, BN

1625 Galen, Opera [9th ed. See 1541].
Venice, heirs of L. A. Junta, fol. BM, Bod.

1627   Galen, De morbis et symptomatis (de symptomatum differentiis, de symptomatum causis. Ed. J. F. Rossellus). Barcelona, S. & I. Mathevat, fol.   BM

1715   Linacre, Rudimenta grammatices (tr. G. Buchanan). *In* Buchanan (G.), *Opera omnia*, vol. 2 [separate pagination and signatures. 28 pp.]. Edinburgh, R. Freebairn, fol.   BM, BN, Bod.

1725   Linacre, Rudimenta grammatices (tr. G. Buchanan). *In* Buchanan (G.), *Opera omnia*, ii. 646–98. Leyden, J. A. Langerak, 4°.   BN, Bod.

1881   Galen, De temperamentis et de inaequali intemperie (ed. J. F. Payne). Cambridge, A. Macmillan and R. Bowes, 4°. Osler 385. Facsimile of 1521 edition. Introduction (pp. 5–46) by J. F. Payne.   BM, Bod.

1968   Linacre, De emendata structura Latini sermonis. Menston, Scolar Press (English Linguistics, 83), 4°. Facsimile of the Huntington Library copy of the 1524 edition.   BM, Bod.

1971   Linacre, Rudimenta grammatices. Menston, Scolar Press (English Linguistics, 312), 8°. Facsimile of the British Museum copy of *STC* 15636, here dated [1525].   BM, Bod.

Index of editions (excluding those in Galen's *Opera*).

Linacre, Progymnasmata grammatices vulgaria. [Text in English]
    [1511?], [1515?]
   Rudimenta grammatices. [Text in English]
    [1523], [1525], 1971
   Rudimenta grammatices (Text translated into Latin by G. Buchanan).
    1533(×2), 1536, 1537(×2), 1538, 1539(×2), 1540, 1541(×2), 1542(×3), 1543(×2), 1544, 1545, 1546(×2), 1547, 1548(×2), 1550, 1551, 1552, 1556, 1558, 1559, 1566, 1578, 1715, 1725
   De emendata structura Latini sermonis.
    1524, 1527, 1530, 1531, 1532(×3), 1533(×2), 1537, 1539(3), 1540, 1541(×2), 1542, 1543(×5), 1544, 1545, 1548, 1549, 1550, 1551(×2), 1552, 1553, 1555(×3), 1556, 1557(×2), 1559(×2), 1560, 1564, 1569, 1573, 1580, 1591, 1968

—— Index 1529.
—— Corpus 1554.
—— Syntaxis 1600.

Galen, De naturalibus facultatibus.

1523, 1528, 1537, 1541, 1546, 1547, 1548, 1550, 1560, 1561
De pulsuum usu.

1523/4, 1528, 1532, 1537, 1541, 1549, 1550
De sanitate tuenda.

1517, 1523, 1526, 1530, 1538, 1540, 1541, 1547, 1548, 1549, 1559
De symptomatum differentiis.

1524, 1528, 1627
De temperamentis et de inaequali intemperie.

1521, 1523, 1527, 1528, 1537, 1538($\times$2), 1539, 1540, 1545, 1547, 1549($\times$3), 1553, 1558, 1565, 1592, 1593, 1594, 1596, 1881
Methodus medendi.

1519, 1526, 1527, 1530($\times$2), 1538($\times$2), 1546, 1547, 1549, 1553, 1580, 1597, 1598, 1609

Paulus Aeginetae, De crisi & diebus decretoriis.

1528, 1529($\times$2), 1548, 1563, 1583

Proclus, De sphaera.

1499, 1502, 1503, [1503/4], [1510?], 1511, 1512, 1515, 1522, 1523, 1525, 1534, 1535, 1536, 1539, 1543, 1544, 1547, 1549, 1553, 1554, 1556, 1560, 1561, 1562, 1570, 1578, 1579, 1585, 1589, 1593, 1608

3. *Items associated with Thomas Linacre*

A. *Preface by Linacre*

1. GALEN, Claudius. Claudii Galeni Pergameni de motu musculorum libri duo Nicolao Leoniceno interprete.
London, R. Pynson, 12°. 1522.
STC 11532
Linacre's preface occupies sig. A2 recto. Linacre had attended the lectures of the long-lived and well-known Leoniceno (1428–1524) in Vicenza and must have known his translations of Galen. The manuscript of this work was apparently sent to him by a friend in Italy.

B. *Other works ascribed to Linacre*

Both the following works were published, after Linacre's death, by Robert Wyer who succeeded the author's last printer, Pynson.

1. MACER, Aemilius. Macers herbal practysyd by Doctor Lynacro. Translated out of laten in Englisshe, whiche shewinge theyr Operacyons and Vertues, set in the margent of this Boke, to the intent you myght knowe theyr Vertues.
London, R. Wyer, 8°. [1530?]
STC 17172
See F. R. Johnson, '*A Newe Herball of Macer* and Banckes's *Herball*: Notes on Robert Wyer and the Printing of Cheap Handbooks of Science in the Sixteenth Century', *Bulletin of the History of Medicine*, xv (1944), 246–60.

2. [BORDE, Andrew.] A compendyous Regyment or Dyatorye of healthe. Used at Montpylour, Compyled by Doctour Lynacre, and other Doctours in Physycke.
(London), R. Wyer, 8°. [1542.]
STC 3379
See J. L. Thornton, 'Andrew Boorde, Thomas Linacre and the "Dyetary of Helth"', *Bulletin of the Medical Library Association*, xxxvi (1948), 204–9.
Also later editions in 1567 [1547], 1562, 1576.

3. Rudimenta Latinogallica, cum accentibus, Paris, C. Estienne, 1555, 8°, sometimes ascribed to Linacre, is now attributed to Charles Estienne. See E. Lau, *Charles Estienne* (Inaug. Diss.), Leipzig, 1930, pp. 41, 58.

4. The entry for Linacre in T. Tanner, *Bibliotheca Britannico-Hibernica* (London, 1748, p. 482) ascribes to him, besides a fairly correct list of works, two items which have not been identified or otherwise traced. The entries read: *Epistolas ad diversos*, lib. i. Pr. 'Cum multi tibi quotidie, vir.' *Diversi generis carmina*, lib. i. The absence of bibliographical references, present in the entries for his other works, suggests that the compiler had not actually seen the works in question (see Editors' Introduction, pp. xlv–xlvi, n. 58). There is also a reference later to the translations of Simplicius and Alexander of Aphrodisias mentioned in the opening paragraph of this present survey.

c. *Work dedicated to Linacre*

1. POLLUX, Julius.
ΙΟΥΛΙΟΥ ΡΟΛΙΔΕΥΚΟΥΣ ΟΝΟΜΑΣΤΙΚΟΝ.
Iulii Pollucis Vocabularium (edited by A. Francino).

Florence, B. Junta, folio. 1520.

The undated dedication, which appears on sig AAI, is headed 'Antonius Francinus Varchiensis Thomas Linacro regis Angliae medico. s.' and refers to his translations of the *Methodus medendi*, the *De sanitate tuenda*, and the *De pulsuum usu* and also mentions More's *Utopia*, Pace, and Tunstal. It appears that Francino was induced to dedicate this work to Linacre by their mutual friend Giampiero Machiavelli.

D. *Books from Linacre's library*

No contemporary list of the works in Linacre's library, or in his possession, appears to have survived but the following manuscripts and printed books bear his signature, in a very recognizable thin and precise hand (Liber Thomi Linacri), or have some other mark of possession suggesting his ownership. The following descriptions have been taken from the catalogues cited.

1. ALEXANDER OF APHRODISIAS (and others)

Alexandri Aphrodisiensis commentarius in Aristotelis librum de sensu et sensibilibus; Michaelis Ephesii commentarius in Aristotelis librum de memoria et reminiscentia; Procli Diadochi institutio physica, sive de motu.

Sixteenth-century manuscript on paper.

Now in the Bibliothèque nationale, Paris, MS. Suppl. Gr. 340.

See H. Omont, *Inventaire sommaire des manuscrits grecs de la Bibliothèque nationale*, iii, 1888, p. 251.

2. ALEXANDER OF TRALLES (and others)

Alexandri Tralliani therapeuticon libri XII; Rhazae liber de pestilentia; Aretaei Cappadocis de morborum diuturnorum curatione liber II; ejusdem de causis et signis morborum acutorum libri II; Procli Diadochi commentariorum in Euclidem libri II; Alexandri Aphrodisiensis commentarius in Aristotelis meteorologicorum librum III.

Sixteenth-century manuscript on paper.

Now in the Bibliothèque nationale, Paris, MS. Gr. 2202.

Already associated with Linacre by Montfaucon (*Palaeographia Graeca*, 1708, p. 108). See also Omont, *Inventaire*, ii (1888), p. 213, and J. H. Cotton, 'Materia medica del Poliziano', *Il Poliziano e il suo tempo*, Atti, IV Convegno internazionale di studi sul Rinascimento (Florence, 1957), pp. 241–2.

3. ARISTOTLE

Aristotelis de partibus animalium liber viii; de anima libri iii; de animalium incessu: de sensu et sensibilibus libri ii; de memoria et reminiscentia; de somno et vigilia; metaphysicorum libri xiv.
Fifteenth-century manuscript on paper.
Now in the Bibliothèque nationale, Paris, MS. Suppl. Gr. 333.
See Omont, *Inventaire . . . supplément* (1883), p. 40.

4. ARISTOTLE (and others)

[Works. Greek. Edited by Aldus Manutius, with the assistance of Alessandro Bondini. With tracts by Theophrastus, Philo, and others.]
Venice, A. Manutius, 1495–8. Five volumes, folio.
Now in New College, Oxford, shelfmark Ω.7.1–6.

5. CEDRENUS, G.

Georgii Cedreni compendii historiarum fragmentum.
Sixteenth-century manuscript.
Now in the Bibliotheek der Rijksuniversiteit, Leyden, MS. B.P.G. 10.
See Leyden University Library, *Codices manuscripti*, viii (1965), p. 13.

6. CICERO, M. T.

[Opera. Edited A. Minuziano.]
Milan, Guillaume Le Signerre, 1498[9]. Four volumes, folio. Inscribed by Linacre and also 'Liber ecclesie cathedralis Dunelm', 'Jo. Milner Custos Biblioth. May 4°—1703.' Part of Royal Library, 1715.
Now in the University Library, Cambridge.
See J. C. T. Oates, *A Catalogue of the fifteenth-century printed books in the University Library Cambridge* (1954), no. 2323.

7. CICERO, M. T.

De officiis.
Early thirteenth-century manuscript on vellum.
Formerly belonged to St. Augustine's, Canterbury. Inscribed 'Linacrus emit octo denariis'.
Now in the British Museum, Royal MS. 15 A. VI.
See G. F. Warner and J. P. Gilson, *Catalogue of Western manuscripts*, xi (1921), p. 143.

8. CICERO, M. T. [and other items]
Rhetorica.
Manuscript. Whereabouts unknown.

Presumably inherited by Linacre from his friend John Mower whose will, written in 1489, includes: 'item lego eidem domino Thome studenti Florencij libros subscriptos uidelicet Magistrum Sentenciarum impressum, Thucideni historiarum Peloponencium impressum, Tullium in Noua Rhetorica, in pargameno scriptum. Item eidem duos libros grecos unum impressum, alterum pargamento scriptum'.

See R. Weiss, 'Notes on Thomas Linacre', *Miscellanea Giovanni Mercati*, Studi e testi, 124 (Vatican City, 1946), p. 374.

9. COLUMELLA, L. J. M.

Opera agricolationum Columellae Varronis Catonisque necnon Palladii cum ex scriptionibus ac commentariis D. Philippi Beroaldi. Reggio, D. Bertochus, 1496. Folio.

Apparently given by Cuthbert Tunstal to Richard Sparcheford and by him to Richard Langford in 1551. Later in Thomas Bulkley's possession and presented to the College in 1733 by William Woodford because of its Linacre connections. (See Fig. 3.)

Now in the library of the Royal College of Physicians, London.

FIG. 3. Linacre's signature in Latin on his copy of *Opera agricolationum Columellae Varronis Catonisque necnon Palladii cum ex scriptionibus ac commentariis D. Philippi Beroaldi*, Reggio, 1496, now in the Library of the Royal College of Physicians, London (no. 9 above)

10. EROTIAN (and others)

Erotiani lexicon medicum; Galeni lexicon Hippocratum, [anonymi] theorica spherae; Claudii Ptolomaei geographia libri i–iii.

Sixteenth-century manuscript on paper. Linacre's signature on items one, three, and four.

Now in the Bibliothèque royale, Brussels, MS. Gk. 45.

See H. Omont, *Catalogue des manuscrits grecs de la bibliothèque royale de Bruxelles* (1885), p. 18.

11. GALEN, C.

Galeni anatomica libri i–iv (imperfect).

Sixteenth-century manuscript on paper, inscribed by Linacre with his name in both Latin and Greek. Now in the Bibliotheek der Rijksuniversiteit, Leyden, MS. Vulcaniani 57. (See Fig. 4.)

See H. Diels, 'Die Handschriften der antiken Aerzte', *Abhandlungen der k. preussischen Akademie der Wissenschaften*, 1905/6, p. 66, and Leyden University Library, *Codices manuscripti*, i, *Codices Vulcani* (1910), p. 25.

FIG. 4. Linacre's signature in Greek on his sixteenth-century manuscript copy of *Galeni anatomica libri i–iv*, now in the Bibliotheek der Rijksuniversiteit, Leyden, MS. Vulcaniani 57 (no. 11 above)

12. GALEN, C.

Galeni de simplicium medicamentorum temperamentis ac facultatibus.

Now in the Bibliotheek der Rijksuniversiteit, Leyden, MS. B.P.G. 16 (now 759 C24).

See Leyden University Library, *Codices manuscripti*, viii (1965), p. 15.

13. MAFFEIUS, R.

[Commentariorum urbanorum libri 38. Item Oeconomicus Xenophontis ab eodem latio donatus.]

Paris, J. Petit & J. Bade, 1511. Folio.

Contemporary leather binding by Claude Chevallon.

Now in the Wellcome Historical Medical Library, London; see their *Catalogue of Printed Books*, i (1962), no. 3940.

14. PAULUS AEGINETAE

Pauli Aeginetae de re medica libris sex; de lapidibus et figurae astrologicae.

Fourteenth-century manuscript on paper.

Now in the Bibliothèque nationale, Paris, MS. Suppl. Gr. 338.

See Omont, *Inventaire . . . supplément* (1883), p. 41.

15. PETRUS, LOMBARDUS, bishop of Paris

Liber Sententiarum.

Presumably one of the Venice editions of 1477, 1486, or 1489. Bequeathed to Linacre by John Mower. Whereabouts unknown. See entry D8.

16. PICO DELLA MIRANDOLA, G. F.

Ioannis Francisci Pici Mirandulae domini Concordiaeque comitis liber de providentia dei contra philosophastros.
Novi [di Modena], B. M. Dulcibellus, 1508. Folio.
Written by the younger Pico della Mirandola, the life of whose uncle was translated by More.
This copy was also R. Sparcheford's, then presented by him to the Ludlow parish library in 1557 and by John Selden's executors to the Bodleian in 1659.
Now in the Bodleian Library, Oxford, shelfmark D.2.13 Art. Seld.

17. PLUTARCH

Sapientissimi Plutarchi parallelum vitae Romanorum et Graecorum quadraginta novem.

Florence, P. Junta, 1517. Folio.

This copy, in a typical, plain, early sixteenth-century English binding with the title inscribed on the upper and lower edges, bears the name of Robert Throckmorton 1684 and the book-labels of the third (1662–1721) and fourth (1702–91) baronets of the same name.
Now in the library of the Royal College of Physicians, London.

18. SENECA, L. A.

Epistolae. Opera philosophica. [*With*] Controversiae. Suasoriae.
Venice, B. de Chonis, 1492. Folio.
Now in the Wellcome Historical Medical Library; see their *Catalogue of Printed Books*, i (1962), no. 5918.

19. THEOPHYLACT, archbishop of Achrida

Theophylactii Bulgariae archiepiscopi Enarrationes in quatuor evangelistas, praevie SS. Lucae et Johannis evangeliis capitulorum tabula. Fifteenth-century manuscript on vellum and in Greek. Inscribed on folio 4 'Magister Grocinus' and 'Linacrus emit a vivo Grocino eodem pretio, quo Grocinus emerat' and on folio 5 'Orate pro anima Joannis Claimondii, primi praesidis collegii Corporis Christi, qui hunc librum eidem condonavit'.
Now in Corpus Christi College, Oxford (MS. 30).
See H. O. Coxe, *Catalogus codicum MSS. qui in collegiis aulisque Oxoniensibus hodie adservantur*, Pars II, *Catalogus Codicum MSS. Collegii Corporis Christi* (Oxford, 1852), pp. 8–9.

20. THUCYDIDES

Historiarum Peloponnensium liber primus (–octavus). [Tr. L. Valla. Ed. B. Parthenius.]
[Treviso, J. Vercellensis, 1483?] Folio.
Bequeathed to Linacre by John Mower in 1489. Whereabouts unknown. See entry D8.

FIG. 5. Historiated capital letter from George Buchanan's introduction in the first edition of his translation of Linacre, *Rudimenta grammatices*, Paris, 1533. (See p. 314)

Published References to Thomas Linacre

MARGARET PELLING*

IN THE BIBLIOGRAPHY WHICH FOLLOWS, THE ITEMS
are arranged in alphabetical order within centuries. At no point is
the list intended to be exhaustive, but as many references as possible
from the period before 1600 have been included, since these provide
almost the only basis in fact for the later items. These early references are unexpectedly few in number, and usually very brief. This
naturally means that many of the later items, especially those dating
from between 1600 and 1800, merely repeat each other, at least in
essentials. Repetition has not been used as a criterion for exclusion,
because it is not intended that this bibliography will serve simply
as a reading list. It should also show what notice was taken of
Linacre at different times (as either a particular or a representative
figure), and for what reasons; that this is possible with respect to
the modern, as well as earlier periods perhaps indicates how little
attention has been paid to Linacre by historians in general.

No attempt has been made to indicate the comparative merits of
the items listed. Older works must obviously be approached with
caution, but it should also be noted that many of the more recent
items are inferior in quality as well as repetitious.

Early references are listed under the author and title of the work
in which they were first published. In many cases, a reference made
its first appearance in a work which was issued under a name other
than that of the author of the reference itself; for example, a letter
by Guillaume Budé which refers to Linacre was first published by
Erasmus in the *Epistole elegantes* of 1517, and was not included in a

* Research Assistant, Wellcome Unit for the History of Medicine, Oxford
University.

work by Budé until 1531. Where possible in such cases, cross reference is made to a modern edition of the relevant text. Some letters
to Erasmus which refer to Linacre (by, for example, John Colet,
Thomas More, Thomas Lupset, William Latimer, Josse Bade, Girolamo Aleandro) were not published until the modern period, or until
Leclerc's edition of Erasmus's works (1703–6); these do not appear
under the names of their authors but may be located in P. S. Allen's
edition of Erasmus's letters (1906–58).[1]

References to Linacre which appear in prefaces to works or translations which are wholly his do not appear in this section of the
bibliography.

In some of the earlier works either Linacre's name is not indexed
or there is no index. In such cases the page references are recorded
on the cards on which this list is based; these, together with xero-
graphic reproductions of the more interesting or less readily available items, are now on deposit in the Library of Linacre College,
Oxford. Locations, and some indication of the nature of references,
as well as some items of peripheral interest, may also be found in
this card index.

Linacre is mentioned in most histories of his period and these, as
well as the usual reference works, have generally been omitted. The
reader will observe that Linacre's name appears in a sufficient number of early biographical dictionaries and similar works, and in
encyclopaedias from Moréri (1674) and the second edition of Bayle
(1702). Linacre's name also tends to appear in Harveian Orations
and on other prescribed occasions. Most of the 'Linacre Lectures'
make some mention of their founder, but, as in all such cases, these
are included only if Linacre is a subject of particular concern. Most
of the Lectures (not all of which have been published) may be found
in the Library of the Royal College of Physicians, London.

Lastly, in all doubtful cases, both names and titles follow the
practice of the British Museum General Catalogue of Printed Books.

REFERENCES BEFORE 1600

Afineus, Henricus. *Quaestiones tres . . . de reductione medicinarum ad actum
. . . de correctione calendarii . . .*, Antwerp, 1517. See Erasmus, D.,
1906–58, vol. ii, no. 542.

---

[1] A very few omissions from the entry for Linacre in the index volume of
the Allen edition are recorded in the card index mentioned below.

Bale, John. *Illustrium maioris Britanniae scriptorum, hoc est, Angliae, Cambriae, ac Scotiae summarium* [Wesel], 1548. See also Bale, J., 1902.

Idem. *Scriptorum illustrium maioris Brytannie . . . Catalogus*, Basle, [1557, 1559].

Barth, Michael. *Oratio de Thoma Linacro Britanno conscripta et habita in academia Lipsica*, Leipzig, 1560.

Bildius, Beatus, Hutten, U. von, Hattstein, M. von [and others]. *Epistolae aliquot eruditorum virorum, ex quibus perspicuum quanta sit Eduardi Lei virulentia*, Basle, 1520.

Budé, Guillaume. *Epistolae G. B. Regii Secretarii*, Paris, 1520. For Budé see Delaruelle, L., 1907. See here also Johnson, J. N., 1835, pp. 252–4, 309–11.

Idem. *G. B. R. S. Epistolae*, Basle, 1521.

Bullein, William. *Bulleins Bulwarke of defence againste all Sicknes, Sorenes, and woundes . . . (Here after insueth a little Dialogue, betwene twoo men, the one called Sorenes, and the other Chyrurgj . . .)*, London, 1562.

Caesarius, Joannes. *Dialectica*, Paris, 1538. Cf. the editions of [1525], 1532, 1551, in which there is respectively no reference, minimal, and diminished reference to Linacre.

Caius, John. *De libris propriis, liber unus*, London, 1570. For Caius, see Caius, J., *Works*, 1912.

Idem. *J. C. . . . De pronunciatione Grecae et Latinae linguae cum scriptione nova libellus*, London, 1574.

Idem. *Historiae Cantebrigiensis Academiae ab urbe condita*, London, 1574.

Champier, Symphorien. *Claudii Galeni Pergameni historiales campi per D. S. C. . . . in quatuor libros congesti et commentariis non poenitandis illustrati . . . Clysteriorum camporum secundum Galeni mentem . . .*, Basle, 1532.

Cheke, John. *J. C. . . . De pronuntiatione Graecae potissimum linguae disputationes cum Stephano Wintoniensi Episcopo . . .*, Basle, 1555.

Croke, Richard. *Orationes R. Croci duae, altera a cura, qua utilitatem laudemque Graecae linguae tractat, altera a tempore, qua hortatus est Cantabrigienses, ne desertores essent eiusdem* [Paris, 1520].

Crusius, Martinus. *Germanograeciae libri sex*, Basle, 1566.

Erasmus, Desiderius. *Aliquot epistole sanequam elegantes E. R. . . .*, Louvain, 1517. For the letters of Erasmus see Erasmus, D., 1906–58; letters to Erasmus are included. See here ibid., vol. ii, no. 435.

Idem. *Apophthegmatum sive scite dictorum libri sex . . .*, Paris, 1531.

Idem. *Auctarium selectarum aliquot epistolarum E. R. ad eruditos, et horum ad illum*, Basle, 1518.

Idem. *De recta Latini Graecique sermonis pronuntiatione D. E. R. dialogus. Eiusdem dialogus cui titulus, Ciceronianus . . .*, Paris, 1528.

Idem (ed.). *Divi Joannes Chrysostomi, quod multae quidē dignitatis, sed difficile sit Episcopum agere, dialogi sex*, Basle, 1525. (Greek. See Erasmus, D., 1906–58, vol. vi, no. 1558.)

Idem. *Epistolae . . . ad diversos*, Basle, 1521.

Idem. *D. E. . . . Epistolarum floridarum liber unus, antehac nunquam excusus*, Basle, 1531.

Idem. *Epistole aliquot illustrium virorum ad E. R. et huius ad illos*, Louvain, 1516. See Erasmus, D., 1906–58, vol. ii, no. 388.

Idem. *E. R. Apologia, refellens suspiciones quorundam dictitantium dialogum D. Iacobi Latomi de tribus linguis & ratione studii Theologici, conscriptum fuisse adversos ipsum . . .*, Basle, 1519.

Idem. *Farrago nova epistolarum . . .*, Basle, 1519. See also Erasmus, D., 1906–58, vol. i, nos. 221, 243; ibid., vol. ii, no. 520.

Idem. *Omnia Opera D. Erasmi . . . quaecunque ipse autor pro suis agnovit . . . Cum praefatione B. Rhenani Selestadiensis, vitam autoris describente . . .*, 9 vols., Basle, 1540, etc. See esp. Erasmus, D., 1906–58, vol. i, nos. III and IV; ibid., vol. iii, no. 664.

Idem. *Omnium operum Divi Eusebii Hieronymi . . . tomus primus . . . una cum argumentis et scholiis D. Erasmi . . .*, Basle, 1516.

Idem. *Opus epistolarum . . .*, Basle, 1529.

Fuchs, Leonhart. 'Reverendo in Christo Patri ac Domino D. Nicolao Biechnero Abbati . . . Leohartus Fuchsius, S. P. D.', Dedicatory letter in *Claudii Galeni . . . de sanitate tuenda libri sex, a Thoma Linacro Anglo latinitate donati . . .*, Tübingen, 1541.

Furio Ceriol, Federico. *Bononia, sive de libris sacris in vernaculam linguam convertendis libri duo*, Basle, 1556.

Gesner, Conrad. *Bibliotheca universalis*, Zürich, 1545.

Idem. 'Prolegomena tripartita, De vita Galeni, eiusque libris et interpretibus', *C. Galeni Pergameni omnia, quae extant, in latinum sermonem conversa*, vol. i, 5 vols., Basle, 1561–2. There is no such introduction in the edition of 1550.

Giovio, Paulo. *Elogia doctorum virorum ab avorum memoria publicatis ingenii monumentis illustrium*, Antwerp, 1557. See also idem, *Elogia virorum literis illustrium, quotquot vel nostra vel avorum memoria vixere*, Basle, 1577. See also Johnson, J. N., 1835, pp. 147–8.

Hakluyt, Richard. *The Principal Navigations, Voyages, Traffiques and Discoveries of the English Nation, made by Sea or over-land . . . at any time within the compasse of these 1600 yeres . . .*, 3 vols., London, 1599–1600.

Holinshed, Raphael. *The Last Volume of the Chronicles of England, Scotlande, and Irelande, with their descriptions* (London, 1577).

Hutten, Ulrich von. *U. H. . . . Aula dialogus. Phalarismus Huttenicus. Dialogus febris . . .*, Basle, 1519. See More, T., 1947, no. 67.

Jobst, Wolfgang. *Chronologia*, Frankfurt, 1556.

Joubert, Laurent. *In Galeni libros de facultatibus naturalibus annotationes...* A.D. *MDLXIII,* in *Operum Latinor.,* 2 tom., Lyons, 1579.

Lascarus, J. *De Romanorum militia, et castrorum metatione liber utilissimus, ex Polybii historiis . . . Eiusdem A. J. L. epigrammata . . .,* Basle, 1537.

Le Coq, Pascal. *Bibliotheca medica,* Basle, 1590.

Leland, John. *Principum, ac illustrium aliquot et eruditorum in Anglia virorum, encomia, trophaea, genethliaca et epithalamia . . .,* London, 1589.

[Lily, William, *et al.*]. *Institutio compendiaria totius grammaticae, quam et eruditissimus atque idem illustrissimus Rex noster hoc nomine evulgari iussit, ut non alia que haec una per totam Angliam pueris praelegeretur,* London, 1542.

Longolius, Christophorus. *C. L. Orationes duae pro defensione sua . . .,* Florence, 1524.

Lyly, George. 'Virorum aliquot in Britannia, qui nostro seculo eruditione, et doctrina clari, memorabilesque fuerunt, elogia', in Paulo Giovio, *Descriptio Britanniae, Scotiae, Hyberniae, et Orchadum,* Venice, 1548.

Manutius, Aldus. [Prefatory epistle, to Alberto Pio] in *Aristoteles Stagyris, Philosophus. Opera, Graecè . . .* [Works. Edited by Aldus, with Alexander Bondinus. With tracts by Theophrastus, Philo, *et al.*], 5 vols., Venice, 1495–8, vol. i, Part II.

More, Thomas. *Ad lectorem. Habes candide lector opusculum illud vere aureū Thomae Mori nō minꝰ utile q̃ elegās de optimo reipublicę statu, deꝗ nova Insula Utopia . . .* [Paris, 1517]. See Delaruelle, L., 1907, no. 12; Lupton, J. H., *The Utopia of Sir Thomas More,* Oxford, 1895, pp. lxxx–xcii.

Idem. *T. M. . . . Lucubrationes . . . quibus additae sunt duae aliorum Epistolae . . .,* Basle, 1563.

Neander, Michael. *Graecae linguae erotemata . . .,* Basle, 1565. Linacre is mentioned in a preface by Neander which does not occur in the edition of 1561.

Newton, Thomas. [Prefatory poem] in *A Niewe Herball, or Historie of Plantes: wherin is contayned the whole discourse and perfect description of all sortes of Herbes and Plantes . . . First set foorth in the Doutche or Almaigne tongue, by that learned D. Rembert Dodoens . . . and nowe first translated out of French into English, by Henry Lyte Esquyer,* London, 1578.

Pace, Richard. *R. P. . . . De fructu qui ex doctrina percipitur, liber,* Basle, 1517.

Rabelais, F. *Le Quart Livre des faicts & dictz heroiques du bon Pantagruel,* Lyons, 1552.

Reuchlin, Johann. *Illustrium virorum epistolae, Hebraicae, Graecae et Latinae, ad I. R. . . .,* Hanau, 1519. See Erasmus, D., 1906–58, vol. ii, no. 471.

Stapleton, Thomas. 'D. Thomae Mori Angliae quondam Cancellarii vita', *Tres Thomae* . . ., Douai, 1588. See also Erasmus, D., 1906–58, vol. iii, no. 907; More, T., 1947, no. 3.

Vives, J. L. *De disciplinis libri XX*, Antwerp, 1531. See Vives, J. L., 1913.

Idem. *I. L. V. V. Epistolarum, quae hactenus desiderabantur, farrago* . . ., Antwerp, 1556.

Idem. *J. L. V. . . . Opera* . . ., Basle, 1555.

Idem. *Opuscula aliquot vere catholica* . . . *De ratione studii puerilis epistolae II*, Strasburg, [1521]. Cf. the edition of 1527.

Whittington, Robert. *Vulgaria R. W. L. et de institutione grammaticulorum Opusculum* . . ., London, [1521].

Zasius, Johannes Udalricus. *Lucubrationes*, Basle, 1518. See Erasmus, D., 1906–58, vol. iii, no. 862.

1600–99

Baillet, Adrien. *Jugemens des sçavans sur les principaux ouvrages des auteurs*, 4 tom. (9 vols.), Paris, 1685–6.

[Baker, Thomas.] *Reflections upon Learning*, London, 1699.

Bernier, J. *Essais de médecine*, 3 pts., Paris, 1689.

Blount, Thomas Pope. *Censura celebriorum authorum*, London, 1690.

[Burton, Robert.] *The Anatomy of Melancholy*, Oxford, 1621.

Castellanus, Petrus. *Vitae illustrium medicorum*, Antwerp, 1617. (On British Museum copy, date of imprint altered by hand to 1618.)

Dugdale, William. *The History of St Paul's Cathedral in London* . . ., London, 1658. (See above, Editors' Introduction, pp. xxv–xxvi and xlviii, nn. 78 and 79.)

Fuller, Thomas. *The History of the Worthies of England*, London, 1662. (Bodleian copy has notes in MS. by R. Thoresby and Oldys.)

Gaddius, Jacobus. *De scriptoribus non ecclesiasticis, Graecis, Latinis, Italicis* . . ., vol. i, Florence, 1648.

Goodall, Charles. *The Royal College of Physicians of London, founded and established by law* . . ., London, 1684.

Hayne, Thomas. *Grammatices compendium, anno 1637* . . ., London, 1640.

Hentzner, Paul. *Itinerarium Germaniae, Galliae; Angliae; Italiae*, Nuremberg, 1612.

Huet, Pierre Daniel. *P. D. H. De interpretatione libri duo: quorum prior est, de optimo genere interpretandi: alter, de claris interpretibus*, Paris, 1661.

Koenig, Georg Matthias. *Bibliotheca vetus et nova*, Altdorf, 1678.

Linden, J. A. van der. *De scriptis medicis libri duo*, Amsterdam, 1662. This reference does not appear in the two earlier editions of 1637 and 1651.

Magirus, Tobias. *T. M. Eponymologium criticum, complectens cognomina, descriptiones, elogia, et censuras* . . . Ed. C. W. Eubenius, Frankfurt/

Leipzig, 1687. There is no reference to Linacre in the edition of 1644.

M[ilton], J[ohn]. *Accedence Commenc't Grammar, Supply'd with sufficient Rules, for the use of such as, Younger or Elder, are desirous, without more trouble then needs, to attain the Latin Tongue . . .*, London, 1669.

Moréri, Louis. *Le Grand Dictionaire historique*, Lyons, 1674.

Moufet, Thomas. *Insectorum sive minimorum animalium theatrum* [ed. T. Turquet de Mayerne], London, 1634.

Neander, J. *Antiquissimae et nobilissimae medicinae natalitia, sectae earumque placita . . .*, Bremen, 1623.

Opmeer, Pieter van. *Opus chronographicum orbis universi . . .*, Antwerp, 1611.

Philipot, Thomas. *Villare Cantianum: or Kent surveyed and illustrated*, London, 1659.

Pirckheimer, W. *V. illustriss. B. P. . . . Opera politica, historica, philologica et epistolica . . .*, ed. M. Goldast, Frankfurt, 1610. See Erasmus, D., 1906–58, vol. vi, no. 1603.

Pitseus, Joannes. *J. P. A. . . . Relationum historicarum de rebus Anglicis . . .*, tom. i, Paris, 1619. (Running title of work: *De illustribus Angliae scriptoribus*.)

Selden, John. *I. S. De synedriis et praefecturis iuridicis veterum Ebraeorum*, 3 Bks., London, 1650–5.

Vives, J. L. *Epistolarum D. Erasmi . . . libri xxxi . . . Quibus adjiciuntur . . . L. V. epistolae*, London, 1642.

Vossius, Gerardus. *G. I. V. De quatuor artibus popularibus, de philologia, et scientiis mathematicis . . . libri tres* [ed. F. Du Jon], Amsterdam, 1650.

Weever, John. *Ancient Funerall Monuments*, London, 1631.

Wood, Anthony. *Athenae Oxonienses . . . From . . . 1500 to the end of the year 1690 . . . To which are added, the Fasti or Annals of the said University . . .*, 2 vols., London, 1691. See also Wood, A., 1813–20.

[Idem.] *Historia et antiquitates universitatis Oxoniensis*, Oxford, 1673. See also Wood, A., 1792–6.

1700–99

Aikin, J. *Biographical Memoirs of Medicine in Great Britain from the Revival of Literature to the time of Harvey*, London, 1780.

Baker, George. *Oratio ex Harveii instituto habita in Theatro Collegii Regalis Medicorum Londinensis, Octob. 19, MDCCLXI*, London, 1761.

Bayle, Pierre. *Dictionaire historique et critique*, 2nd edn., revd. corrected and enlgd. by the author. 3 vols., Rotterdam, 1702. There is no reference to Linacre in the 1st edn., 1697. See also Chauffepié, J. G. de, 1750–6.

Biographia Britannica: or, the lives of the most eminent persons who have flourished in Great Britain and Ireland . . ., 6 vols., vol. 6 in 2 pts., London, 1747–66.

Boerner, C. F. C. F. B. *De doctis hominibus Graecis litterarum Graecarum in Italia instauratoribus liber*, Leipzig, 1750.

Caius, Thomas. *Vindiciae antiquitatis Academiae Oxoniensis contra Joannem Caium, Cantabrigiensem* . . ., 2 vols., Oxford, 1730.

Chauffepié, J. G. de. *Nouveau dictionnaire historique et critique, pour servir de supplément ou de continuation au Dictionnaire historique et critique de Mr. Pierre Bayle*, 4 vols., Amsterdam, etc., 1750–6. See also Bayle, P., 1702.

Clarmundus, Adolphus [pseud. J. C. Ruediger]. *Vitae clarissimorum in re literaria virorum*, Wittenberg, 1704.

Davies, Myles. *Athenae Britannicae: or, a Critical History of the Oxford and Cambridge writers and writings*, Part i, London, 1716.

Idem. [as above]: Vol. vi, *Containing the Present and Former State of Physick* . . ., 5 pts., n. p., [1719].

Éloy, N.-F.-J. *Dictionnaire historique de la médecine, contenant son origine, ses progrès, ses révolutions*, . . . *l'histoire des plus célèbres médecins* . . ., Liège/Frankfurt, 1755. Cf. 2nd edn., 1778.

Fabricius, J. A. *Bibliotheca Graeca*, 14 vols., Hamburg, 1705–28.

Freind, John. *The History of Physick; from the time of Galen, to the beginning of the Sixteenth Century. Chiefly with regard to practice*, 2 vols., London, 1725–6.

Idem. *J. F. . . . Opera omnia medica* [ed. . . . J. Wigan, etc.], London, 1733.

Haller, Albrecht von. *Bibliotheca medicinae practicae* . . ., Berne/Basle, 1776–88.

Hasted, E. *The History and Topographical Survey of the County of Kent*, 4 vols., Canterbury, 1778–99.

Hoadly, B. *Oratio anniversaria in Theatro Collegii Medicorum Londiniensium, ex Harveii instituto habita, die 18 Oct. A.D. MDCCXLII*, London, 1742.

Hutchinson, Benjamin. *Biographica medica*, 2 vols., London, 1799.

Jones, David. *Some Remarks upon Modern Education. A Sermon preach'd in the Cathedral-Church of Canterbury . . . at the Anniversary Meeting of the Gentlemen Educated at the King's School There*, London, 1729.

Jortin, J. *The Life of Erasmus*, 2 vols., London, 1758, 1760.

Knight, Samuel. *The Life of Dr. John Colet, Dean of St. Paul's* . . ., London, 1724.

Leland, John. *Commentarii de scriptoribus Britannicis*. Ed. from Leland's MS. by A. Hall, Oxford, 1709.

Maittaire, M. *Annales typographici ab artis inventae origine ad annum MD* . . ., 3 vols., vols. 2 and 3 in 2 pts., The Hague, 1719–25.

Idem. 'Viro doctissimo J. Freind, . . . M. M.' [a life of Linacre]. See Freind, J., *The History of Physick*, 1725–6.

Mencke, Friedrich Otto, *F. O. M. . . . Historia vitae et in literas meritorum Angeli Politiani . . .*, Leipzig, 1736.

Montfaucon, B. de. *Palaeographica Graeca*, Paris, 1708.

Morhof, Daniel Georg. *D. G. M. Polyhistor, in tres tomos, literarium . . . philosophicum et practicum . . .*, ed. and enlgd. by J. Möller, Lübeck, 1708. There is no reference to Linacre in the editions of 1688 and 1695–8.

[Niceron, J. P., and others.] *Mémoires pour servir à l'histoire des hommes illustres dans la république des lettres avec un catalogue raisonné de leurs ouvrages*, 43 vols., Paris, 1727–45.

Relhan, Anthony. *Oratio ex Harveii instituto*, London, 1771.

Ruediger, J. C. See Clarmundus, A., 1704.

Rymer, Thomas. *Foedera, conventiones, literae et cuiuscunque generis Acta publica inter Reges Angliae . . .*, 20 vols., London, 1704–35.

Saxe, Christoph. *C. Saxii Onomasticon literarium, sive nomenclator historico-criticus praestantissimorum omnis aetatis, populi, artiumque formulae scriptorum . . .*, 8 vols., Utrecht, 1775–1803.

Schoettgen, Christian. *J. A. Fabricii . . . Bibliotheca Latina mediae et infimae aetatis . . . Quos post fata viri summi addidit C. S.*, vol. 6, Hamburg, 1746.

Tanner, Thomas. *Bibliotheca Britannico-Hibernica: sive, de scriptoribus qui in Anglia, Scotia, et Hibernia ad saeculi XVII initium floruerunt . . .*, London, 1748.

Wood, Anthony. *The History and Antiquities of the University of Oxford*, ed. J. Gutch, 2 vols., vol. 2 in 2 pts., Oxford, 1792–6. See also Wood, A., 1673.

Zedler, J. H. *Grosses vollständiges Universal Lexicon . . .*, vol. xvii, Halle/Leipzig, 1738.

1800–99

Anonymus. 'Bygone Medical Worthies: I. Thomas Linacre M.D.', *Medical Times and Hospital Gazette*, xxiv, 1896, 89.

Idem. '*The Life of Thomas Linacre . . .* by John Noble Johnson . . .', *Medical Quarterly Review*, iv, 1835, 337–41.

Idem. 'The Life of Thomas Linacre, by S. M. [*sic*] Johnson, M.D. Edited by R. Graves', *The Gentleman's Magazine*, N.S. III, 1835, 633–4.

Baker, Thomas. *History of the College of St. John the Evangelist, Cambridge*, ed. J. E. B. Mayor, 2 vols., Cambridge, 1869.

Bayle, A.-L.-J., and Thillaye, A.-J. *Biographie médicale par ordre chronologique d'après Daniel Leclerc, Éloy, etc.*, 2 vols., Paris, 1855.

Bennett, James Risdon. 'Thomas Linacre, M.D.', *Leisure Hour*, xxxvii, 1888, 546–8.

Bettany, G. T. *Eminent Doctors: their Lives and their Work*, 2 vols., London, [1885–6].

Bridgeman, G. T. O. *The History of the Church and Manor of Wigan in the County of Lancaster*, 4 vols. Chetham Society, N.S. xv–xviii, Manchester, 1888–90.

Burrows, Montagu. 'Linacre's Catalogue of Books belonging to William Grocyn in 1520, together with his Accounts as Executor, followed by a Memoir of William Grocyn', *Collectanea*, ed. M. Burrows, 2nd Ser., Oxford Historical Society, Oxford, 1890, pp. 319–80.

Idem. *Worthies of All Souls*, London, 1874.

Cabanis, P. J. G. *Coup d'œil sur les révolutions et sur la réforme de la médecine*, Paris, 1804.

Encyclopaedia Britannica, 9th edn., vol. xiv, Edinburgh, 1882. Article on Linacre by J. F. P[ayne], q.v.

Gasquet, F. A. 'The Notebooks of William Worcester, a Fifteenth Century Antiquary' in *The Old English Bible, and other Essays*, London, 1897, pp. 286–318.

Haase, Friedrich. *Vorlesungen über lateinische Sprachwissenschaft*, ed. F. A. Eckstein, 2 vols., Leipzig, 1874.

Jeaffreson, J. C. *A Book about Doctors*, 2 vols., London, 1860.

Johnson, John Noble. *The Life of Thomas Linacre*, ed. R. Graves, London, 1835.

Linacre Reports. Vols. i–iii, 1893–7. Ed. E. Ray Lankester.

[MacMichael, W.] *Lives of British Physicians*, London, 1830. The Family Library, No. XIV.

Manning, Joseph. 'Linacre's "Three Parts of Medicine"', *Notes and Queries*, 8th ser. iv, 1893, 146.

Munk, W. *The Roll of the Royal College of Physicians of London: compiled from the annals of the College . . . by W. Munk*, 2 vols., London, 1861.

Payne, J. F. *Galeni Pergamensis de temperamentis, et inaequali intemperie libri tres Thoma Linacro interprete . . . Impressum . . . per J. Siberch, anno MDXXI*, facsimile edn., with introduction by J. F. Payne, Cambridge, 1881. See also *Encyclopaedia Britannica*, 1882.

Idem. *Harvey and Galen*, London, 1897. Harveian Oration, 1896.

Idem. 'Linacre', *Dictionary of National Biography*, xxxiii, ed. Sidney Lee, London, 1893, pp. 266–71.

Pettigrew, T. J. *Medical Portrait Gallery. Biographical memoirs of the most celebrated physicians, surgeons . . .*, 4 vols., London, [1840].

[Public Record Office.] *Letters and Papers, Foreign and Domestic, of the Reign of Henry VIII . . .*, vols. 1–4 arranged and catalogued by J. S. Brewer; vol. 5, etc., by J. Gairdner; vols. 14–21 by J. Gairdner and R. H. Brodie. 34 pts., London, 1862–1932. See also the 2nd edn., revd. and gtly. enlgd. by R. H. Brodie, 3 pts., 1920.

Richardson, B. W. 'The Inter-relationships of Clerical and Medical Functions', *The Clergyman's Magazine*, iv, 1877, 1–19. A Trophy Room Lecture to the Homilectical Society.

Robertson, C. Grant. *All Souls College*, London, 1899. University of Oxford College Histories.

Seebohm, F. *The Oxford Reformers of 1498: being a History of the Fellow-Work of John Colet, Erasmus, and Thomas More*, London, 1867. See also the 3rd edn., 1887.

Sherwood, G. F. T. 'Early Berkshire Wills, from the P.C.C., ante 1558', *Berks, Bucks and Oxon Archaeological Journal*, N.S. i, 1895, 89–92 [part of article].

Simson, J. *Eminent Men of Kent*, London, 1893.

Wood, Anthony. *Athenae Oxonienses*, ed. and contd. by P. Bliss, 4 vols., London, 1813–20. See also Wood, A., 1673.

REFERENCES AFTER 1900

Allen, C. G. 'The Sources of "Lily's Latin Grammar": A Review of the Facts and Some Further Suggestions', *The Library*, 5th Ser. ix, 1954, 85–100.

Allen, P. S. *Erasmus: Lectures and Wayfaring Sketches*, Oxford, 1934.

Idem. 'Linacre and Latimer in Italy', *English Historical Review*, xviii, 1903, 514–17.

Anonymus. 'Contributors to the Science of Medicine. Thomas Linacre', *Medical Journal and Record*, New York, cxxi, 1925, 432–3.

Idem. 'Dr. Thomas Linacre. "Restorer of Learning"', *Clinical Medicine and Surgery*, xlii, 1935, 118–19.

Idem. 'The Founder of the Royal College of Physicians. Rector of Wigan from 1519–1524', *Wigan Observer and District Advertiser*, 6 March 1920.

Idem. 'Heroes of Medicine. Thomas Linacre', *Practitioner*, lxiv, 1900, 75–8.

Idem. 'Memorial to Thomas Linacre', *Lancet*, 1938 (ii), p. 1533.

Idem. 'The Selection of the Term "The Linacre Quarterly"', *Linacre Quarterly*, i, 1932, 1.

Idem. 'Thomas Linacre', *British Medical Journal*, 1960 (ii), pp. 1724–5.

Idem. 'Thomas Linacre', *Central African Journal of Medicine*, vii, 1961, 64.

Idem. 'Thomas Linacre and the First Public School in Wigan', *Wigan Observer*, 22 November 1952.

Idem. 'Thomas Linacre: Royal Physician', *Linacre Quarterly*, xxvii, 1960, 73–4.

Idem. *Thomas Linacre School, Wigan. Official Opening, 24 November 1953.* *Commemorative Brochure,* Wigan, [1953].

Bale, John. *Index Britanniae scriptorum quos ex variis bibliothecis non parvo labore collegit Ioannes Balęus, cum aliis. John Bale's Index of British and other writers.* Ed. R. L. Poole and M. Bateson. Anecdota Oxoniensia, Mediaeval and Modern Series, Part IX, Oxford, 1902. See also Bale, J., 1548.

Barraud, G. 'Le Premier Grand Médecin humaniste anglais: Linacre (1460–1524)', *Mémoires de la Société française d'Histoire de la Médecine,* iii, 1947, 105–7.

Bashford, H. H. *The Harley Street Calendar,* London, 1929.

Bassler, A. 'Thomas Linacre', *Linacre Quarterly,* i, 1933, 50–1. Also pr. in *The Apollonian,* xvii, 1942, 91–2.

Bennett, J. W. 'John Morer's Will: Thomas Linacre and Prior Sellyng's Greek Teaching', *Studies in the Renaissance,* xv, 1968, 70–91.

Blach, Samuel. *Die Schriftsprache in der Londoner Paulsschule zu Anfang des XVI. Jahrhunderts (bei Colet, Lily, Linacre, Grocyn),* Halberstadt, 1905.

'B. J.' 'A Letter and Linacre', *The Cantuarian,* xxvi, 1956, 410–11.

Bolgar, R. R. *The Classical Heritage and its Beneficiaries,* Cambridge, 1954, repr. 1973.

Bosatra, A. 'British Doctors at Padua University', *Acta Medicae Historiae Patavina,* ii, 1955–6, 1–14.

Brown, T. J. 'English Scientific Autographs I. Thomas Linacre 1460?–1524', *Book Collector,* xiii, 1964, 341.

Budé, G. See Delaruelle, L., 1907.

Caius, John. 'The First Book of the Annals of the Royal College of Physicians, London, compiled by John Caius, comprising the years 1518–1572. Printed for the first time, 1911', *The Works of John Caius, M.D.,* ed. E. S. Roberts, Cambridge, 1912. From a MS. in the Royal College of Physicians Library: 'Annalium Collegii medicorum Londini liber', etc.

Cameron, Roy. 'Thomas Linacre at the Portal to Scientific Medicine', *British Medical Journal,* 1964 (ii), pp. 589–94. Linacre Lecture.

Cawadias, A. P. 'Thomas Linacre and the First Scholar-Physicians of Oxford', *British Medical Journal,* 1936 (ii), pp. 550–2.

Charlton, K. *Education in Renaissance England,* London, 1965.

Clark, George Norman. *A History of the Royal College of Physicians,* 2 vols., Oxford, 1964.

[Idem.] 'Thomas Linacre', *British Medical Journal,* 1960 (ii), pp. 1728–9. See also *Lancet,* 1960 (ii), p. 1356.

Copeman, W. S. C. *Doctors and Disease in Tudor Times,* London, 1960.

Cotton, Juliana Hill. 'Materia Medica del Poliziano', *Il Poliziano e il suo tempo*, Atti del IV Convegno internazionale di studi sul Rinascimento, Florence, 1957, pp. 237–45.

Craneveldius, Franciscus. *Literae virorum eruditorum ad Franciscum Craneveldium 1522–1528*, ed. H. de Vocht, Louvain, 1928.

Cushing, H. *The Life of Sir William Osler*, 2 vols., Oxford, 1925.

Delaruelle, L. *Répertoire analytique et chronologique de la correspondance de Guillaume Budé*, Toulouse/Paris, 1907.

Denton, Sydney. 'Thomas Linacre, M.D. 1460–1524. A Mediaeval Master of Medicine', *Temple Bar*, cxxviii, 1903, 536–46.

Donnelly, J. H. 'The Thomas Linacre Medical Guild', *Linacre Quarterly*, xx, 1953, 128–9.

Durling, R. J. 'A Chronological Census of Renaissance Editions and Translations of Galen', *Journal of the Warburg and Courtauld Institutes*, xxiv, 1961, 230–305.

Emden, A. B. *A Biographical Register of the University of Oxford to A.D. 1500*, 3 vols., Oxford, 1957–9.

Erasmus, Desiderius. *Opus Epistolarum Des. Erasmi Roterodami denuo recognitum et auctum per P. S. Allen* [and others], 12 vols., Oxford, 1906–58.

Fletcher, C. R. L., and Walker, Emery. *Historical Portraits. Richard II to Henry Wriothesley, 1400–1600*, Oxford, 1909.

Flynn, V. J. 'Englishmen in Rome, 1450–1510', *Times Literary Supplement*, 12 September 1935.

Idem. 'Englishmen in Rome during the Renaissance', *Modern Philology*, xxxvi, 1938–9, 121–38.

Francis, W. W. 'Linacre and Aldus', *Journal of the History of Medicine*, viii, 1953, 329–30.

Franklin, A. W. 'Osler Transmitted—A Study in Humanism', *Medical History*, xvi, 1972, 99–112.

Fulton, J. F. 'Early Medical Humanists: Leonicenus, Linacre and Thomas Elyot', *New England Journal of Medicine*, ccv, 1931, 141–6, 158–9.

Idem. 'Medicine and the Humanities—Linacre and Allbutt', *Transactions of the American College of Cardiology*, vii, 1957, 24–38. Groedel Lecture.

Gasquet, F. A. *Cardinal Pole and His Early Friends*, London, 1927.

Idem. *A History of the Venerable English College, Rome*, London, 1920.

Gee, J. A. *The Life and Works of Thomas Lupset*, New Haven, 1928.

Gemmill, C. L. 'Thomas Linacre and John Caius', *Virginia Medical Monthly*, lxxxix, 1962, 15–18.

Germani, G. M. 'Un inglese, educato in Italia, fondatore del "Royal College of Physicians" di Londra', *Rivista di storia delle scienze mediche e naturali*, xxvii, 1936, 429–30.

Gilroy, J. F. 'Who is Thomas Linacre?', *Linacre Quarterly*, xxii, 1955, 86–9.

Greenwood, M. *Authority in Medicine: Old and New*, Cambridge, 1943. Linacre Lecture.

Himsworth, H. 'The Integration of Medicine: the endeavour of Thomas Linacre and its present significance', *British Medical Journal*, 1955 (ii), pp. 217–22. Linacre Lecture.

Hogrefe, P. *The Life and Times of Sir Thomas Elyot, Englishman*, Iowa, 1967.

Idem. *The Sir Thomas More Circle: A Program of Ideas and their Impact on Secular Drama*, Urbana, 1959.

Hyma, A. 'The Continental Origins of English Humanism', *The Huntington Library Quarterly*, iv, 1940–1, 1–25.

'J. Y.' 'Linacre', *New Zealand Medical Journal*, xxi, 1922, 115–19.

King, Ethel. *Dr. Linacre 1460–1524*, Brooklyn, N.Y., 1968.

Lakin, C. E. *Our Founders and Benefactors*, London, [1947]. Harveian Oration.

Linacre. Quarterly Journal of the United Hospitals Catholic Society (University of London). Nos. 1–16, January 1948–November 1951.

The Linacre Quarterly. 'A journal of the philosophy and ethics of medical practice.' National Federation of Catholic Physicians' Guilds, Wisconsin. No. 1– , 1932– .

Lupset, T. See Gee, J. A., 1928.

McConica, J. K. *English Humanists and Reformation Politics under Henry VIII and Edward VI*, Oxford, 1965.

MacNalty, A. S. 'Sir Thomas More as student of medicine and public health reformer', in *Science, Medicine and History. Essays on the Evolution of Scientific Thought and Medical Practice, written in honour of Charles Singer*, ed. E. A. Underwood, 2 vols., London, 1953, i. 418–36.

Malloch, A. 'Browning's copy of Linacre's Latin grammar', *Proceedings of the Charaka Club*, New York, Columbia University Press, viii, 1935, pp. 171–6.

Marcel, Raymond. 'Les "Découvertes" d'Érasme en Angleterre', *Bibliothèque d'Humanisme et Renaissance*, xiv, 1952, 117–23.

Marc' Hadour, G. 'Thomas More and Thomas Linacre', *Moreana*, iv, 1967, 63–7.

M[artin], J[ohn] M[iller]. 'An Unpublished Letter from Linacre to Claymond', *Pelican Record*, Oxford, xvii, 1925, 34–7. Based on material supplied by Dr. P. S. Allen.

Michael, Ian. *English Grammatical Categories and the Tradition to 1800*, Cambridge, 1970.

Mitchell, R. J. 'Thomas Linacre in Italy', *English Historical Review*, l, 1935, 696–8.

Moore, Norman. *Books of the Time* [and from the library of] *Linacre*, n. p., [May 8, 1913].

Idem. *The Friends of Erasmus whose Names appear in the Letters Patent founding our College* [Royal College of Physicians, London], *September 25, 1518*, n. p., [March 17, 1913].

Idem. *The History of the Study of Medicine in the British Isles*, Oxford, 1908.

More, Thomas. *The Correspondence of Sir Thomas More*, ed. E. F. Rogers, Princeton, 1947.

Newman, Charles. 'Thomas Linacre', *London Hospital Gazette*, lxiv, 1961, 20–4. Talk given to the Osler Club.

Newman, George. 'Linacre's Influence on English Medicine. Linacre Lecture delivered at St. John's College, Cambridge, May 5, 1928', *Lancet*, 1928 (ii), pp. 947–53.

O'Donovan, W. J. 'Thomas Linacre' in *Great Catholics*, ed. C. Williamson, London, 1938, pp. 130–8.

Idem. 'Thomas Linacre: Doctor and Priest 1460–1524', *Linacre*, ii, 1948, 4–6.

Idem. 'Thomas Linacre: Physician and Priest', *Linacre*, xvi, 1951, 17–18. Repr. of part of the previous item.

O'Malley, C. D. *English Medical Humanists. Thomas Linacre and John Caius*. Logan Clendening Lectures on the History and Philosophy of Medicine, 12th Ser., Lawrence, Kansas, 1965.

Idem. 'Thomas Linacre', *Dictionary of Scientific Biography*, ed. C. C. Gillispie, vol. 8, New York, 1973.

Idem. 'Tudor Medicine and Biology', *The Huntington Library Quarterly*, xxxii, 1968, 1–27.

Osler, W. *Thomas Linacre*, Cambridge, 1908. Linacre Lecture.

Parks, George Bruner. *The English Traveler to Italy*, vol. i, Rome, 1954.

Payne, J. F. 'Linacre and the "Grammarian's Funeral"', *British Medical Journal*, 1909 (ii), p. 1010.

Poynter, F. N. L. 'The Medical Society of London's Library', *Transactions of the Medical Society of London*, lxxxii, 1965–6, 153–65.

Pye, J. P. *Thomas Linacre. Scholar, Physician, Priest (1460–1524)*, London, 1912. Catholic Men of Science Series.

Raven, Charles E. *English Naturalists from Neckam to Ray*, Cambridge, 1947.

Redfern, Roger. 'Land of a Tudor Doctor: the Linacre Valley', *Country Life*, 5 December 1974.

Reed, A. W. 'The Regulation of the Book Trade before the Proclamation of 1538', *Transactions of the Bibliographical Society*, xv, 1920, 157–84.

Rhodes, D. E. 'Two Early German Editions of Proclus', *Beiträge zur*

Geschichte des Buches und seiner Funktion in der Gesellschaft: Festschrift für Hans Widmann, Stuttgart, 1974, pp. 178–82.

[Rogers, D. M.] *Erasmus and His English Friends. Catalogue of an Exhibition Held at the Bodleian Library to Commemorate the Fifth Centenary of the Birth of Erasmus, May 1969*, Oxford [forthcoming].

Rolleston, H. D. *The Cambridge Medical School: A Biographical History*, Cambridge, 1932.

Rook, Arthur (ed.). *Cambridge and its Contribution to Medicine*, London, 1971.

Royal College of Physicians. '. . . And Beginning with Linacre'. An Exhibition of Books, etc. on the Occasion of the Presidential Election, 1953 [duplicated typescript].

Idem. 'Thomas Linacre 1460?–1524. 8 December 1960' [exhibition catalogue, duplicated typescript].

Sandys, J. E. *A History of Classical Scholarship*, 3 vols., Cambridge, 1903–8.

Schirmer, W. F. *Der Englische Frühhumanismus*, Leipzig, 1931.

Sharpe, W. D. 'Thomas Linacre, 1460–1524: An English Physician Scholar of the Renaissance', *Bulletin of the History of Medicine*, xxxiv, 1960, 233–56.

Talbot, C. H., and Hammond, E. A. *The Medical Practitioners in Medieval England: A Biographical Register*, London, 1965.

Taylor, F. M. 'Thomas Linacre. Humanist, Physician, Priest', *Linacre Quarterly*, xxix, 1962, 176–83. Repr. ibid. xxxviii, 1971, 82–9, 198–205. From an address before the Osler Society, Baylor University College of Medicine, The Texas Medical Centre, 6 Jan. 1961.

Thornton, John L. 'Andrew Boorde, Thomas Linacre and the "Dyetary of Helth"', *Bulletin of the Medical Library Association*, xxxvi, 1948, 204–9.

Topley, W. W. C. *Authority, Observation and Experiment in Medicine*, Cambridge, 1940. Linacre Lecture.

Vives, J. L. *Vives: On Education. A Translation of the* De tradendis disciplinis *of Juan Luis Vives . . .*, by Foster Watson, Cambridge, 1913.

Walsh, J. J. 'An English Physician Priest at the Eve of the Reformation', *The Ecclesiastical Review*, xxix, 1903, 144–61.

Idem. 'Linacre, the Priest', *Linacre Quarterly*, iii, 1935, 50–1.

Watson, Cecil J. 'Linacre and Locke: Pillars of Medical Humanism', *California Medicine*, cvii, 1967, 413–19. William J. Kerr Gold-Headed Cane Lecture.

Weiss, Roberto. 'Un allievo inglese del Poliziano: Thomas Linacre', *Il Poliziano e il suo tempo*. Atti del IV Convegno internazionale di studi sul Rinascimento, Florence, 1957, pp. 231–6.

Idem. 'Letters of Linacre', *Times Literary Supplement*, 26 September 1936.

Idem. 'Notes on Thomas Linacre', *Miscellanea Giovanni Mercati*, vol. iv, Studi e Testi, 124, Vatican City, 1946, pp. 373–80.

Wenkebach, E. *John Clement: ein englischer Humanist und Arzt des sechzehnten Jahrhunderts* . . ., Studien zur Geschichte der Medizin herausgegeben von der Puschmann-Stiftung an der Universität Leipzig, Heft 14, Leipzig, 1925.

Williamson, R. T. *English Physicians of the Past*, Newcastle, 1923.

Wohlfarth, P. 'Thomas Linacre', *Deutsches medizinisches Journal*, viii, 1957, 501–3.

N

An Iconography of Thomas Linacre

MAUREEN HILL*

IT APPEARS THAT NO CONTEMPORARY PORTRAIT OF Thomas Linacre, painted either from the life or within living memory, exists. Indeed, the few facts we have concerning his life, and the considerable knowledge we have of the development of painting and sculpture in western Europe during his lifetime, suggest that he is an unlikely candidate for such pictorial record. In 1487, probably in William Sellyng's[1] company, Linacre travelled through France to Italy. He visited Florence, Rome, Padua, and Venice at a time of immensely significant artistic activity. But the fine arts were still under the control and patronage of Court, Church, or State. It is as incredible that the young grammarian-physician should have considered commissioning his own portrait whilst on his travels as it is that any individual or institution would have

* Late of the National Portrait Gallery, London.

Acknowledgements. In the preparation of a study of this nature it is necessary to seek the help and take up the time of a large number of people. I am greatly indebted to the following: Monsignor J. L. Alston; Miss Margaret Andrews; Dr. R. Burgess; Professor Sir Richard Doll; Miss A. Scott Elliot; the late Professor E. F. Jacob; the Revd. J. D. James; Mr. A. T. Linacre; Sir Oliver Millar; Miss Margaret Pelling; Mr. Colin Sizer; Mr. G. E. S. Turner; Miss E. B. Wells; Mrs. S. A. Williamson; the Rt. Hon. Richard Wood, M.P. Mr. Giles Barber, Librarian of the Taylor Institution, Oxford, initiated research into the iconography of Thomas Linacre and generously placed his notes and correspondence at my disposal. Dr. Roy Strong, formerly Director of the National Portrait Gallery, London, made invaluable suggestions during the course of the work and kindly read the typescript.

[1] William Sellyng or Celling, d. 1494, prior of Christ Church, Canterbury, 1472–94, and envoy to Rome, 1486.

wished to commission it at this date and at this period in Linacre's life.

If, as may be likely, Linacre returned to England through Flanders, the bourgeois character of Flemish society makes it more plausible that a portrait of him might have been painted, perhaps in Antwerp. There is, however, not a single precedent for a portrait of an English traveller being painted in the Low Countries before 1500, and Linacre's age and station in life seem to rule out the possibility. In addition, what is known of his retiring character and single-minded scholarship weighs against it.

On his return to England Linacre's life followed a tranquil course in London, and later at Court. The list of works produced by him between 1499 and his death is formidable in the context of the age.[1] Such biographical information as we have presents Linacre as a man with many preoccupations. One can detect no suggestion of egotism. There is therefore no good reason for a portrait, and what is known of the state of artistic production in Tudor England seems to preclude the existence of one. Few works of art survive from the first quarter of the sixteenth century in England; among them portraits of commoners are all but non-existent. The names of one or two of the King's Serjeant Painters, who were more precisely decorators and craftsmen, are known from before 1526 when Hans Holbein (1497/8–1543) arrived for his first short visit.[2] It is from Holbein and his connection first with the family of Sir Thomas More (1478–1535), and subsequently with the Court, that the tradition of modern portraiture begins to grow. But Thomas Linacre had died in 1524.

However, if portraits from life do not exist, posthumous representations can be invented when required by succeeding generations. The iconography, that is the list of known representations of Thomas Linacre, spans more than three centuries: from *circa* 1500 to 1968. It comprises paintings, drawings, engravings, and sculpture. Some of these works are derived in good faith from earlier images; a few are intentional fakes—both as portraits and as works of art. None has an unshakeable claim to reflect the features of Thomas Linacre.

The portrait in the Royal Collection at Windsor Castle (Catalogue No. 1, Plate VII) is the most widely disseminated of the

---

[1] J. N. Johnson, *The Life of Thomas Linacre*, ed. R. Graves, London, 1835, p. 239 n.   [2] See E. Auerbach, *Tudor Artists*, London, 1954.

Linacre images. The name of Thomas Linacre appears to have become attached to it towards the middle of the eighteenth century. By 1937 it appears, in C. H. Collins Baker's *Catalogue*, once more as a portrait of an unknown man. This picture seems to have entered the Royal Collection at the time when Charles I, as Prince of Wales, was laying the foundations of his collection of works of art, a collection of very great quality later to be dispersed under the Commonwealth. Charles's seal, with the cipher *CP*, is attached to the back of the panel.

The picture is undoubtedly Flemish, a statement based on stylistic grounds; and can be accepted as dating from the second or third decade of the sixteenth century, depending on how the date on the paper in the sitter's hand is deciphered. In the *James II–William III Catalogue* the picture is described as 'An Old Man, a letter in his hand . . .'. In the *George III Kensington Catalogue* (1778) it appears as 'Dr Linacre by Matsys'. George Vertue (1684–1756), when he visited Kensington Palace in 1734, recorded 'Dr Linacer [*sic*] painted by Quintin. 1521' (i.e. Quintin Matsys, 1466?–1530). The identification of the portrait as Linacre in the *George III Kensington Catalogue* may well stem from Horace Walpole's statement: 'Quintin Matsys too painted Ægidius with which Sir Thomas More was so pleased that he wrote a panegyric on the painter. . . . Ægidius held a letter in his hand from Sir Thomas, with his hand-writing so well imitated, that More could not distinguish it himself. Quintin too in the year 1521 drew the picture of the celebrated physician Dr Linacre.'[1]

The attribution of the Windsor picture to Matsys can be ruled out on stylistic grounds and by comparison with portraits known to have come from his hand, such as the Ægidius mentioned by Horace Walpole.[2] In Walpole's defence, it should be stated that the facilities for this kind of check or comparison were not available to him; nor were they available to the compilers of eighteenth- and nineteenth-century catalogues. It is only during the past half-century that the growth of photographic collections, such as the Witt Library (Courtauld Institute of Art, London), and the publication

[1] H. Walpole, *Anecdotes of painting in England . . . collected by the late Mr. George Vertue; and now digested and published from his original MSS.*, 2nd edn., 3 vols., Strawberry Hill, 1765, i, p. 68. Petrus Ægidius (Pierre Gilles), Town Clerk of Antwerp, was a friend and correspondent of Sir Thomas More.

[2] Helen, Countess of Radnor, and W. B. Squire, *Catalogue of the Pictures in the Collection of the Earl of Radnor*, 2 pts., privately printed, London, 1909, i. 44–45 rep. no. 80.

of illustrated catalogues of many collections, public and private, have allowed methods of comparative analysis to be brought to bear on the attribution and identification of portraits. There is also a contributory factor in refuting the suggestion that Matsys painted the portrait: his path and Linacre's can have crossed only once, if Linacre returned to England from Italy by way of Antwerp.[1]

Some time, therefore, between the compilation of the *James II– William III Catalogue* and 1734, when Vertue noticed the portrait at Kensington, the name of Thomas Linacre became attached to it. It is possible, and in character for George Vertue, that the suggestion was his own; but there is no certain proof that it was. Horace Walpole presumably bases his statement that Quintin drew Linacre in 1521 on his knowledge of the royal collections or on Vertue's note. (Walpole acquired Vertue's *Notebooks* from the latter's widow, and drew on them for his *Anecdotes of Painting*.)

It is the date on the paper in the sitter's hand which forms the core of the argument as to whether the portrait represents Thomas Linacre or not. It can be read as 1521, 1527, 1531, or 1537. A definite pronouncement is impossible because of the condition of the panel. An opaque film of paint and varnish covers the tails of the last two digits in the inscription. It is possible that this repaint dates from the time when the picture was placed in its present frame, which bears tablets inscribed: 'Linacre / Founder of the College of Physicians' and 'Dr Thomas Linacre / Quintin Matsys'. In 1810, when the painting was copied by William Miller for the Royal College of Physicians (see Catalogue No. 2, Plate VIII), the date was apparently read and copied as 1521. The present state of the paint appears to reveal 1527 or possibly 1537.

Allowing that the date 1521 is correct, the Windsor picture still cannot represent Linacre, an Englishman, aged about 60, doctor of medicine and priest. The creation of such a portrait would have been so without precedent that some event of major importance must have occasioned it. Of Cardinal Wolsey himself, probably the most powerful man in England during the last decade of Linacre's life, the few portraits that were made, and have survived, are stiff hieratic images, medieval in feeling.[2] The strong-featured Fleming

[1] Linacre finally returned to England in 1499; there is, however, a possibility that he made a return visit at an earlier date.

[2] For portraits of Wolsey, see R. C. Strong, *National Portrait Gallery: Tudor and Jacobean Portraits*, 2 vols., London, 1969.

of the Windsor portrait belongs to the Renaissance side of the artistic watershed. In 1521 his English contemporaries had hardly broken with the stultifying visual conventions of the Middle Ages.

If the date is deciphered as 1527, 1531, or 1537 Thomas Linacre was by then dead, and the portrait has none of the qualities of a posthumous likeness, since in this case it would almost certainly be inscribed with the sitter's dates of birth and death, and possibly some description of the offices he had held.

If the identification of the Windsor picture as Thomas Linacre cannot be accepted today, its acceptance as such during the early eighteenth century, and its propagation as a likeness of Linacre, make an interesting study. This is an excellent illustration of the unquestioning and uncritical attitude so often extended in the past to works of art, and to portraits in particular.

The portrait in the possession of the Royal College of Physicians, London (Catalogue No. 2, Plate VIII) is probably the first painted copy of the Windsor picture. It was made in 1810 for the College by William Miller. The College was, presumably, unhappily aware that it possessed no portrait of its founder and first president, for its splendid collection of portraits dates predominantly from the eighteenth century. (The College's premises at Amen Corner were destroyed in the Great Fire of 1666.) William Miller, a member of the College staff, was a competent copyist. Sir William Osler states that Sir Lionel Cust,[1] then director of the National Portrait Gallery, and Sir Walter Armstrong,[2] then director of the National Gallery of Ireland, both considered that the portrait could have been painted by an 'old master'.[3] The College records, however, as quoted by David Piper, establish the authorship of, and record the payment to, William Miller.

The appearance of the Royal College of Physicians picture gives some idea of the deterioration of the panel at Windsor since 1810, when the copy was made. In the Royal College of Physicians painting the background is considerably lighter than in the Windsor panel; the contrast in texture between fur collar and dark stuff

[1] Sir Lionel Cust (1859–1929), Director of the National Portrait Gallery, London, 1895–1909. Surveyor of the King's Pictures, 1901–27.

[2] Sir Walter Armstrong (1850–1918), critic and art historian, Director of the National Gallery of Ireland, 1892–1914.

[3] W. Osler, *Thomas Linacre*, Linacre Lecture, 1908, Cambridge, 1908, p. 61.

gown is much more obvious; the pattern on the shirt neck-band is more clearly defined. To sum up: the Windsor picture must have darkened considerably during the past two hundred years and the paint in the areas of hair, face, shirt and hands has been rubbed. The decoration on the neck-band has been rubbed almost out of existence. As stated above, William Miller appears to have copied the date on the paper as 1521.

The Royal College of Physicians picture was first engraved by H. Cook in 1838 for Pettigrew's *Medical Portrait Gallery* (1840) (Plate IX). Impressions of the engraving are fairly common.

Thomas Linacre was a fellow of All Souls College, Oxford, from 1484. It has not been possible to discover exactly when the All Souls copy of the Windsor portrait (Catalogue No. 3, Plate X) entered the College collection. Professor E. F. Jacob[1] believed that it was between 1815 and 1840, but knew of no actual record of its acquisition. C. Grant Robertson, in his history of All Souls, states that 'between 1815 and 1840 a splendid start was made with the collection of portraits, Wren, Sydenham, Linacre . . .' and goes on to comment that the College records for the period 1800–50 are even more meagre in quantity than those of the preceding century. It seems likely that the All Souls portrait was copied from the Windsor portrait some years later than the Royal College of Physicians portrait. There are three main reasons for this assumption: the background of the All Souls portrait is dark in tone; the neck-band of the shirt is without ornament, and the date inscribed on the paper was copied as 1527. Robertson, in his list of College portraits, describes it as a 'Replica of the original in Kensington Palace attributed to Quentin Matsys'.

Mrs. Lane Poole states that the All Souls portrait was engraved for the *Medical Portrait Gallery*, but the date, 1521, on the paper in the sitter's hand, and the elaborate decoration on the neck-band depicted in the engraving, appear to me to disprove this.

It is interesting to note that the All Souls portrait was lent to the Oxford Exhibition of Historical Portraits in 1904 (and to the Royal Academy in 1902), when it was presumably accepted as an old master painting.

The portrait of Thomas Linacre at 13 Norham Gardens, the residence of the Regius Professor of Medicine in Oxford (Catalogue

[1] Ernest Fraser Jacob (1894–1971), Fellow and Librarian (1960–71) of All Souls College; Professor Emeritus, 1961.

No. 4, Plate XI.*a*), is stated by Mrs. Lane Poole to be a copy of the All Souls portrait. It was made for Sir Henry Acland, Regius Professor 1858–94, and was originally placed, together with copies of portraits of Thomas Sydenham and William Harvey, in the three panels of the overmantel in the library at 13 Norham Gardens. A photograph mounted in an album in the possession of Professor Sir Richard Doll shows the three paintings in this position. They were subsequently removed from the panels over the fireplace, and now hang, framed together, in the adjacent office. It is very likely that the Royal College of Physicians portrait, as well as the All Souls portrait, was known to the copyist, for the background of the Acland painting is green, as in the former, and the paper is inscribed 1521.

Sir Henry Acland's copy of the All Souls painting was itself copied for Sir William Osler (1849–1919) (Catalogue No. 5, Plate XI.*b*). This copy was made as a birthday present for Osler from his wife some time between 1894 and 1897.[1] Cushing, in his *Life of Sir William Osler*, describes Osler's delight at first seeing the three paintings over the fireplace in Acland's study when he and his wife visited Oxford *circa* 1894: 'He made such an ado about it that Mrs Osler subsequently asked Sir Henry if they might not be copied for him as a birthday present. This was done, and in turn the triumvirate came to adorn the mantel of his own library and office at 1 West Franklin Street [Baltimore, U.S.A], a familiar sight to countless students, friends, and patients. This same panel, moreover, was to dominate Osler's library in Oxford, for though his teacher Burdon Sanderson came between, it would almost seem as though Acland had knowingly handed on an emblem of the Regius Professorship to the man destined, in the whirligig of time and place, to become his successor.'[2]

Osler's own set of three copies passed into the possession of McGill University as part of the Osler Library.

The portrait belonging to the English College in Rome (Catalogue No. 6, Plate XII.*a*) is of a rather different category from those paintings discussed above, in that it is not an exact copy and cannot be connected definitely with any one of the others. Thomas Linacre was admitted to the English Hospice, from which the English

[1] Information from Miss E. B. Wells, Associate Osler Librarian, McGill University.

[2] H. Cushing, *The Life of Sir William Osler*, 2 vols., Oxford, 1925, i. 401.

College grew, in 1490 and became a *custos* in 1491.[1] The portrait was presented in 1920 by Lady Allchin who stated that it had been bought at a sale at an old house in Ware about 1885. It had hung in the consulting-room of her husband, Sir William Allchin (1846–1912). In a letter of 29 November 1920 to Cardinal Gasquet, Cardinal Protector of the English College (copy in the Royal College of Physicians Library),[2] suggesting that she should present the portrait to the College, Lady Allchin referred to it as a water-colour and described the background as dark green.

The figure is placed lower than in the other paintings of this type and more of the body is seen. The modelling of the hands, while technically inexpert, appears to be based on the Royal College of Physicians picture and that picture is also likely to be the source of the dark green background. The nose, mouth, and chin appear larger than in other paintings of the Windsor type. This may possibly reflect a knowledge of the British Museum drawing (Catalogue No. 10, Plate XV). All in all the painting is a fairly elaborate water-colour version of this portrait type. Such water-colour copies of paintings in oil are typically Victorian. It is very likely that this particular example dates from the 1860s when the series of National Portrait Exhibitions held at the South Kensington Museum (now the Victoria and Albert Museum) aroused new interest in historic portraits. The Windsor painting was itself included in the 1866 exhibition.

Only one of the three so-called Linacre portraits in the collection of the Wellcome Institute of the History of Medicine (Catalogue No. 7, Plate XII.*b*) derives from the Windsor type, and, like the picture belonging to the English College, it is a somewhat hybrid derivative. The painting is executed on an extremely thick and heavy panel. The Curator states that an X-ray provides evidence of another painting underneath: apparently a Madonna and Child. The portrait itself is crude and very unattractive in handling. It has the appearance of a deliberate fake—a conscious attempt to deceive; while those versions of the Windsor picture discussed above appear all to have been made in good faith. The use of an early panel, better described as a hunk of wood with a tendency to convexity, and not of a type generally found in English painting of the early sixteenth

---

[1] Information from the Rector.
[2] London, Royal College of Physicians Library, 92. Lin. (uncatalogued material).

century, is immediately suspect. The painter has also employed various elements from the Windsor and Royal College of Physicians paintings and has circumvented the awkward question of date by leaving out both hands and paper.

The Linacre image represented by the Windsor portrait has been accepted without critical appraisal until quite recently. The pattern was used for the figure of Linacre which appears in one of the lower lights of the oriel window of the Hall at Christ Church, Oxford (Catalogue No. 9, Plate XX.*a*). The Linacre window was presented to the College by Archdeacon Charles Carr Clerke (1798–1877) in memory of the residence of the Prince of Wales (Edward VII) and of that of the Crown Prince of Denmark. Linacre is seen at full length so the lower part of the figure must be the invention of the window designer, as also the purple gown.[1]

The case of the 'Fuller Maitland' portrait once called Thomas Linacre (Catalogue No. 10, Plate XIV) is somewhat similar to that of the Windsor picture, but the period of its masquerade as Linacre was very much shorter, under thirty years, and as a Linacre image it is therefore less widely known. The portrait was acquired by the National Gallery, London, from William Fuller Maitland in 1878. It is now catalogued as Netherlandish School, and described as a 'Man with a Pansy and a Skull'. Fuller Maitland had purchased the picture from the trade in 1849, probably as a portrait of Linacre. It was exhibited as such in 1852, 1868, and 1872. The identification must have been in doubt at the time of its acquisition by the nation, for it has never been described as Thomas Linacre in National Gallery catalogues. The unknown Dutch sitter might well have been a doctor of medicine, though the National Gallery draws attention to the equal possibility that the skull is merely a *memento mori*. Of the paintings included in this study, this portrait is the finest in quality and the most aesthetically pleasing. The paint is in good condition, especially the head, while the costume is sufficiently defined for the fairly precise description of 'Dutch, *circa* 1535' to be attached to it.

The drawing in the Cracherode Collection at the British Museum (Catalogue No. 11, Plate XV) is, after the Windsor picture, the

---

[1] Miss Margaret Pelling has drawn my attention to G. Lyly, '. . . elogia' in P. Giovio, *Descriptio Britanniae Scotiae, Hyberniae, et Orchadum*, Venice, 1548, fol. 49, where Linacre is described as in *toga purpurea*; *cf.* 'Editors' Introduction', above, pp. xvii, and xxxvi n. 21.

most widely diffused Linacre image. Clayton Mordaunt Cracherode (1730–99), bibliophile and print collector, bequeathed his collections to the British Museum. The drawing of Linacre was first engraved in 1794,[1] and was therefore known and recognized as a representation of Linacre before it entered the British Museum. It is unfortunate for the purpose of this study that nothing is known of its history before Cracherode acquired it. On the reverse of the drawing the following note appears, written, according to British Museum sources, by the late A. E. Popham:[2] 'D. Lincoln[3] in a letter of October 28th 1949, suggests that this drawing is by the same hand as the original studies for the engravings in Thevet's *Hommes illustres*, 1594[4] which are in an interleaved copy of the work in the Bibliothèque Nationale.' Mr. Giles Barber, Librarian of the Taylor Institution, Oxford, has kindly allowed me to see some correspondence which he had in 1965 with Mlle Jeanne Veyrin-Forrer of the Bibliothèque Nationale. Mlle Veyrin-Forrer states that the drawings in the volume referred to by Mr. Lincoln are probably not Thevet's originals, but reduced copies of his engravings destined to be used for a later edition. To support this theory she points out that the series includes a drawing of Thevet himself inscribed 'mourut Ian. 1592 . . .'.

Whether or not the British Museum drawing of Thomas Linacre was made as a study for an engraving to be included in a later, enlarged edition of *Hommes illustres* must remain entirely conjectural. It is, however, a very plausible suggestion. The drawing is undoubtedly French; A. E. Popham accepted it as such and Sir Sidney Colvin,[5] as quoted by Sir William Osler in Osler's 1908 Linacre Lecture,[6] stated that 'the drawing is by a French hand, of about A.D. 1600'. Thevet included two Englishmen in his work, Sir Thomas

---

[1] Line engraving, $3\frac{5}{8}$ inches diameter. Head in profile to right. Inscribed: 'Thomas Linacre M.D. / was born in Canterbury 1460 and died in London 1524 / from a very curious old drawing in the collection of the Rev. Mr. C. M. Cracherode / London Pub. Sept. I. 1794 by J. Thane. Spur Street, Leicester Square'.

[2] Arthur Ewart Popham (1889–1970). Keeper of the Department of Prints and Drawings, British Museum, from 1945.

[3] David Lincoln, then of 16 Longwall Street, Oxford.

[4] André Thevet (1504–92), engraver. *Les Vrais pourtraits et vies des hommes illustres . . .*, Paris, 1584.

[5] Sir Sidney Colvin (1845–1927). Keeper of the Department of Prints and Drawings, British Museum, 1883–1912.

[6] Osler, op. cit., p. 63.

More (1478–1535) and John Fisher (1459–1535). Neither of these engravings agrees well with established portraits of these sitters and the quality of the engravings themselves is less impressive than that of the engravings of contemporary Frenchmen. From a close study of the Linacre drawing it seems possible that the head was copied from an earlier image, perhaps a medal, and the body drawn, rather more clumsily, to fit. The head is in profile, the body turned slightly to front, while the scale of the hand clasping his gown does not agree well with the scale or handling of the head. The buttoned doublet is too late in style for Linacre's lifetime. If these points are admitted, then the possibility that the head in the British Museum drawing derives from an earlier image with some claim to represent Thomas Linacre cannot be ruled out.

The earliest image of Linacre (it cannot be considered a portrait) must be the figure on the title-page of his translation of Galen's *De sanitate tuenda* (Paris, 1517) (Catalogue No. 19, Frontispiece).[1] Two nearly identical figures about 1½ inches high, labelled Galen and Linacre, face each other from the spandrels above the cartouche inscribed with the title. Galen is in profile to right, and Linacre, in profile to left, holds a scroll in his right hand to which he points with his left. The treatment of the figure is as a decorative motif incorporated within a piece of late medieval illumination. It is interesting to note, however, that the tradition of the paper in the hand, which descends through the Windsor picture and its dependent copies, appears to begin here.

The three-dimensional images of Thomas Linacre recorded at present are all posthumous and display the artistic characteristics of their own day. By far the most important of these pieces of sculpture is the bust usually attributed to Sir Henry Cheere (1703–81) and made for All Souls College *circa* 1749 (Catalogue No. 12, Plate XVI.*a*). This bust is one of a series placed on the cornice in the Codrington Library. Mrs. M. I. Webb records a document in the college archives[2] dated 6 November 1749, which reads: 'Agreed that Mr Blackstone when he goes to Town shall give Orders to Mr Cheere at Piccadilly to send down to College one Bust and one Vase

[1] The existence of the title-page is noticed by the late Professor C. D. O'Malley in unpublished material on Thomas Linacre. Professor O'Malley's reference was drawn to my attention by Mr. F. R. Maddison.

[2] It has not been possible to trace either of the documents cited by Mrs. Webb.

as specimens.' In due course Blackstone[1] ordered twenty-five vases and twenty-four busts. Mrs. Webb points out that it was Henry Cheere's younger brother, John (born 1709), who had premises in Piccadilly, so it is presumably he who executed the busts. Another entry in the College MSS. quoted by Mrs. Webb states: 'Mr Cheere had made diligent Enquiry after a picture of Dr Godolphin in order to make a Bust of him according to ye College order . . . but had not been able to procure one. It was therefor agreed that Dr Godolphin's Bust be deferred till some future Opportunity, and that instead therof Mr Cheere do make a Bust of Sir Anthony Sherley.' This suggests that some trouble was taken to produce faithful portraits of contemporary figures. For the Linacre bust the sources available to the Cheere brothers would have been the Windsor portrait and, perhaps, the British Museum drawing. No particular use appears to have been made of either. One can only conclude that they were not accessible, or that 'Mr Cheere' was less concerned with verisimilitude in a likeness so far beyond living memory.

The Cheere brothers were responsible for a large body of decorative and commemorative sculpture. Neither specialized in portraits, though Henry certainly produced some, among them the statue of Christopher Codrington which dominates the library. The All Souls bust of Linacre has much of the character of a library ornament, a genre very popular in the eighteenth century. The broad handling of the features is designed to be seen from some distance. There is no noticeable attempt at characterization. The long hair and the treatment of costume, in particular the plain collar and tasselled draw-strings, are a typical eighteenth-century conception of sixteenth-century dress. The bust is, in this way, more a memorial in the Cheere brothers' tradition than a portrait.

The second piece of sculpture commemorating Thomas Linacre is, or was, the near-monumental figure designed by Henry Weekes (1808–77) for the portico of the old building of the Royal College of Physicians in Pall Mall (Catalogue No. 14, Plate XVII). The library of the Royal College of Physicians contains a scrap-book of photographs, etc., connected with the history of the institution and this includes a photograph of the façade of the Pall Mall building.[2]

---

[1] Sir William Blackstone (1723–80), Fellow of All Souls College 1744, first Vinerian Professor of English Law.

[2] London, Royal College of Physicians Library, MS. Catalogue (1928), no. 119: Frederic John Farre, 'An Album containing maps, plans, engravings,

Three statues, Thomas Sydenham (1624–89), William Harvey (1578–1657), and Thomas Linacre, were set in niches behind the Ionic colonnade.

When demolition work on the old building began in 1965, Mrs. Constance Linacre, who had always been interested in the history of the Linacre family, became anxious about the probable fate of the statues. She passed by them daily on her way to work. When at length they disappeared her son, Mr. A. T. Linacre, made inquiries of the College authorities and traced the statue of Linacre to a stone-breaker's yard in Maidstone. The firm agreed to perform one cut on the statue (such operations are quite costly) and transformed it into an over life-size bust, approximately 24 inches high. It was taken back to London by Mr. Linacre and placed in his front garden in Peckham.

Henry Weekes was a sculptor of some eminence. He was a pupil of Behnes and an assistant of Sir Francis Chantrey.[1] The Linacre statue was a professional piece of work. It was designed to be seen in an architectural setting. The deep undercutting gives rise to a variety of light and shade, producing a liveliness which the greater than life-size features would otherwise have lacked. This late-nineteenth-century conception of the founder and first President of the Royal College of Physicians was an impressive piece of monumental sculpture; an embodiment of dignity, and a founder-figure image, but in no sense a portrait.

Among the references to portraits of Thomas Linacre in the National Portrait Gallery archive is a slip of paper with the cryptic reference: 'Windsor, Raphael Collection. An early engraving of the British Museum picture attributing the picture to Raphael' (Catalogue No. 15, Plate XIII.*b*). The Raphael Collection comprises mainly portrait engravings. Of the entire collection only one small etching appears likely to be connected with the note in the National Portrait Gallery. It is inscribed in faded ink: 'R. d'Urbino'. It is difficult to date but is certainly post-1700. It appears to portray a cleric. It has not been possible to equate the type with a portrait by Raphael: the subject is almost certainly later in date. Comparison with the head

photographs and drawings to illustrate Dr. Farre's History of the College', 1883, p. 47.

[1] For Henry Weekes, William Behnes (1795–1863), and Sir Francis Chantrey (1781–1841) see R. Gunnis, *Dictionary of British Sculptors 1660–1851*, London, 1953.

in the British Museum drawing shows distinct similarities, certainly sufficient to make a connection appear possible, were there no photograph to hand of the drawing. When the two images are closely compared the similarities in shape of nose and head-dress appear to be fortuitous. The costume, too, of the man in the Windsor print is of a type too late and too Italianate for a connection with Thomas Linacre to be possible.

The Royal Library also contains another, tiny print (Catalogue No. 16, Plate XX.*b*), inscribed with the name *Thom. Lynacer*. This engraving comes from one of three sets of minute portraits prefixed to the three parts of Johann Christian Ruediger, *Vitae clarissimorum in re literaria virorum* (Wittenberg, 1704). The print is seventeenth-century in feeling; it depicts a Laudian cleric with moustache but no beard. There is no apparent connection with any other Linacre portrait type. Its main interest for the purpose of this study is as an image of Linacre cast in the mould of a seventeenth-century cleric. Engraved portraits of notable English divines would presumably have been the sole reference point for the German printmaker.

The final images in this study are both of the 19th century and can be classed as fakes; that is, deliberate attempts to deceive with a made-up portrait image not based on a reputable, known portrait type. Both paintings are in the possession of the Wellcome Institute of the History of Medicine.

Catalogue No. 17, Plate XVIII.*a*, is technically a poor piece of work. It employs elements from the Flemish tradition of the fifteenth and early sixteenth centuries and borrows directly from Holbein. The two wall brackets and the panelling background with papers tucked behind transverse members are copied from Holbein's portrait of the Hanseatic merchant George Gisze, painted in 1532 (Plate XVIII.*b*).[1] The *cartelino*, with its inscription *Thomas Linacrus . . .* nailed up behind the sitter's head, can hardly have looked convincing to the forger himself. Indeed, the calligraphy of these, the first two words of the inscription, appears to be copied directly from the facsimile signature appended to Henry Cook's engraving for the *Medical Portrait Gallery* (Plate IX).

The figure is based upon the image in the Windsor portrait.

[1] The portrait is in the Staatliche Museen Preussicher Kulturbesitz, Gemäldegalerie, Berlin (West). See P. Ganz, *The Paintings of Hans Holbein the Younger. First Complete Edition*, London, 1950, Pl. 98.

However, the painter became confused when he had to invent; the sleeves (not seen in the Windsor picture) are quite improbable, while the awkwardly drawn inner garment is copied from the Holbein of Gisze.

The second picture (Catalogue No. 18, Plate XIX.*a*) is a close copy of Holbein's portrait of Dirk Tybis, merchant of Duisberg, painted in 1533 and now in the Kunsthistorisches Museum, Vienna (Plate XIX.*b*).[1] Additions to Holbein's design are the skull, and the banner inscribed *Qui Patitor Vincit*, together with the background inscription *Thomas Linacre | M.D. | ANNO DM | MDVII*. The seal lying by Tybis's left hand is omitted, as also the coins in the round metal box. The Wellcome panel measures $13 \times 10\frac{1}{2}$ inches; the Holbein is stated to be $19 \times 13\frac{7}{8}$ inches. The paint in the Wellcome picture is unattractive, and has a nineteenth-century quality. The drawing of details such as the shirt, fur collar, and right hand, is crude.

Mr. Colin Sizer, Curator of the Wellcome Collection, kindly pointed out that Mr. Henry Wellcome is known to have been a target for persons wishing to dispose of spurious and doubtful works of art with a medical flavour, and the three portraits called Linacre in the collection (Nos. 7, 17, and 18) illustrate this unfortunate state of affairs very vividly.

The main purpose in attempting to clarify the iconography of an individual is to clear away confusion and to reveal truth, or attempts to portray truth, as far as may be possible. In a study of this kind the question of truth can never be entirely resolved. Where a portrait is concerned it is easier by far to define deliberate deceit. Thomas Linacre was a man of many parts. His many friends must have known different facets of his character, appreciated different qualities and, in short, seen him differently. The greatest portrait, even while acclaimed as an important work of art, can only represent a man in a moment of time, as he appeared to the artist. Its success is qualified always by the artist's technical ability. The sitter's intimates may disagree with the painter's view of the man they know. Alternatively, a portrait can strike a chord of intense recognition, and present an aspect of the sitter with which the spectator is instantly familiar. Subjectivity in portraiture is an incalculable quality. In conclusion I suggest that no contemporary portrait of Thomas Linacre survives, and that the images that have

[1] Ganz, op. cit., Pl. 105.

come down to us are at best the tributes of later generations to his qualities of mind and to his use of them in his work, which remains his most objective memorial.

Catalogue

Catalogue No. 1

Plate VII

Painting. Royal Collection, Windsor Castle.

Oils on panel, $18\frac{5}{8} \times 13\frac{3}{4}$ inches. Artist unknown.

Collections: Probably acquired by Charles I when Prince of Wales; at Kensington Palace (when seen by G. Vertue) 1734; at Windsor from *c*. 1860 when seen by Sir G. Scharf.

Exhibitions: National Portrait Exhibition, 1866, no. 96; British Institution, 1820, no. 82.

Literature: C. H. Collins Baker, *Catalogue of Pictures in the Royal Collection at Windsor*, London, 1937, p. 235; Sir George Scharf, Notebooks, Windsor i. 20, Windsor ii. 59, National Portrait Gallery Archives; George Vertue, *Notebooks*, Oxford, Walpole Society, 1930–47, iv. 6, 66, 94; *James II–William III Catalogue* (MS. list in Royal Library, Windsor), p. 18, Whitehall no. 258; *George III Kensington Catalogue*: Catalogue of Pictures in His Majesty's Apartments at Kensington Palace, 1778 (commonly called *Geo. III Ken. Cat.*; copies in British Museum and at Windsor), p. 11, Queen's Dining Room, no. 23.

Apparently engraved in woodcut when at Kensington Palace. The print is reproduced on the title-page of *The Linacre Quarterly*. A version of this portrait type is reproduced in *Medical Journal and Record*, cxxi, April 1925, 432. The upper part of the figure closely follows the design of Catalogue No. 1. The foreground details and background curtain derive from some Jacobean, rather than Tudor, prototype.

Catalogue No. 2

Plates VIII and IX

Painting. Royal College of Physicians, London.

Oils on canvas, 19×15 inches.

Collections: Copied from the Windsor picture (Catalogue No. 1) by William Miller, 1810, for the Royal College of Physicians. Engraved by H. Cook for T. J. Pettigrew's *Medical Portrait Gallery*, 4 vols., London, (1840,) i, no. 14. Impressions are fairly common: Ashmolean Museum, Oxford (Hope Collection); National Portrait Gallery Library; Department of Zoology, University of Oxford; etc.

Literature: David Piper, *Catalogue of Paintings . . . Royal College of Physicians*, London, 1963, p. 260.

Catalogue No. 3

Plate X

Painting. All Souls College, Oxford.

Oils on panel, 18 × 14 inches. Artist unknown.

Collections: A copy of the Windsor painting (Catalogue No. 1) thought to have been presented to the College between 1815 and 1840.

Exhibitions: Oxford Exhibition of Historical Portraits, 1904, no. 10; Royal Academy of Arts, *Exhibition of Works by the Old Masters*, etc. (1902), no. 165.

Literature: Mrs. Reginald Lane Poole, *Catalogue of Portraits in the Possession of the University . . .*, 3 vols., Oxford, 1912–25, ii. 181; C. Grant Robertson, *All Souls College*, London, 1899, pp. 193, 212.

Catalogue No. 4

Plate XI.*a*

Painting. Residence of the Regius Professor of Medicine, 13 Norham Gardens, Oxford.

Oils on panel, 20¼ × 16½ inches. Artist unknown.

Collections: Stated by Mrs. Lane Poole to be a copy of the All Souls portrait (Catalogue No. 3). Made for Sir Henry Acland, Regius Professor of Medicine 1858–94.

Literature: Mrs. R. Lane Poole, op. cit. i. 231; H. Cushing, *Life of Sir W. Osler*, Oxford, 1925, i. 401.

Catalogue No. 5

Plate XI.*b*

Painting. Osler Library, McGill University, Montreal.

Oils on canvas, 20¼ × 16½ inches. Artist unknown.

Collections: Copy of the painting in the residence of the Regius Professor of Medicine, Oxford (Catalogue No. 4), made for Sir William Osler between 1894 and 1897. Osler in turn had his copy (Catalogue

No. 5) copied for the William Pepper Laboratory, Philadelphia, *circa* 1898.

Literature: Cushing, op. cit. i. 401, 444.

Catalogue No. 6

Plate XII.*a*

Painting. Ven. Collegio Inglese, Rome.

Water-colour on paper, $17\frac{1}{2} \times 13\frac{1}{4}$ inches. Artist unknown. Recorded as a copy of the Windsor painting (Catalogue No. 1).

Collections: Purchased by Sir William Allchin, *circa* 1885, and presented to the English College by his widow, Lady Allchin, November 1920.

Catalogue No. 7

Plate XII.*b*

Painting. Wellcome Institute of the History of Medicine, London.

Oils on panel, $21\frac{1}{2} \times 16\frac{1}{2}$ inches. Artist unknown.

An apparent fake, or deceptive copy, based upon the Windsor painting (Catalogue No. 1) or on copies of it.

Collections: Sold Robinson & Fisher, 15 October 1924, lot 97.

Catalogue No. 8

Plate XIII.*a*

Copy of the All Souls painting (Catalogue No. 3) made by Mrs. Marcelle Young for Linacre College, Oxford, 1966.

Catalogue No. 9

Plate XX.*a*

Oriel window in the Hall, Christ Church, Oxford.

The figure of Linacre appears in one of the lower lights on the left side of the window.

Presented by Archdeacon C. C. Clerke in memory of the residence of the Prince of Wales (Edward VII) and of the Crown Prince of Denmark.

Literature: Mrs. R. Lane Poole, op. cit. iii. 109.

Catalogue No. 10

Plate XIV

Painting. National Gallery, London, 'Man with a Pansy and a Skull', no. 1036.

Oils on panel, 10¾ × 8½ inches. Netherlandish School, *c.* 1535.

Collections: Bought from Farrer, 1849, by W. Fuller Maitland, and purchased from him by the National Gallery, 1878.

Exhibitions: (as Linacre by Holbein) British Institution, 1852, no. 118; Leeds, 1868, no. 553; Royal Academy, 1872, no. 214.

Literature: M. Davies, *Early Netherlandish School*, National Gallery Catalogues, 3rd edn., London, 1968, pp. 137–8.

Reproduced (as Linacre): *Wigan Parish Church Magazine*, December 1903, frontispiece; *Wigan Observer*, 6 March 1920.

The authenticity of the identification as Linacre appears to have been in doubt before the picture was purchased by the National Gallery.

Catalogue No. 11

Plate XV

Drawing. British Museum, London, Department of Prints and Drawings, Cracherode Collection.

Ink and wash on paper, 13⅝ × 8¼ inches. Artist unknown. Engraved by John Thane, 1794; for inscription see above, p. 363 n. 1.

Collections: Bequeathed by Clayton Mordaunt Cracherode (1730–99). *Literature*: W. Osler, *Thomas Linacre*, Linacre Lecture, Cambridge, 1908, p. 61.

A tracing of Catalogue No. 11 exists in the Hope Collection, Ashmolean Museum, Oxford (Erasmus Exhibition, Bodleian Library, Oxford, 1969, no. 54); a water-colour copy belongs to the Wellcome Institute of the History of Medicine, London. A copy drawn in pen and ink by A. Litchfield belongs to the Royal College of Physicians, London.

Catalogue No. 12

Plate XVI.*a*

Bust. Codrington Library, All Souls College, Oxford.

Bronze cast of a bust attributed to Sir Henry Cheere, *c.* 1749.

One of a series of twenty-four busts of Fellows of All Souls commissioned by the College from the Cheere brothers from 1749.

Literature: Mrs. R. Lane Poole, op. cit. ii. 205; Mrs. M. I. Webb, 'Henry Cheere . . . and John Cheere', *Burlington Magazine*, July 1958, pp. 232–40.

Catalogue No. 13

Plate XVI.*b*

Small-scale bust. All Souls College, Oxford.

Plaster, painted black. Artist unknown.

No record appears to survive of its date or acquisition.

Literature: Mrs. R. Lane Poole, op. cit. ii. 182.

There is an obvious connection with the bust in the Codrington Library (Catalogue No. 12). The two are very close in design, apart from the difference in shape of cap. Catalogue No. 13 is immeasurably coarser in execution. It may possibly have been produced as a model or sketch for No. 12.

Catalogue No. 14

Plate XVII

Monumental figure of Thomas Linacre by Henry Weekes, 1876.

Collections: Given to the Royal College of Physicians, London, by subscription of the Fellows, 1876, and placed behind the portico of the College's old building in Pall Mall; cut down to head and shoulders, 1965, when acquired by Mr. A. T. Linacre, Peckham, London.

Literature: *List of the Portraits and other Works of Art in the Royal College of Physicians of London*, London, 1900.

Catalogue No. 15

Plate XIII.*b*

Etching, *c.* 1700. Raphael Collection, Catalogue no. 1876, Royal Library, Windsor Castle.

$7 \times 5\frac{5}{8}$ inches. Artist unknown. Inscribed, bottom left: *F R V R* and, faintly, in ink, *R d' Urbino*.

Catalogue No. 16

Plate XX.*b*

Woodcut. $1\frac{1}{4} \times \frac{7}{8}$ inches. Inscribed *Thom. Lynacer* (*sic*).

This small print comes from one of three sets of portrait engravings prefixed to the three parts of Adolphus Clarmundus (*pseud.* J. C. Ruediger) *Vitae clarissimorum in re literaria virorum* (Wittenberg, 1704). The Linacre portrait is included in the third set.

Catalogue No. 17

Plate XVIII.*a* and *b*

Painting. Wellcome Institute of the History of Medicine, London.

Oils on panel, 14¼ × 12 inches. Artist unknown.

A fake, or deceptive copy, probably of nineteenth-century origin.

The design of the background is based on Holbein's portrait of George Gisze, 1532 (Berlin (West), Staatliche Museen Preussicher Kultur-besitz, Gemäldegalerie). The figure is copied from the Windsor painting (Catalogue No. 1).

Catalogue No. 18

Plate XIX.*a* and *b*

Painting. Wellcome Institute of the History of Medicine, London.

Oils on panel, 13 × 10½ inches. Artist unknown.

A fake, or deceptive copy, probably of nineteenth-century origin.

Almost an exact copy of Holbein's portrait of Dirk Tybis, merchant of Duisberg, 1533 (Vienna, Kunsthistorisches Museum).

Catalogue No. 19

Frontispiece

Title-page. Thomas Linacre's translation of Galen, *De sanitate tuenda*, Paris, 1517. Nearly identical figures, approximately 1½ inches high, labelled *Galenus* and *Linacrus*, face each other from the spandrels above the cartouche inscribed with the title.

Catalogue No. 20

Plate XX.*c*

Fresco. Sala dei Quaranta, University of Padua.

By Giacomo del Forno, 1942.

The figure of Thomas Linacre forms one of a group of distinguished scholars who have worked at the University of Padua. The portrait is imaginary but the design indicates that the British Museum draw-ing (Catalogue No. 11) may have been known to the artist.

Reproduced by A. Bosatra in 'British Doctors at Padua University', *Acta Medicae Historiae Patavina*, ii, 1955–6, p. 7.

Medical Humanism—A Historical Necessity in the Era of the Renaissance

WALTER PAGEL[*]

THE SIXTEENTH CENTURY IS COMMONLY ACCEPTED as the period of decision—when ancient and medieval tradition, and naturalist and medical lore were converted into science and medicine of the 'modern' stamp. This was accomplished, or so it seems, almost at one single stroke and in the same year. Customarily, 1543 is regarded as the turning-point—the year, that is, in which the Copernican revolution and Vesalius's new Anatomy were communicated through the new mass-medium of printing. This view may be basically correct, but it cannot be accepted without considerable qualification.[1] No single event dispelled the proverbial 'medieval darkness'; the development was gradual and slow. The Middle Ages had seen several periods of 'renaissance'. Some of the 'modern' outlook in physics had been that of medieval commentators on Aristotle. Cardinal Nicolaus Cusanus (1401–64) rejected the geocentric cosmos, and held a view of the universe that was free of the limitations imposed by the Copernican system. The astoundingly successful anatomy of Vesalius (1514–64) was the first concerted exercise in representing the human body naturalistically,

* M.D., Hon. D.Litt. (Leeds), etc., Professor Emeritus of the History of Medicine, University of Heidelberg.

[1] See W. P. D. Wightman, *Science and the Renaissance. An Introduction to the Study of the Emergence of the Sciences in the Sixteenth Century*, 2 vols., Edinburgh and London, 1962, i. 1–44, and idem, 'Science and the Renaissance', *History of Science*, iii, 1964, 1–19. Concerning the development of humanist medical translation, see R. J. Durling, 'A Chronological Census of Renaissance Editions and Translations of Galen', *Journal of the Warburg and Courtauld Institutes*, xxiv, 1961, 230–305.

accurately, in detail, and at the same time artistically. Though deliberately correcting errors of the apish anatomy of Galen (A.D. 129–99), it largely submitted to Galenic physiology and medicine. Nearly another century, and another *Zeitgeist*, were needed before what today may appear to be the decisive step into modernity could be taken—through Harvey's (1578–1657) discovery of the circulation of the blood (1628).

Two years before the great works of Copernicus and Vesalius were published, there had died in wretched circumstances Theophrastus Paracelsus (1493–1541). He was a man radically different from the creators of the new greater and lesser cosmos and yet no less, perhaps more, destructive of tradition. He was active in many fields that today look foreign to medicine and science, such as theology, or natural and supernatural magic; he attempted a synthesis of human knowledge and wisdom based on symbolism and analogy between the greater and the lesser worlds. And yet it is he to whom the most modern and durable trend in scientific medicine must be traced: the chemical interpretation of organ function, normal and morbid, and the systematically reasoned and tested introduction of chemical medicines. After almost a century of bitter quarrel Paracelsus's aims may be said to have been achieved, through the inclusion of chemical remedies in the first London Pharmacopoeia of 1618.[1] Rapid developments in all other fields of scholarship and social life took place between Vesalius and the appearance of the London Pharmacopoeia.

We started by looking at the great scientific and medical innovations as products of the closing decades of the Renaissance when there were signs of transition to a new period: the Baroque. In popular and somewhat chivalrous terms it has been said that this was the time when movement and change replaced the static and the statuesque. In a similarly superficial appraisal, the spirit of the time has been summed up as the final abolition of the Aristotelian 'substances' and 'forms', and their replacement by atoms and the synthesis and dissolution of the atomic clusters. With this, it is said, has been associated a general rejection of substantial forms in favour of functional relationships—a movement away from a view of things as beings in their own right ('ontology') towards a

---

[1] College of Physicians of London, *Pharmacopoeia Londinensis in quo medicamenta antiqua ut nova usitatissima*, London, 1618 (facsimile reprint with an introduction by G. Urdang, Madison, 1944).

conception of energetic interplay, or dynamism. Again, such a sweeping view calls for drastic revision. Aristotle was by no means 'dead', nor had he to be killed when modern science developed. Indeed, the so-called scientific revolution remains unthinkable without him. This is true not only in the negative sense of his having inspired criticism and thereby the search for new ways, but also in the positive and essential role which he played in the full bloom of biology and comparative anatomy from Rondeletus (1507–66) via Harvey to Francis Glisson (1597–1677). This even applies to such a (rather rhetorically) professed anti-Aristotelian as Johann Baptista van Helmont (1579–1644), and the very discovery by which he is remembered in textbooks of chemistry today, namely that of gas. The latter, as van Helmont understood it, embodied all the attributes of Aristotelian *entelecheia*—the inseparable unit of matter and form that is responsible for the specificity and perfection of an individual object—with the difference that it was a concept with Aristotle, but believed by van Helmont to be demonstrable *in vitro*.[1] So Aristotle remained alive, and perhaps more so Galen, the medical methodist and therapist, until far into the seventeenth and even the early eighteenth centuries.[2]

Perhaps the best example to illustrate this is the chequered career of the liver in the history of physiology. To Galen it had been a centre of vital function of the highest order and, in particular, the organ which formed the blood. Vesalius had no objection to this, although he doubted Galen's opinion that blood began to be formed in the portal vein. Harvey, a staunch Aristotelian throughout his life and consequently a defender of the primacy of the heart (and blood), showed little interest in the lymphatic and chylus vessels. But it was the discovery of the latter which led Thomas Bartholinus (1616–80) to issue his famous funeral orations on the liver—'How far the Burial of the Liver calls for a Reform of the Method of Healing' (1653), 'On the Liver Deceased' (1661), and 'The Difficulties of [its] Resurrection' (1661). This, and the triumph of Harvey's discovery of the circulation of the blood, detracted from the liver the functional principate allotted to it by Galen, and its consequent

---

[1] W. Pagel, 'William Harvey revisited', *History of Science*, viii, 1969, 1–31; ix, 1970, 1–41; idem, 'Chemistry at the Cross-Roads. The Ideas of Joachim Jungius', *Ambix*, xvi, 1969, 100–8.

[2] See now the definitive account of the topic in Owsei Temkin, *Galenism. Rise and Decline of a Medical Philosophy*, Ithaca and London, 1973, esp. pp. 126–7.

importance in pathology. However, apart from morbid-anatomical observations and the ideas of G. E. Stahl (1660–1734) on the portal vein as the *porta malorum* (1698), the liver was 'resurrected' in the nineteenth century through the great works of K. B. Reichert, E. H. Weber, and Th. Kölliker on blood formation in the embryo, of Tiedemann and Gmelin on the way in which gastro-intestinal products are transmitted to the blood (1820), and, above all, of Claude Bernard (1855) and contemporary and subsequent bio-chemists and clinicians such as, notably, Theodor Frerichs (1858–61).[1]

Galen's idea of diastolic attraction of venous blood by the heart —so much deprecated by Harvey—seems to be borne out by the research of early-nineteenth-century and much more recent authors, as Lord Cohen of Birkenhead has shown.[2] Galen's knowledge of the movements of the chest and their significance in respiration was certainly far in advance of the ideas of Harvey and van Helmont who, because they thought the bird's lung analogous, believed in a penetration of air into the chest in inspiration. Galen had rightly emphasized the differences between arterial and venous blood. Harvey ignored them. This was a 'retrogressive' step in that he thus revived the Aristotelian tradition of the singleness (*henotes*) of the blood, and yet a *felix culpa*, for it was in harmony with the concept of blood preservation and circulation.[3]

It is well known that the zoological observations of Aristotle still stimulate and enjoy the admiration of zoologists, just as much as they impressed Cuvier, Owen, Darwin, and Huxley, before and after the rediscovery of viviparous birth and placental attachment to the mother in such fishes as the smooth galeus (*Mustelus laevis*) by Johannes Müller (1839). As Ogle found in 1882, not a few of Aristotle's generalizations have stood the test of time and some, restated by moderns in ignorance of his works, have been claimed as original by them or by their modern admirers. Thus, the law of organic equivalents—perfectly recognized and stated by Aristotle —has been attributed to Geoffrey St. Hilaire and Goethe.[4]

[1] Fried. Th. Frerichs, *Klinik der Leberkrankheiten*, 2 vols. and Atlas, Braun-schweig, 1858–61.

[2] Lord Cohen of Birkenhead, 'On the Motion of Blood in the Veins. The Harveian Oration for 1970', *British Medical Journal*, ii, 1971, 551–7.

[3] W. Pagel, 'Harvey revisited', p. 8.

[4] W. Ogle, *Aristotle on the Parts of Animals*, London, 1882, pp. xii, xvi, and note 9 to book II, cap. 9.

Again, Johannes Müller (1801–58) must be praised. Not only did he rediscover a brilliant piece of Aristotelian zoology, but he also showed himself deeply imbued with the first principles of Aristotle's biological philosophy. He saw in all organization an idea and a plan in which purpose and necessity coincide and, in generation, the *cyclical* transmission of an identical form.[1]

It is true, however, that Galenic and Aristotelian bastions were progressively falling, and ancient tradition became progressively diluted. Nevertheless, the soil from which the Vesalian as well as the Paracelsian reform emerged was *humanism*. Paracelsus certainly was indifferent to textual criticism and hermeneutics; nor was he interested in the beautiful. Vesalius, however, was an aestheticist of the first order. He would argue at length and, as his quarrel with his room-mate John Caius at Padua shows, quibble bitterly and cantankerously about a single Galenic word and its tradition. We shall return again to humanism in the life and work of Paracelsus.

Vesalius had been an alumnus of the Trilingual College at Louvain. Ever after, he could not help exercising his elegant Ciceronian style, and being engrossed in and showing off his knowledge of Hebrew terms (though his knowledge of this tongue is adversely criticized today). The three languages which had been the buttresses of the humanistic curriculum of his old school—Latin, Greek, and Hebrew—remained essential tools to him, in the true Erasmian tradition. His academic teachers had been two staunch humanistic Galenists: Jacobus Sylvius (1478–1555) and Johann Winther (Guintherus) of Andernach (1487–1574). Vesalius's first literary assignment was an edition of Winther's *Anatomicarum institutionum a Galeni sententia libri IV* (Basel, 1536). His *Tabulae anatomicae* of the same year were still Galenic. In 1541 he contributed to the Latin edition of Galen printed by the Giunta press in Venice. Galen's treatises on the dissection of nerves, veins, and arteries, and the *Anatomical Procedures*, came under his editorship.[2] In spite of all criticism, Galen remained to him 'the foremost among the teachers of anatomy', the 'author of all good things' and the prince of physicians, from whom

---

[1] Johannes Müller, *Handbuch der Physiologie des Menschen*, vol. ii, part 3 (6. Buch. Vom Seelenleben, 1. Abschnitt: Natur der Seele. Verhältnis der Seele zur Organisation und Materie), Coblenz, 1840, pp. 505 ff.

[2] H. Cushing, *Bio-Bibliography of Andreas Vesalius*, Hamden, Conn., 1962, pp. 65–6.

he, in his own words, did not dare to deviate by as much as a nail's breadth in the matter of cardio-vascular function.[1]

There was a further humanist motive professed by Vesalius: the search for the traces of a pristine medicine and anatomy obscured and lost through the triumph of the traditional classics. He believed it to have been known by the ancients, but lost from view after the 'Gothic invasions'. It furnished Vesalius with a standard for judging the medicine of his own time and its decline since of old. He felt himself to have come as a restorer of this pristine tradition rather than as a destroyer. The empiricism needed at his time was, to Vesalius, the return to a *prisca anatomia*.[2] This he achieved by taking the dissecting knife into his own hand and demonstrating and teaching not from the height of the teacher's desk, but sharing the floor with his pupils and the cadaver. He thus went back to the pre-Galenic anatomy of the great masters of Alexandria in the third century.

Another example of an anatomist of outstanding merit, who can claim the laurels of a medical humanist of the first order, is Vesalius's great critic Bartolomeo Eustachi (1524–74). In 1564 Eustachi signed the preface to his annotated edition and translation of the Hippo-crates-Lexicon of Erotianus, published by the Giunta Press in Venice in 1566. He had been the first to discover and to recognize the importance of this book, but the first edition of the Greek text was printed in 1564 without his being consulted. His annotations contain a collation of all the Hippocratic *loci* with the interpretations of Galen and his own observations. They are invaluable even today, and yet not mentioned in any of the standard textbooks of medical history, so much were his humanist activities overshadowed by his brilliant anatomy. He shows himself a faithful Galenist—in opposition to Vesalius. In his work *De multitudine* (appended to the edition of Erotianus), however, he paraphrases Galen with a considerable note of criticism. Here he describes his position succinctly: 'If I appear not to acquiesce completely in the *dicta* of Galen and throw doubt on some of them, nobody should suspect that I disapprove of his authority or doctrine, particularly with reference to what he

---

[1] W. Pagel, 'Vesalius and the Pulmonary Transit of Venous Blood', *Journal of the History of Medicine*, xix, 1964, 335–6; idem, *William Harvey's Biological Ideas*, Basle and New York, 1967, p. 162.

[2] W. Pagel and P. M. Rattansi, 'Vesalius and Paracelsus', *Medical History*, viii, 1964, pp. 322–6.

explains about *Plethora*. How much I appreciate the man clearly emerges from my anatomical work.' A desire to contradict not Galen, but rather those who interpreted him wrongly, and the search for the truth, have actuated him in writing—as Galen himself admonished us to weigh, after his own example, the force of reason rather than the authority of anybody.[1]

In the truly humanist search and nostalgic yearning for a pre-Galenic, pristine medicine, Vesalius was on common ground with Paracelsus. The latter invokes the secret tradition of the *Kabbala*, whereby he envisages much of that hermeticism which had been rejuvenated in the humanist activities of the Florentine School, notably through the work of Marsilio Ficino (1433–99), Giovanni Pico della Mirandola (1463–94), and Johann Reuchlin (1455–1522). Paracelsus left an extensive commentary on the *Aphorisms* of Hippocrates, whom he professedly venerated whilst reviling Aristotle and Galen in his customary ribald terms. Ficino, the humanist physician and priestly savant, is the only contemporary for whom he found words of unqualified admiration and approval. And rightly so, for Paracelsus's analogical natural philosophy and medicine are broadly based on Neoplatonism and the subterranean secret tradition of Hellenistic hermeticism and alchemy. Perhaps the most conspicuous feature in this respect is the unlimited hegemony which Paracelsus allowed the spiritual to enjoy, and its conversion into material substance at an instant's notice through the power of meditation and imagination. In this field Gnostic ideas come to the surface in the Paracelsian *Corpus*, in the non-authentic treatises as well as, somewhat diluted, in the genuine treatises. We recall the position of Prime Matter—which is the word *Fiat*, uncreated and spiritual, the *logos* of the Gospel—as witness more than one of Paracelsus's genuine pronouncements. There is as well the idea of the conjunction, the 'marriage' of the four celestial elements, the *vulcani*, with the four lower, the traditional elements on earth, both forming together the 'Eight Mothers'. There are the inept creator-gods, astral demiurges, 'celestial apprentices and not grown-up masters' who are responsible for the creation of man and notably of fools. There are also the 'elementary spirits'—subhuman, but

[1] B. Eustachi, *Erotiani Graeci scriptoris vetustissimi vocum, quae apud Hippocratem sunt, collectio* (Venice, 1566). See fol. 125, cap. I, 'De occasione scribendi Libellum de Multitudine', and also dedication and preface to the whole work, sigs. 1, 2 ff.

man-like and soul-less beings which people water, earth, air, and fire. All this is in the best Hellenistic, Neoplatonic and Gnostic tradition, just as a classical, mostly Galenic, root can be demonstrated for many Paracelsian concepts, even such an original doctrine as that of *tartarus*.

It has been said that the Renaissance 'discovered man' and turned from the medieval *universalia* to the 'Book of Nature' and its *singularia*: that is individuals in general, and man, the centre of the world, in particular. Precisely this *anthropocentric* view was that of Paracelsus. Man, the last to be created, was the quintessence of all that went before and contained the virtues of every previous creation. Paracelsus, though uncompromising and rough of manners especially towards his colleagues, showed warm humanity towards his patients and notably the mentally sick. These included the fool (*stultus*) who, he thought, was closer to God than anybody else, because of his lack of complacent human reason, a gift of the malicious astral demi-gods (the 'administrators' (*dioiketeis*) in Gnostic–Hellenistic parlance). It is true that Paracelsus was not quite consistent, nor prepared to go to extremes in humanitarianism towards the lunatic, but the trait was there and may well be correlated with the similar views of a humanist such as Agrippa of Nettesheim (1487–1535), with whom he has many ideas in common.

Perhaps the most conspicuous connections of Paracelsus with humanism were his movements in humanist circles throughout his chequered life and career. There are the teachers of his youth, humanist bishops and the abbot Johannes Trithemius (1462–1516), the master of *philosophia adepta* which uncovers the deeper sense hidden behind phenomena, makes visible what is occult, and elucidates the secret coherence of all objects throughout the greater world and the lesser world of man (*pansophia*). There are the academic studies through which Paracelsus must have obtained his thorough knowledge of the whole medical syllabus. It is not unlikely that he sat at the feet of the venerable Niccolò Leoniceno (1428–1524), the foremost medical humanist, translator and interpreter of Galen, at Ferrara. There is the climax of his life, his short-lived academic preferment at Basle. He owed this status to the humanist circle around the publisher Johann Froben (1460–1527), to Erasmus and the Amerbach brothers, as also to the humanist Reformers Oecolampadius, Hedio, Gerbelius, and, notably, the humanist polymath Capito. Later, at St. Gall, he dedicated his famous *Opus Paramirum* to the influential classicist Joachim Vadianus (1484–1551), although his personal relationship with Vadianus remained tenuous and not altogether satisfactory. Johannes Oporinus (1507–68), at one time professor of Greek and better known as the publisher of Vesalius and a galaxy of humanist books, had been Paracelsus's pupil and amanuensis. We owe to him a realistic and lively pen-portrait of the somewhat overpowering master.

If it was not the quest for new and pure manuscript sources of the classics and notably of Galen, or textual criticism, or the yearning for beauty, the contempt for scholasticism and Arabism, for logic and rhetoric was surely the ground which Paracelsus had in common with the humanists. He deserved the humanist sentiment which actuated his father in calling him Theophrastus.[1]

The examples given so far may suffice to make plausible our thesis of the historical necessity of medical humanism during the Renaissance. Test cases to that effect could be increased in number. Moreover, there are different ways of approaching this matter. One way, I believe, would be an examination of humanist botany in depth. Diligence and philological acumen were lavished not only on Galen, but even more so, and earlier, on Pliny and Dioscorides. It is well known how much of a stir was created by Leoniceno's exposition of the 'Errors of Pliny' (1492) against the slavish belief in *verba magistri* shown by such humanist and meritorious fundamentalists as Ermolao Barbaro (died 1493). Leoniceno had rightly insisted on a collation of Pliny with such Greek *exemplaria* as Theophrastus, Aristotle, and Dioscorides, but had hardly envisaged a confrontation of Plinian lore with the facts of nature, or even the reports of such facts. Indeed, his criticism of Pliny largely remained within the con-

---

[1] W. Pagel, *Paracelsus. Introduction to Philosophical Medicine in the Era of the Renaissance*, Basle and New York, 1958; idem, *Das medizinische Weltbild des Paracelsus. Seine Zusammenhänge mit Neuplatonismus und Gnosis*, Wiesbaden, 1962; idem, 'Paracelsus and the Neo-Platonic and Gnostic Tradition', *Ambix*, viii, 1960, 125–66; idem, 'The Prime Matter of Paracelsus', *Ambix*, ix, 1961, 117–35; idem, 'Paracelsus: Traditionalism and Mediaeval Sources' in *Medicine, Science and Culture. Historical Essays in honour of O. Temkin*, ed. L. G. Stevenson and R. P. Multhauf, Baltimore, 1968, pp. 51–75; idem and Rattansi, 'Vesalius and Paracelsus' (see above, p. 380 n. 2); idem and M. Winder, 'The Eightness of Adam and related "Gnostic" Ideas in the Paracelsian Corpus', *Ambix*, xvi, 1969, 119–39; idem et eadem, 'The Higher Elements and Prime Matter in Renaissance naturalism and the Paracelsian Corpus', *Ambix*, xxi, 1974, 93–127; K. Goldammer, *Paracelsus, Humanisten und Humanismus*, Salzburger Beiträge zur Paracelsusforschung, iv, Salzburg, 1964.

fines of nomenclature. It thus had no real answer to such defenders of Pliny as Pandolf Collenuci of Pesaro. The latter claimed first-hand naturalist knowledge, expressly condemning authority and books as against study of the natural object itself. His performance was all the more remarkable as he was not a 'qualified' expert but a statesman and lawyer. This may, of course, have helped him, in acquiring knowledge of rare and outlandish specimens on ambassadorial journeys and in gaining an insight into the truthfulness of ancient plant-lore from mediterranean countries which could not so easily have come to botanists in northern places.[1] Nevertheless, much of the knowledge of early botanists derived primarily from what they could glean from texts then becoming available in an ever-increasing number and of improved textual quality. But how far was the opposite course taken: primary excursions into nature with a view to utilizing what it could teach for the improvement of the traditional texts and the 'invention' of the most acceptable readings? A detailed examination of this question can be expected to lead to spectacular results in illuminating the merit of 'philological medicine' in general and that of Linacre, Leoniceno, and their numerous fellow interpreters in particular. In this respect, a study in depth of Valerius Cordus (1515–44) and Konrad Gesner (1516–65) should be specially rewarding. Moreover, an inquiry of this nature would be of acute interest for the background to the new 'Vesalian' naturalistic and advanced iconography as embodied in the *Historia stirpium* of 1542 of Leonhart Fuchs (1501–66). It was Fuchs who more vociferously than anybody else gave the call to liberate medicine from the *faeces Arabum melle Latinitatis conditae*—the Arabic dung dressed with the honey of Latinity. 'I declare', he said, 'my implacable hatred for the Saracens and as long as I live shall never cease to fight them. For who can tolerate this pest and its ravings among mankind any longer—except those who wish for the Christian world to perish altogether. Let us therefore return to the sources and draw from them the pure and unadulterated water of medical knowledge.'[2]

---

[1] See K. Sprengel, *Versuch einer pragmatischen Geschichte der Arzneykunde*, 3rd edn., Halle, 1827, iii. 41 with ref. also to Manardus and his first-hand knowledge of botany. Ernst H. F. Meyer, *Geschichte der Botanik*, vol. iv, Königsberg, 1857; repr. A. Asher, Amsterdam, 1965, iv. 232, rather critical of Collenuci and his largely rhetorical criticism of Leoniceno, as against L. Thorndike's eulogy in *History of Magic and Experimental Science*, New York, 1934, iv, chap. 66, pp. 593–610 with a detailed account of the 'Attack on Pliny'.

[2] Sprengel, op. cit., pp. 151 and 189.

The same Fuchs, who stood in the first rank of philological and critical translators of Hippocratic and Galenic treatises, founded one of the first and famous botanical gardens and greatly enriched our knowledge of plants. His great book appeared one year before Vesalius's *Fabrica*. It was inspired by the same spirit, and the proximity of the two works in time expressed the *Zeitgeist* and was not by any means accidental. At the same time, the motives which actuated his interest in philology and hermeneutics were the same as those of Linacre and Leoniceno. The two aspects of his activity—progressive botany and antiquarian restoration of sources—gave him a world of his own in which all aspects were joined into one organic whole.[1]

The *pragmatic view* by which Fuchs was actuated, the imperative to help suffering mankind directly by providing a purified text of the Greek classics and notably of Galen, was eloquently expressed by Linacre. He speaks about an *arcanum naturae* which Galen has brought forth from darkness into light. One of Galen's great achievements was, in Linacre's opinion, the preservation and transmission of Hippocrates, who would otherwise have been lost, to the detriment of mankind. There is little in medicine that Galen had not covered inimitably, but there is much that had been misunderstood or wrongly arrogated. Galen's efforts in prophylaxis—the *sanitas tuenda*—are of immortal merit to all periods of time and indispens-

---

[1] Compare with this some observations on the relationship between Renaissance medicine and classical terminology by Dietlinde Goltz, *Studien zur Geschichte der Mineralnamen in Pharmazie, Chemie und Medizin von den Anfängen bis Paracelsus*, Wiesbaden, 1972. Here the humanist endeavour towards clarifying medical nomenclature and in particular the position of Manardus, Fuchs, Sylvius, and Andreas Alpago Bellunensis have been accorded a whole section (vii. 334–65, esp. chap. 2, pp. 338–48). According to Goltz, Avicenna should be vindicated and the 'errors' of which he was accused by Manardus and Fuchs laid at the doorsteps of his translators. With regard to the hostile attitude of Fuchs to Arabic medicine: 'neither Mesue nor Avicenna issued their prescriptions for the pharmacists of sixteenth century Tübingen' (p. 342). Some of the humanists seem to have forgotten that they wrote in Arabic, as well as that medieval Persia was productive of drugs different from those of ancient Greece. It was thus that Arabic physicians were denied originality and pilloried as 'barbarians'. This prejudice was repeatedly expressed, for example by Sprengel in 1794. Nevertheless, the polemical attitude of the humanists was admittedly legitimate—methodical return to the ancient texts was the only way out of terminological chaos. It was a salutary reaction and meant to benefit mankind. For further detail see W. Pagel, essay-review of Goltz's work in *History of Science*, xii, 1974, 69–76.

able as the 'soldiers at peace', to prevent war (Prooemium, *De sanitate tuenda*, 1517).

In conclusion, yet a further instance of the vigour of medical humanism should be recorded. Sanctorius Sanctorius (1561–1636) is chiefly remembered today for his discovery (or rather rediscovery) of insensible perspiration by means of a magnificent device for weighing the whole body and careful measurement of its gains and losses, other than through intake and excretion (1614). In addition, and obviously under the influence of Galileo, he designed a pulse-watch and other mechanical devices for use in the sick-room. These tokens of 'modern' mechanical inventiveness are embedded in commentaries on Avicenna and Galen respectively. Surely a detailed study of their context is called for. It would promise further information on our subject, all the more because Sanctorius shows himself as an orthodox and traditional Galenist and Arabist, in spite of his spectacularly progressive discoveries and inventions.[1]

So far we have discussed the importance, the historical necessity, of medical humanism in the life, development, and work of the luminaries of the sixteenth century. But what has all this to do with Linacre, the medical philologist and Galenist—who had no share in any of their achievements and left in his own work nothing comparable? The answer is: a good deal. For it should lift up his memory from the level of the few small-print lines which are customarily given to him if he is mentioned at all. The studies incorporated in this volume should go far to implement this.

When all this is said and done, however, we should consider that we are the beneficiaries of a hindsight of four and a half centuries. In other words we judge Linacre against modern standards of progress in scientific medicine, and select from his work what seems to be 'relevant' today. Instead, we should write the history of events as they 'really were' and thereby raise the literary genius of a past age, as if by a magic formula, from the dead. No historian who is worth his salt can ignore this call. He will endeavour to forget modern standards and progress altogether or at least as far as he conceivably can. He will then reach Pisgah and find himself in possession of the master-key that admits him to a wonderland of surprising fertility, the world which Linacre shared with nobody but himself.

---

[1] See Temkin, *Galenism*, p. 160, on Sanctorius and his doubtful success in supporting Galen.

Index

I. Letter from Linacre to John Claymond, President of Magdalen College, Oxford, 1507 to 1516; Corpus Christi College, Oxford, MS. 318, fol. 135. (See p. xlv, n. 58, & p. 71)

II. Letter from Linacre to Giampiero Machiavelli, Florence, 13 December 1512 or 1513; British Library, London, MS. Add. 12107, fol. 10ᵛ (letter) and 10ʳ (address). (See p. xlv, n. 58, & pp. 71–2)

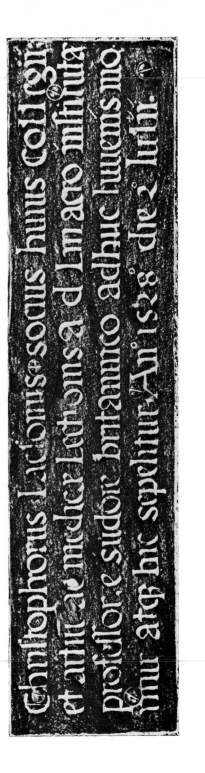

III. Rubbing of a memorial brass recording the death and burial in 1528 of Christopher Jackson, Linacre lecturer at Cambridge, who died of the sweating sickness. Now on the south wall of the chancel of the chapel of St. John's College, Cambridge; moved from the old chapel about 1869. The inscription reads: *Christophorus Iacsonus socius huius collegii et artium ac medicae Lectionis a d Linacro institutae professor, e sudore britannico adhuc Iuuenis moritur atque hic sepelitur. An° 1528° die 2° Iulii.* (See pp. 136 & 228)

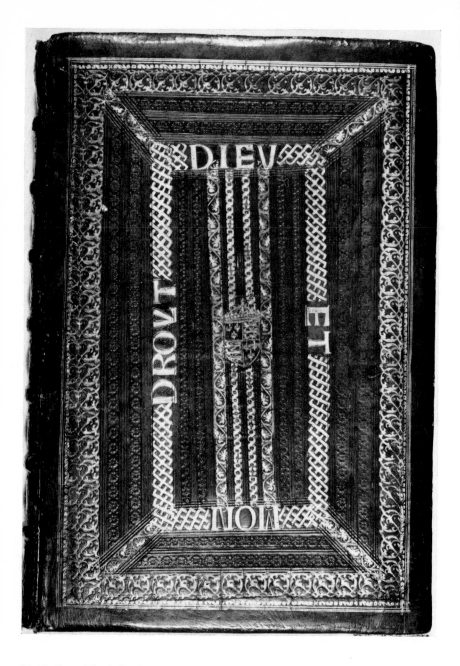

IV. Binding of the dedication copy presented to Henry VIII of Linacre's translation of Galen, *Methodus medendi*, Paris, 1519. The binding is ascribed to the French 'Louis XII–François I' bindery, possibly that of the publisher, Simon Vostre. British Library, London, C 19 e. 17. (See pp. 297–9)

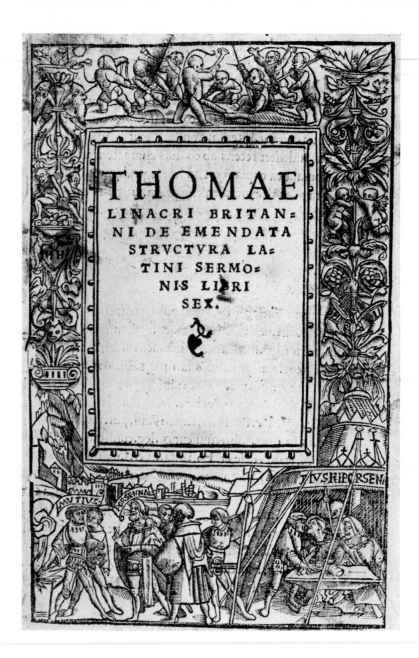

V. Title-page of the first edition of Linacre, *De emendata structura latini sermonis libri sex*, London, 1524. The woodcut border is copied from a design by Hans Holbein and bears his initials. (See pp. 303-4)

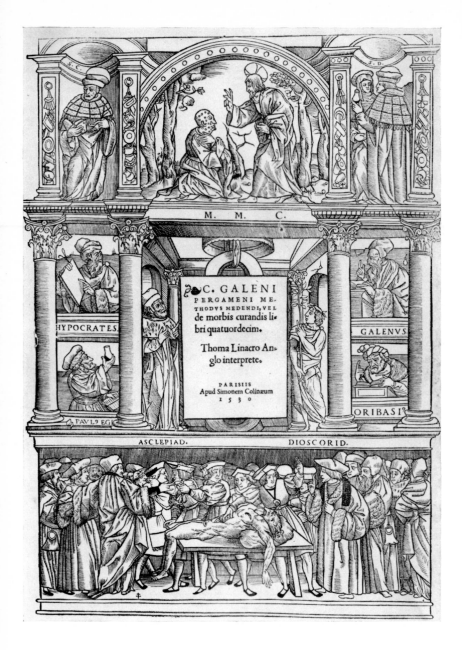

VI. Title-page of Linacre's translation of Galen, *Methodus medendi*, Paris, 1530. The patron saints of physicians, St. Cosmas and St. Damian, are depicted in the panels on the left and the right at the top, and indicated by the initials 'S.C.' and 'S.D.'. (See pp. 312-13)

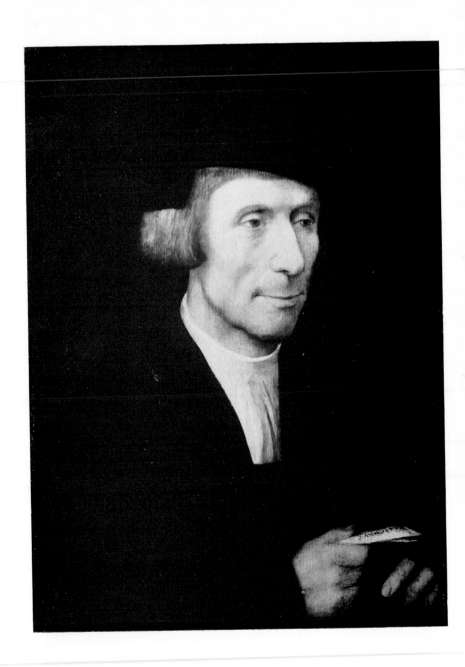

VII. Painting, oils on panel; artist unknown. Royal Collection, Windsor Castle. Reproduced by gracious permission of Her Majesty the Queen. *Catalogue no. 1.* (See pp. 355–9, 361–2, 364, 367–8 & 369)

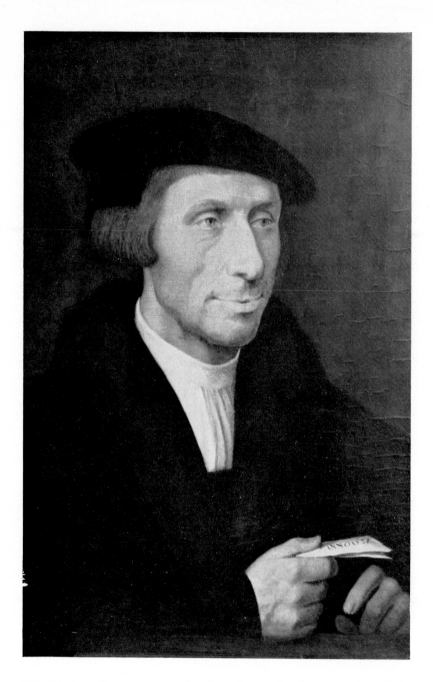

VIII. Painting, oils on canvas; copied, from the painting shown on Plate VII, by William Miller, 1810. The Royal College of Physicians, London. *Catalogue no. 2.* (See pp. 357, 358–9 & 369–70)

Engraved by H. Cook.

THOMAS LINACRE, M.D.

First President of the Royal College of Physicians.

Thoмs Linacrus Medicus

IX. Engraving by H. Cook, 1838, of the painting shown on Plate VIII, for T. J. Pettigrew, *Medical Portrait Gallery*, 4 vois., London, 1840, i, no. 14. *See under Catalogue no. 2.* (See pp. 359, 367 & 369-70)

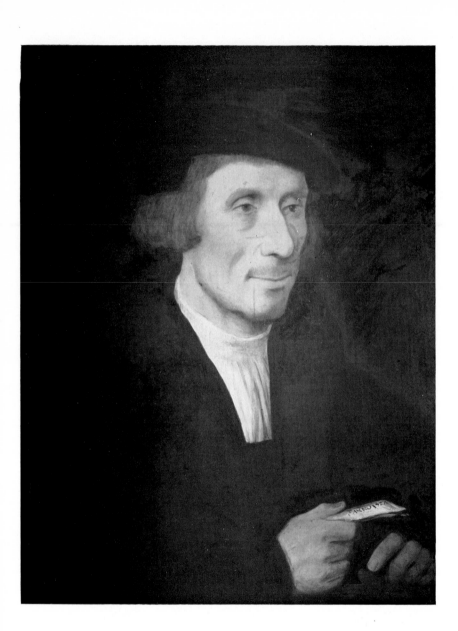

X. Painting, oils on panel; copied from the painting shown on Plate VII, artist unknown, early nineteenth century. All Souls College, Oxford. *Catalogue no. 3.* (See pp. 359 & 370)

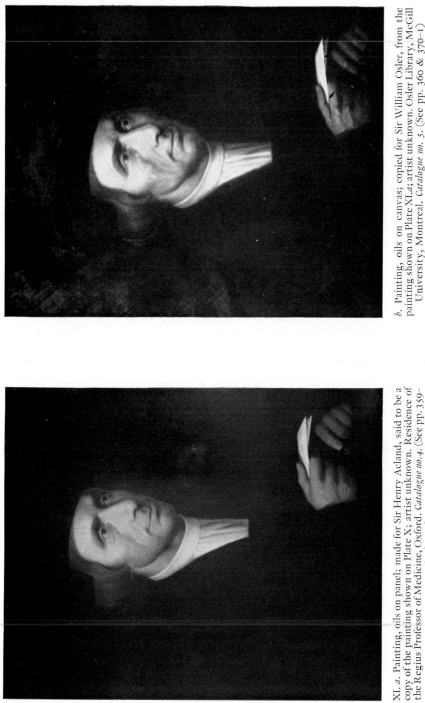

XI. *a.* Painting, oils on panel; made for Sir Henry Acland, said to be a copy of the painting shown on Plate X; artist unknown. Residence of the Regius Professor of Medicine, Oxford. *Catalogue no. 4.* (See pp. 359–60 & 370)

b. Painting, oils on canvas; copied for Sir William Osler, from the painting shown on Plate XI.*a*; artist unknown. Osler Library, McGill University, Montreal. *Catalogue no. 5.* (See pp. 360 & 370–1)

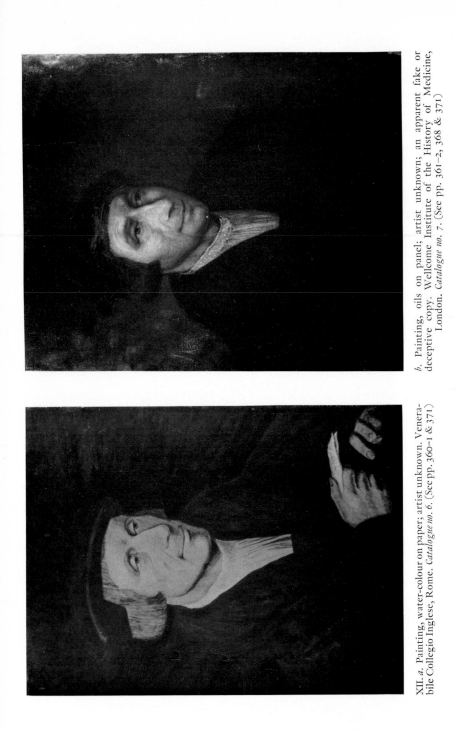

XII. *a*. Painting, water-colour on paper; artist unknown. Venerabile Collegio Inglese, Rome. *Catalogue no. 6*. (See pp. 360–1 & 371)

b. Painting, oils on panel; artist unknown; an apparent fake or deceptive copy. Wellcome Institute of the History of Medicine, London. *Catalogue no. 7*. (See pp. 361–2, 368 & 371)

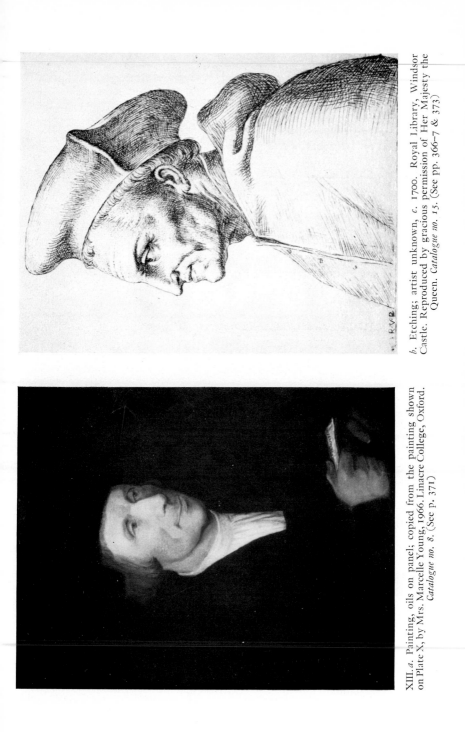

XIII. *a.* Painting, oils on panel; copied from the painting shown on Plate X, by Mrs. Marcelle Young, 1966. Linacre College, Oxford. *Catalogue no. 8.* (See p. 371)

b. Etching; artist unknown, *c.* 1700. Royal Library, Windsor Castle. Reproduced by gracious permission of Her Majesty the Queen. *Catalogue no. 15.* (See pp. 366–7 & 373)

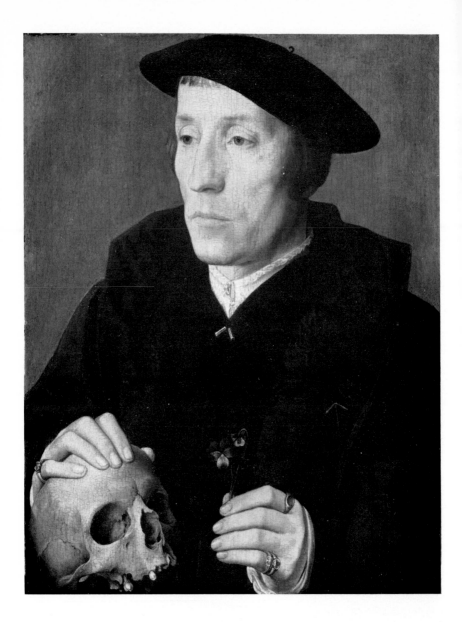

XIV. Painting, oils on panel; Netherlandish School: 'Man with a Pansy and a Skull'. National Gallery, London. *Catalogue no. 10.* (See pp. 362 & 371–2)

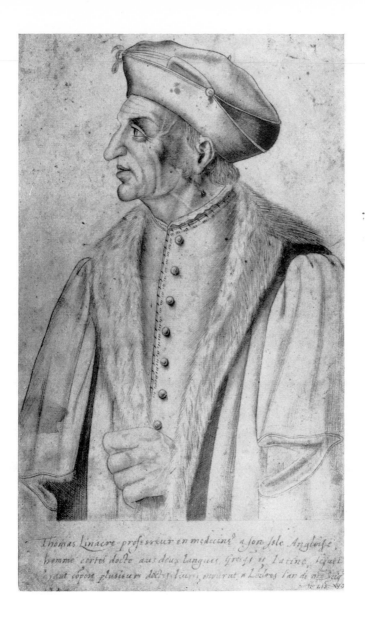

XV. Drawing, ink and wash on paper; artist unknown. Department of Prints and Drawings, British Museum, London. *Catalogue no. 11.* (See pp. 361, 362–4, 365 & 372)

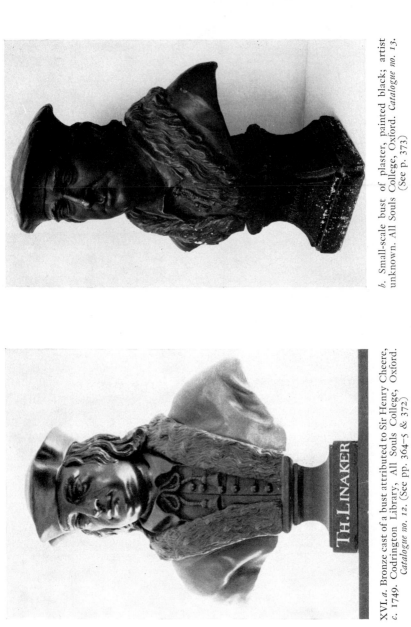

XVI. *a*. Bronze cast of a bust attributed to Sir Henry Cheere, *c*. 1749. Codrington Library, All Souls College, Oxford. *Catalogue no. 12*. (See pp. 364-5 & 372)

b. Small-scale bust of plaster, painted black; artist unknown. All Souls College, Oxford. *Catalogue no. 13*. (See p. 373)

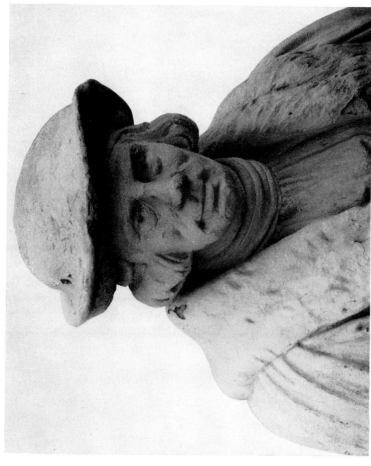

XVII. Monumental stone figure of Thomas Linacre by Henry Weekes, 1876. Formerly behind the portico of the old building of the Royal College of Physicians in Pall Mall, London; cut down to head and shoulders in 1965, and now at Peckham. *Catalogue no. 14.* (See pp. 365–6 & 373)

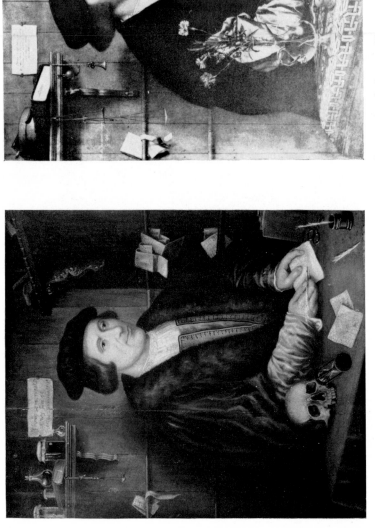

XVIII. *a.* Painting, oils on panel; artist unknown; a fake, or deceptive copy, probably of nineteenth century origin; the figure is copied from the painting shown on Plate VII, the background from that shown on Plate XVIII. *b.* Wellcome Institute of the History of Medicine, London. *Catalogue no. 17.* (See pp. 367–8 & 374)

b. Portrait of George Gisze, 1532, by Hans Holbein. Staatliche Museen Preussicher Kulturbesitz, Gemäldegalerie, Berlin (West). *See under Catalogue no. 17.* (See pp. 367–8 & 374)

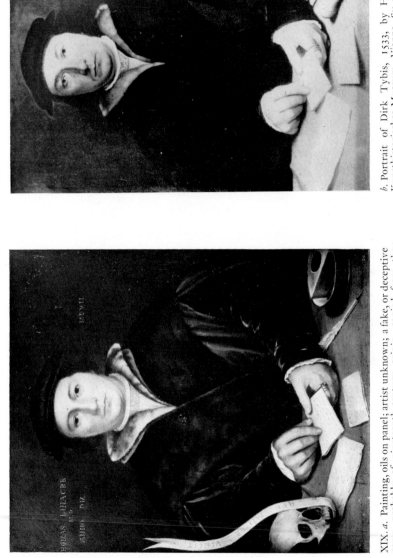

XIX. *a*. Painting, oils on panel; artist unknown; a fake, or deceptive copy, probably of nineteenth-century origin, copied from the painting shown on Plate XIX. *b*. Wellcome Institute of the History of Medicine, London. *Catalogue no. 18.* (See pp. 368 & 374)

b. Portrait of Dirk Tybis, 1533, by Hans Holbein. Kunsthistorisches Museum, Vienna. *See under Catalogue no. 18.* (See pp. 368 & 374)

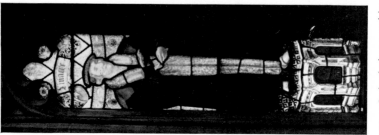

XX. *a*. Stained glass panel in Oriel window in the Hall, Christ Church, Oxford. *Catalogue no. 9*. (See pp. 362 & 371)

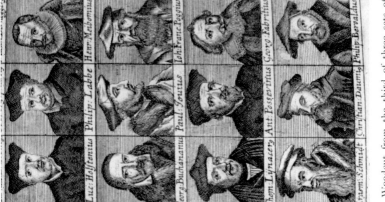

b. Woodcut from the third of three sets of portrait engravings prefixed to the three parts of Adolphus Clarmundus (= J. C. Ruediger), *Vitae clarissimorum in re literaria virorum*, Wittenberg, 1704. *Catalogue no. 16*. (See pp. 367 & 373)

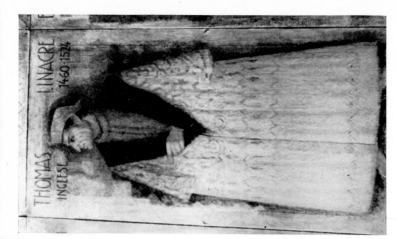

c. Part of a fresco by Giacomo dal Forno, 1942. Sala dei Quaranta, Università di Padova. *Catalogue no. 20*. (See p. 374)